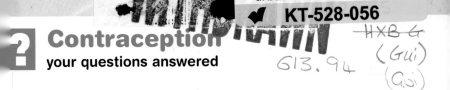

Contraception
your questions answered

Commissioning Editor: Miranda Bromage
Project Development Manager: Rachel Robson
Production Manager: Mark Sanderson

Contraception
your questions answered

THIRD EDITION

John Guillebaud MA FRCSE FRCOG

Professor of Family Planning and Reproductive Health, University College London
Medical Director of the Margaret Pyke Family Planning Centre, London

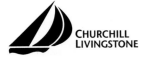

CHURCHILL
LIVINGSTONE

LONDON EDINBURGH NEW YORK PHILADELPHIA SYDNEY TORONTO

CHURCHILL LIVINGSTONE
An imprint of Harcourt Publishers Limited

© John Guillebaud 1985, 1993
© Pearson Professional Ltd 1996
© Harcourt Publishers 1999

◢◗ is a registered trademark of Harcourt Publishers Limited

The right of John Guillebaud to be identified as author of this work has been asserted by him in accordance with the Copyright, Designs and Patents Act 1988.

First edition 1985 (Pitman Publishing Ltd)
Reprinted 1986
Reprinted 1987 (twice)
Reprinted 1988
Revised and reprinted 1989
Reprinted 1991
Reprinted 1992
Second edition 1993
Revised and reprinted 1994
Reprinted 1995 (twice)
Reprinted 1997

Third edition 1999

ISBN 0–443–06153–X

British Library Cataloguing in Publication Data
A catalogue record for this book is available from the British Library.

Note
Medical knowledge is constantly changing. As new information becomes available, changes in treatment, procedures, equipment and the use of drugs become necessary. The editor and the publishers have, as far as it is possible, taken care to ensure that the information given in this text is accurate and up-to-date. However, readers are strongly advised to confirm that the information, especially with regard to drug usage, complies with the latest legislation and standards of practice.

The
publisher's
policy is to use
**paper manufactured
from sustainable forests**

Printed by Grafos, Arte sobre papel, Barcelona, Spain

Contents

Preface to the Third Edition

We have not inherited the earth from our grandparents – we have borrowed it from our grandchildren.

(Attributed to the ancient Chinese)

Although the second edition of this book was adequately revised and brought up to date in 1994, more changes have been required than I expected when I set out to produce this one.

Frighteningly, we have over a billion more humans on the planet since the first edition. Population is *the great multiplier* of those vast problems – the environment, the extinction of other species, poverty, global violence – facing our children as the human race reaches the next millennium.

Several new contraceptive products have arrived since the last edition: Persona, plastic male condoms, subcutaneous implants, the levonorgestrel-IUS and GyneFIX. The contraceptive sponge, C-Film and several other spermicides – and some pill brands – were withdrawn by the distributors for commercial reasons. The levonorgestrel vaginal ring featured in advance of marketing never made it (due to the development of unexplained erythematous patches which our MPC researchers identified in the vaginae of a proportion of users). And we are still waiting for that elusive 'male pill', or more probably, long-acting injection.

The biggest professional crisis of the last 5 years was of course the UK 'pill-scare' generated by the CSM's letter of 18 October 1995: not an easy time for most of us in this business! Sad that a well-meaning attempt at 'fine-tuning' pill-prescribing led to so many young women getting the message that the pill itself had been discovered to be dangerous, and to a documented 8% increase in the number of terminations of pregnancy performed the following year. (The right name for any girl babies born as a consequence would be Prescilla, being an anagram of 'pillscare'!). Even now there remains scientific and regulatory uncertainty in this country regarding the two targeted progestagens (desogestrel and gestodene): but very little concern on the issue in continental Europe. Unsurprisingly, none of the expected new pill formulations were marketed here in the late 1990s.

Contraception has everything to do with sex! Sexuality and communication influence crucially both strong and weak motivation for effective contraception (see Q 8.4), and we forget that whole area, and the other interface of sexually transmitted infections, at our peril – and too often. ... We must be perpetually on the look-out for the relevant verbal and non-verbal clues, particularly at the 'moment of truth' during a genital examination. We must avoid the busy doctor's knee-jerk reaction of reaching for the prescription pad.

In addition to those already acknowledged, who helped particularly with the first edition, I wish to thank Drs Elphis Christopher, Ron Kleinman, Sam Rowlands, also Anne Szarewski and other colleagues at the Margaret Pyke Centre; and for their keyboard skills my secretary Mrs Helen Prime and my son Jonathan. Toni Belfield, Director of Information of the UK FPA, helped particularly in the writing of Chapter 8. Dr. Hilary Luscombe and Joan Walsh assisted with literature searches and lists of the topics about which questions are most commonly asked. Lucy Gardner, Miranda Bromage and Rachel Robson at Churchill Livingstone, now part of Harcourt, turned my efforts into the completed book. All of these are most warmly thanked.

John Guillebaud

1999

Preface to the First Edition

As its title suggests, this book is designed as a ready source of answers to the many questions which are being asked, always with interest and often with a hint of anxiety, both by the consumers and the providers of modern reversible birth control methods. I have acquired experience in answering most of them as a result of lecturing in family planning very widely, in this country and abroad, and also on the postgraduate lecture courses held regularly at the Margaret Pyke Centre. In these, upwards of 600 doctors and 200 nurses are trained each year. The book is intended primarily for general practitioners and family planning doctors, working in a developed country such as Britain, but it will also be of value to other health care professionals, and medical students.

The questions about each method are arranged so far as possible in a logical order. They are mostly based on the questions which doctors ask of a specialist colleague like myself, arising from their clinical experience and the questions they have been asked by patients. In a concluding section of most chapters there is an assortment of the very practical questions which are asked by patients, some of which can be demanding to the unprepared (see, for example, Qs 4.266 and 6.175).

Reasons of space have required me to concentrate almost entirely on answers to questions about the technology of reversible birth control, with little discussion of and male and female sterilization and induced abortion, as well as essential subjects such as counselling, social factors affecting contraceptive use, medico-legal aspects, sexual problems and health screening. Most of these are dealt with in other texts in the Further Reading section, notably the *Handbook of Family Planning* edited by Nancy Loudon and published by Churchill Livingstone.

For reading and commenting on sections of the text, I am most grateful to the following: Walli Bounds, Ken Fotherby, Susan Hatwell, Sam Hutt, Howard Jacobs and Pram Senanayake. Special thanks are due to my deputy at the Centre, Mr Ali Kubba, who has read and constructively criticized the whole book: but I must be held responsible for any errors that remain.

Ray Phillips and his staff of the Middlesex Hospital Department of Medical Photography and Illustration, especially Stuart Nightingale and

Angela Scott, have been most helpful in the preparation of figures – apart from some separately acknowledged in the figure captions and tables. Toni Belfield contributed a list of questions which have been asked of the Family Planning Association's Information Service by the general public. My publishers have been most understanding, notably Katherine Watts and Howard Bailey. I also acknowledge the help of Mr John Adkins, Headmaster of Egerton-Rothesay School, in providing me with a haven of quiet for much of the writing. Last, but not least, I record my thanks to my select team of typists: Margaret Bailón, Diane Berry, Sue Nickells and Georgina Tregoning.

My wife Gwyneth as usual has been enormously supportive. She and our young children have been most tolerant of their recent one-parent family status.

John Guillebaud
September 1985

Glossary

AIDS	acquired immune deficiency syndrome
ALOs	*Actinomyces*-like organisms
AUC	area under the curve – in pharmacokinetic studies
BBD	benign breast disease
BBT	basal body temperature
BMI	body mass index
BP	blood pressure
BTB	breakthrough bleeding
CASH Study	Cancer and Sex Hormones Study
CGHFBC	Collaborative Group on Hormonal Factors in Breast Cancer
CIN	cervical intraepithelial neoplasia
COC	combined oral contraceptive
CSM	Committee on Safety of Medicines
CVS	cardiovascular system
D&C	dilatation and curettage
DES	diethylstilboestrol
DM	diabetes mellitus
DMPA	depot medroxyprogesterone acetate
DVT	deep venous thrombosis
EE	ethinyloestradiol
EC	emergency contraception
ENB	English National Board (of nursing)
Epinephrine	adrenaline
Faculty	Faculty of Family Planning & Reproductive Health Care
of FPRHC	(a faculty of the RCOG formed in 1995 by merger of JCC with NAFPD)
FNH	focal nodular hyperplasia
FOC	functional ovarian cysts
FPA	Family Planning Association
FSH	follicle stimulating hormone
GUM	genito-urinary medicine
HDL–C	high-density lipoprotein–cholesterol
hCG	human chorionic gonadotrophin
HIV	human immunodeficiency virus
HRT	hormone replacement therapy
IMB	intermenstrual bleeding
IPPF	International Planned Parenthood Federation
IUD	intrauterine device
I.U.D.	intrauterine death

LA	local anaesthesia
LH	luteinizing hormone
Lidocaine	lignocaine
LNG	levonorgestrel
LNG-IUS	levonorgestrel-releasing intrauterine system
JCC	Joint Committee on Contraception (see Faculty of FPRHC)
MPA	medroxyprogesterone acetate
MPC	Margaret Pyke Centre
NAFPD	National Association of Family Planning Doctors (see Faculty of FPRHC)
NET EN	norethisterone oenanthate
NFP	natural family planning
NMR	nuclear magnetic resonance
OC	oral contraceptive
PC	postcoital
PCO	polycystic ovary/ovaries
PD	peak day
PFI	pill-free interval
PG	prostaglandins
PGSI	prostaglandin synthetase inhibitor
PID	pelvic inflammatory disease
PMS	premenstrual syndrome
POEC	progestagen-only emergency contraception
POP	progestagen-only pill
PPA	post-pill amenorrhoea
RCGP	Royal College of General Practitioners
RCOG	Royal College of Obstetricians and Gynaecologists
RCT	randomized controlled trial
SAH	subarachnoid haemorrhage
SEM	scanning electron microscope
SHBG	sex hormone binding globulin
SLE	systemic lupus erythematosus
STI	sexually transmitted infection(s)
TSS	toxic shock syndrome
UC	ulcerative colitis
UK NCCS	UK National Case Control Study
US	ultrasound
USA FDA	USA Food and Drug Administration
VTE	venous thromboembolism
WHO	World Health Organization
WHO 1, WHO 2, WHO 3, WHO 4	WHO categories for contraindications, explained at Q 4.130
WTB	withdrawal bleeding

Figures

Tables

? 0

Introduction: The population explosion and the importance of fertility control

See Figure 0.1. According to the 1998 figures of the Population Reference Bureau, there will be 6000 million humans on the planet in October 1999. During the closing months of the 20th century, every 10 seconds there are 43 births and 17 deaths, meaning 26 extra people somewhere on the globe

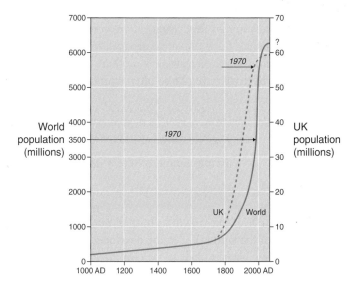

Figure 0.1   Estimated rate of population growth, AD 1750–2000. Q 0.1 *Note*: the UK differs from the rest of the world mainly by having had its population explosion slightly earlier. England too was once covered by forest.

1

every 10 seconds. Those 26 extra births beyond replacement mean approaching 1 million new additions arriving every 4 days, or more than 500 full jumbo jets arriving every day at London Airport. Because most of tomorrow's parents are children already born (Q 0.6), we must expect the arrival of close to a complete new world before the earliest date of stabilization. Yet even now many of the existing 6000 million are grossly deficient in the bare necessities of life: food, clean water, clothing, housing, health care, education and recreation. ... Is it quality of life we are after, or quantity of flesh?

We will never meet human needs on this finite planet until we stabilize human numbers.

0.2 SO HOW IS THE WORLD DOING AT PRESENT?

According to the UN's figures, out of about 185 million pregnancies each year at least 75 million are unwanted, resulting in about 45 million abortions of which 20 million are performed in unsafe circumstances. At least 585 000 women die each year (equalling a jumbo jet crashing every 6 hours) from those pregnancies, through abortion or for lack of the basic requirements for safe delivery. An estimated 200 000 would not die if adequate services and supplies for contraception were available.

What infamous statistics! Such dreadful carnage! When you add the preventable deaths among children as well as mothers when births are too frequent, how can birth planning be so often stigmatized as anti-life! On the contrary:

Family planning could provide more benefits to more people at less cost than any other single 'technology' now available to the human race

(James Grant, UNICEF ANNUAL REPORT, 1992)

0.3 BUT ISN'T THIS PRIMARILY A *DEVELOPING WORLD* PROBLEM?

Certainly, more than 90% of the growth in human numbers is occurring in the poor countries of the world. But in the developed world it has been calculated that every new birth is likely to lead, in the lifetime of that individual, depending on their affluence and the 'greenness' of their technology, to up to 30–200 times more damage to the fragile environment. More humans multiplied by a per capita affluence-plus-effluence factor is leading to climate change and the relentless destruction of the habitats of other animals and plants. According to the Worldwide Fund for Nature, total extinction now proceeds at the rate of several species per day, and rising.

Moreover, as was shown by the two reports of the Brandt Commission, the developed countries of the world cannot consider themselves forever immune to events elsewhere on this small finite planet. No wall will be high enough to stop the flood of 'economic migrants', for one thing. The rich 'north' ought to give far more and far more appropriate aid to the 'south', out of simple humanity. But even without that motivation, their own calculated self-interest should force voters and therefore politicians, worldwide, massively to increase the aid they give to the poor countries – and the proportion of it given to reproductive health and the methods of birth control.

If we are not part of the solution, we are part of the problem.

0.4 WHAT CHANGES BIRTH RATES?

As shown in Figure 0.2, a great deal more is necessary than simply the provision of family planning. Though all are important, some can be highlighted:

1   Better health and fewer child deaths, since it has been calculated that in rural areas of India a couple need to have five children in order to have a

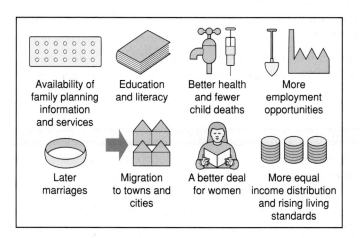

Figure 0.2 What changes birth rates? Q 0.4 (From *The shape of things to come.* 1982 Population Concern)

95% chance of one son reaching maturity. There is a vicious circle here though, as child mortality is itself greater in the absence of effective family spacing, now being exacerbated by the worldwide decline in breastfeeding without enough alternative contraception.

2 A better deal for women. In too many societies worldwide women remain second-class citizens, and have little choice in their destiny or that of their family. They are forced by their male-dominated society in general, and their husbands in particular, as well as by their biology (see Qs 1.1–1.10), to have far more children than they desire. This was clearly shown by the World Fertility Survey and the Reproductive Health Surveys which, in 60 countries of the developing world, found even in the 1980s that almost 50% of married women wanted no more children. So for them at least family planning had become a perceived unmet need – we should, and could (but did not), push at an open door. ...

3 Implicit in the whole of Figure 0.2, are two slogans or sayings. The first is an ancient proverb referring to the inhabitants of rural areas:

Every mouth has got two hands.

In rural poverty the hands are far more noticeable than the mouth, in that the labour and support which a child can give to its parents, especially in their old age or during disease, are far more important to them than the extra cost that may be incurred. It is hard for individuals to see how the macroproblems – burgeoning numbers in large tracts of the Developing World leading to excessive tree-cutting, erosion and floods, desertification, salinization, habitat destruction and ultimately disaster – are in any way their business through decisions about childbearing.

Apart from the regrettable 'Big Brother' Chinese solution – enforcing one-child families – what can be done? Even the Chinese agree that was a draconian and not very successful measure forced on them mainly because they did not bring in a much less restrictive two-child policy when they had half as many people only 50 years ago. The best answer is summarized in another slogan:

Take care of the people and the population will take care of itself.

4 Rising living standards. Poverty should be eliminated, as a matter of social justice (Figure 0.2). But when coupled with (3) above there is a vicious circle. Even if the gross domestic product (GDP) of a country like

Burundi (the land of my birth) or of Rwanda where I was brought up, does increase, the *per capita* GDP goes down if it is shared by more and more people. Ever more hardship results, and violence can be the outcome. When I was a kid there were only 2 million Rwandans. By the time of the appalling genocide in 1994 in which several of my playmates and friends of the 1940s were slaughtered, there were four people to share all available resources where there had been one. This has to be relevant, since 'The stork is the bird of war'.

0.5 DOES THIS MEAN THAT DEVELOPMENT IS THE BEST CONTRACEPTIVE, SO FAMILY PLANNING DOES NOT MATTER?

Far from it; many people have misinterpreted the slogan in this way, claiming for example that improved child survival is a prerequisite for family planning acceptance (though experience in Bangladesh and elsewhere has disproved this). The result is that in large areas of the world, in the slums and rural areas where people actually live, the basic tools for the family planning job are just not available at a price that they can afford. 'Population will take care of itself' only when 'taking care of the people' includes every item in Figure 0.2 as part of an integrated solution. Family planning services must be locally, comprehensively and appropriately provided, as a human right, on an equal basis at least with all the other items illustrated. Instead of 'counting people' the emphasis must be *'people count'*, as highlighted at the UN world population conference in Cairo, 1994. The emphasis must be on reproductive health, education and empowerment for women.

At present the proportion of aid for the Third World spent on the provision of voluntary birth control is around 2%. Family planning is no panacea, the whole answer: but it is surely much more than 2% of the answer!

0.6 IF EVERYTHING WERE DONE THAT COULD AND SHOULD BE DONE, WHAT IS THE MOST LIKELY FUTURE TOTAL WORLD POPULATION AT STABILIZATION?

Realistically, approaching twice its present size. Short of a cataclysm, this is a demographic certainty. Why? Because world population, like a super-tanker, has so much inbuilt momentum. 1700 million of the world's inhabitants are under 15, and that means *very nearly all of tomorrow's parents are already born*. They will be responsible for a doubling even if they have only an average of two children each. To me, this is the most frightening of all alarming ecostatistics.

So everything we must do (and are not doing nearly well enough yet) in the provision of reproductive health is about stopping world number 3 from coming along: world number 2 is all-but inevitable! Scientists can see some chance of a passable if perilous future for around 10–12 billion humans. More than that really does risk collapse of life-support mechanisms in the ecosystem, and deaths and misery on an unheard-of scale.

0.7 IS THE POPULATION CRISIS REALLY THAT BAD?

A frog dropped into boiling water jumps straight out, unscathed. If this (unethical) experiment is repeated with the same water, the same container, the frog and the source of heat, BUT starting from cold, the outcome is a boiled frog. The trouble about the population/development/resources/ pollution story is that it is based on numerous interconnected adverse trends rather than catastrophic events. Very like that frog, we humans have a poor track record for reacting vigorously to serious dangers (take cigarette smoke for instance!) if they are gradual and insidious. But we must.

The crisis is caused much less by wilfulness than by carelessness and ignorance. It happens through millions of people 'doing their own thing'. All of us, whether clearing our forests or driving to the shops, are using technology to improve our families' material environment: oblivious to the fact that, with more and more people doing the same and continuing for long enough, the consequences for our grandchildren could be horrendous. Somehow we must, all of us, learn a 'greener' lesson, that we must stop treating the fragile planet as an inexhaustible 'milch-cow' for our wants and as a bottomless cesspit for our wastes.

In the preface I quoted the saying:

> *We have not inherited the world from our grandparents – we have borrowed it from our grandchildren.*

I believe that our own children's children will brand this generation, living in the last quarter of the 20th century, as the worst ever: in that it was the last to have some chance of preventing the environmental wasteland which they will have inherited, but too little was done and too late. We will be seen as having selfishly mortgaged their future for our present gain.

0.8 SHOULD WE BE APOLOGIZING FOR DAMAGING THIS 'LOAN FROM OUR GRANDCHILDREN'?

Because I felt the need to do just that, I devised the Environment Time Capsule project. Time capsules containing environmentally relevant objects of the year 1994 were buried with letters and poems addressed to people in the year 2044 at strategic sites across the globe: in Mexico, UK, South Africa, the Seychelles and Australia. As well as the apologizing there was the pledge: that all those involved would work tirelessly to ensure that, hopefully, those who dug up each time capsule would wonder what we were on about – i.e. apologies would not be necessary!

NOTE: More details about this ongoing project can be found at http//:www.geocities.com/rainforest/vines/3360timecapsule.htm or in a 'Personal view' article, *BMJ* 1994;308:1377–8.

0.9 IN VIEW OF THE URGENCY, AND THE INBUILT MOMENTUM OF POPULATION GROWTH, WHY IS SO LITTLE BEING DONE?

The main problem is, as the politicians say, 'politics is the art of the possible'. Voters worldwide faced with the challenge of less 'jam' today in order that their children may inherit a tolerable world in the future, invariably vote instead to have at least as much as they currently have, and preferably more. Human perspectives are remarkably insular in terms of space and brief in terms of time. The following sayings summarize things well: 'my car is my car, everyone else's car is traffic'; 'my visit to the seaside is my holiday, but the crowds on the beach!'; and 'my baby is my baby – everybody else's baby is overpopulation'. These attitudes are reinforced by ignorance, by apathy and by a hint of racism: 'the death of one baby, in London, is a tragedy; the death of millions of babies, in Africa, that's a statistic'.

0.10 IS IT ALL DOOM AND GLOOM?

No, there are actually sound grounds for some optimism. Total fertility rates (average family sizes) are falling in almost every country. The money is there. After all, smallpox was eradicated from the face of this planet by an amount of money which was then spent by the world's armed forces every 8 minutes. It has been estimated that the extra money required to provide adequate food, water, education, housing and health for the whole planet, including the means for each woman to control her fertility as she would choose, could be provided for as little as one month's-worth of defence spending!

0.11 AGAINST ALL THE ODDS, ANYTHING I DID WOULD BE JUST A DROP IN THE OCEAN?

True, but

The ocean is made up of drops

As health care professionals, we should not underestimate our influence on those around us, our patients and our peer groups, and through them the politicians. More immediately, knowledge is power. Here we come to the reason why this book has been written: we can ensure that we are so well informed about the whole subject of contraception, that we can answer the questions of the women and the men who come to us for contraceptive advice and help. In so far as we are able to influence events, the aim is simple: 'every child a wanted child'.

0.12 IS IT ENOUGH TO BE ABLE TO ANSWER THE QUESTIONS?

No – 1 g of *empathy* is worth 1 kg of *knowledge*. Moreover:

1 There are *techniques* to be learnt and maintained: counselling skills, and practical skills in the fitting of intrauterine devices, and the fitting and the training for women who wish to use female barrier methods.
2 In reproductive health care, the correct non-directive counselling *attitude* and approach are vital. Couples must decide for themselves what aspects of the list in Q 0.15 below are most important in their situation. It has been well said that in the matter of birth planning: 'we are advisers, we are the suppliers – but we are not the deciders' (see Q8.14).
3 *Time* is always a huge constraint. So doctors should work closely with other professionals, especially (family planning trained) nurses. Appropriate delegation and teamwork ensure the best user-friendly services.

0.13 GIVEN THAT PREGNANCY IS A SEXUALLY TRANSMITTED CONDITION, PRESUMABLY GOOD CONTRACEPTIVE COUNSELLING SHOULD ALWAYS INCLUDE AN ADEQUATE SEXUAL HISTORY?

Absolutely, yet even now too many providers in a family planning context claim to be too rushed (or could they still be too embarrassed?) to do it.

If the request is for 'emergency contraception', by definition a sexually transmitted infection (STI) could have been passed along with the sperm. Indeed, there is increasing evidence that the sperm themselves can be 'bio-vectors' of *Chlamydia* and Gonococci. (But no *Chlamydia* test could yet be positive, it would need doing 5–7 days later).

0.14 WHAT ARE THE BEST QUESTIONS TO ASK?

If asked in a matter of fact way and non-judgementally during the course of a consultation about periods and gynae symptoms, the following questions will almost never cause offence:

- *When did you last have sex?*
- *Was that with your regular partner?*
- *When was your last sex with anyone else?*

Or, faster yet, an initial screening query, followed by more detailed probing only according to the tenor and the body language of the response:

- *Have you had sex with someone different in the last 3 months?* (Note how the question covers both a change of partner during 'serial monogamy' *and* any possible 'one-night stand' within a basically long-term relationship.) And, often very relevant:
- *Do you wonder whether your partner has other partner(s)?*

0.15 WHAT ARE THE FEATURES OF THE IDEAL CONTRACEPTIVE?

The list below is modified from Table 13 in my book *The Pill* (see Further Reading). The ideal method would be:

1 *100% effective*; effective after a single simple procedure, ideally, not thereafter relying on the user's memory. Thus the 'default state' becomes one of staying contracepted, not conceiving! (At present the two commonest methods used by young people, the pill and the

condom, have a completely wrong 'default state'). For the twenty-first century, the IDEAL MODEL has to be to switch off one's fertility at a certain time and then, maybe years later, to switch it on again at will;

2   *100% convenient*, including independent of intercourse;
3   *100% reversible*; reversed very simply, ideally without having to ask permission or get help to stop the method;
4   *100% safe*, without unwanted effects, whether fatal, dangerous or simply annoying;
5   *cheap and easy to distribute*;
6   *independent of the medical professions*, and no follow-up monitoring required;
7   *acceptable*, to every culture, religion and political view;
8   used by or obviously visible to the woman (whose stakes in effective contraception are obviously greatest); but an effective non-condom reversible male option would be welcome!

The ideal contraceptive must also have *beneficial non-contraceptive side-effects*. The most relevant in today's world has to be protection against sexually transmitted infections, including viruses.

Since so far this can only (outside of monogamy) be adequately provided by a condom (male or female), many couples have to be advised to supplement their non-coitally-related pregnancy-preventing method with a condom: the so-called Double Dutch approach.

Couples are almost always ignorant about established non-contraceptive benefits, such as less ovarian cancer with the pill or less blood-loss with the LNG-IUS. Since good news is not 'news'; almost by definition, these get no publicity.

0.16 HOW DO THE AVAILABLE REVERSIBLE METHODS PERFORM WHEN TESTED AGAINST THE LIST IN Q 0.15?

Unfortunately, maximum effectiveness and independence from intercourse tend to go together and, unfortunately, to be inversely linked with freedom from health risk. So in practice, when counselling most couples, one can explain that there is always a dilemma, a 'Hobson's choice', as depicted in Table 0.1.

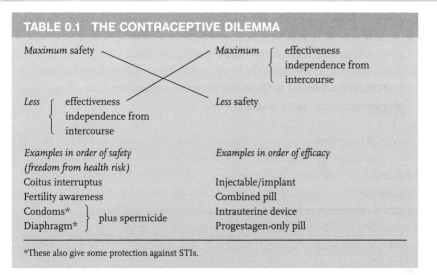

TABLE 0.1   THE CONTRACEPTIVE DILEMMA

Maximum safety

Maximum { effectiveness / independence from / intercourse

Less { effectiveness / independence from / intercourse

Less safety

Examples in order of safety (freedom from health risk)

Coitus interruptus
Fertility awareness
Condoms* }
Diaphragm* } plus spermicide

Examples in order of efficacy

Injectable/implant
Combined pill
Intrauterine device
Progestagen-only pill

*These also give some protection against STIs.

0.17 HOW IS THE EFFECTIVENESS OF ANY METHOD COMMONLY REPORTED?

The data about efficacy, particularly of the non-medical methods, have shown extremely variable results. In clinical investigations an effort is usually made to make the (in practice very difficult) distinction: between pregnancies that occurred despite the fact that the method was used correctly during every act of intercourse (method-failures), and those that resulted from incorrect use or non-use on one or more occasions (user-failures). This process results in estimates of the theoretical or method-effectiveness and of the actual use-effectiveness.

1 Method-effectiveness rates vary because of physiological differences between individuals, notably increasing age which diminishes fertility.
2 Use-effectiveness is a function of the motivation of the study population, the acceptability of another baby, the adequacy of counselling, the difficulty of using the method, the effect of experience through increasing duration of use, and other factors. Hence the findings are even more variable and it is very difficult to compare data from different studies among different populations.
3 Extended use-effectiveness is a measure of all the pregnancies occurring in a large population based on their initial intention to use a particular

method. It includes individuals who abandon the method which they initially set out to use. Failure rates calculated on this basis tend to be very high indeed, even for a highly effective method such as the combined pill, since side-effects or anxiety about side-effects can lead to it being abandoned without any effective replacement, in a large proportion of the initial users.

0.18 HOW ARE THE EFFECTIVENESS RATES MEASURED AND EXPRESSED?

Both method- and use-effectiveness rates are usually expressed as failure rates/100 woman-years of exposure. The basis for many calculations is known as the Pearl pregnancy rate, calculated from the formula:

Failure rate = Total accidental pregnancies × 1200 / Total months of exposure

When applying this formula every known conception must be included, whatever its outcome. The figure 1200 is of course the number of months in 100 years. By convention, 10 months are deducted from the denominator for each full-term pregnancy and 4 months for any kind of abortion.

Trussell (of Princeton, USA) points out that the usual convention of using the same denominator (total number of months) whether the numerator is the number of method-failures or user-failures is wrong. It fails to account for the fact that many contraceptive-users make errors and 'get away with it'. Any such method-failure rate is artificially lowered by the larger denominator. The true 'perfect use' rate would use for the denominator only the months of total compliance. Very few studies, in which all users kept coital diaries, have had any chance of computing this true rate. Because errors in compliance are so common and vary so widely, and the likelihood of 'getting away with it' also varies, this means that standard method- and user-failure rates should not ideally be compared between populations.

The risk of contraceptive failure tends to fall with the duration of use because of changes in the population under study, as women drop out for whatever reason. Long-term users obviously tend to be those who use the method efficiently and also include those of lower fertility (the more fertile ones are likely to leave the study by conceiving!) The life-table method of analysis is an attempt to overcome these problems. This takes into account all the reasons for contraceptive discontinuation, and permits the calculation of failure rates (or the rates for other events such as expulsion of an IUD) for specified intervals of use. The Pearl rate pools the data and can only give one common measurement, not compensating for drop-outs for varying reasons nor different durations of use in different studies.

0.19 WHAT EFFECTIVENESS RATES CAN BE QUOTED, FOR POTENTIAL USERS?

Vested interests (especially by advertisers) and the distinct lack of comparative studies – let alone randomized controlled trials – readily lead to misuse of the data on the effectiveness of particular techniques. Failure rates need to be interpreted by the provider to each potential user, in the context of the woman's age and factors such as the steadiness of the relationship and the frequency of intercourse. See Table 0.2.
Note how modern IUDs and the IUS have entirely comparable efficacy to female sterilization (Q 6.10); vasectomy is also clearly more effective than female sterilization, and injectables and implants beat the remainder (including the combined oral contraceptive [COC]) because of the user-failure problem. Note the considerable overlaps: careful condom-users have been known to do better than poor pill-users. See also the important caveats at Q 3.9 about the Oxford/FPA study, which recruited an untypically good population as regards contraceptive compliance!

In interpreting Table 0.2 to couples at counselling, it is sometimes helpful to divide 100 by the figures given for the rates. This calculation gives the number of years of regular intercourse, carefully using the method, which would be expected to lead to one conception. For example, if per 100 woman-year rates of 10 and 1 were being compared, the couple could be told that regular use of the method would give an 'evens' chance of one pregnancy by the end of 10 years or 100 years of fertility, respectively. This clearly shows the difference, though for a full understanding it is very important to add: 'Of course that one pregnancy could occur in the very first year, with betting odds of 1 in 10 or 1 in 100, respectively'.

It is also helpful to put things in the context of 'the failure rate of no contraception at all'. Among 100 young couples setting out to achieve a pregnancy, that 'failure rate' will be 80–90/100 woman-years. You can halve that when speaking to 40 year olds, meaning that the less effective methods will be 'stronger', for them. This explains why a user-friendly but ordinarily unreliable spermicide method like Delfen foam may usefully be recommended to 50 year olds (Q 8.45).

TABLE 0.2 FIRST-YEAR USER-FAILURE RATES / 100 WOMEN FOR DIFFERENT METHODS OF CONTRACEPTION

	Range in the World literature*	Oxford/FPA Study (Lancet report in 1982; all women married and aged above 25)		
		Overall (any duration)	Age 25–34 (≤2 years use)	Age 35+ (≤2 years use)
Sterilization				
Male (after azoospermia)	0–0.05	0.02	0.08	0.08
Female	0–0.5	0.13	0.45	0.08
Subcutaneous implant				
(Jadelle)	0–0.1			
Implanon	0–0.07			
Injectable (DMPA)	0–1	–	–	–
Combined pills				
50 µg oestrogen	0.1–3	0.16	0.25	0.17
<50 µg oestrogen	0.2–3	0.27	0.38	0.23
Progestagen-only pill	0.3–4	1.2	2.5	0.5
IUD				
Nova-T/Multiload Cu250	1–2			
Nova-T380	0.6			
Multiload Cu 375	0.2–1			
Cu-T 380	0.2–1			
Levonorgestrel IUD-20	0.1–0.2			
Diaphragm	4–20	1.9	5.5	2.8
(Male) condom	2–15	3.6	6.0	2.9
Female condom	5–15			
Coitus interruptus	6–17	6.7	–	–
Spermicides alone	4–25	11.9	–	–
Fertility awareness	2–25	15.5	–	–
'Persona'	6–?	–	–	–
No method, young women	80–90	–	–	–
No method at age 40	40–50	–	–	–
No method at age 45	10–20	–	–	–
No method at age 50 (if still having menses)	0–5	–	–	–

*Excludes atypical studies and all extended-use studies. For sterilization, rates in first column (only) are LIFETIME FAILURE RATES.

Note: 1 First figure of range in first column gives a rough measure of 'perfect use' (but is not the same).

    2 Influence of age: all the rates in the fourth column being lower than those in the third column. Lower rates still may be expected above age 45.

    3 Much better results also obtainable in other states of relative infertility, such as lactation.

    4 Oxford/FPA users were established users at recruitment – greatly improving results for barrier methods (see text Qs 0.19 and 3.9)

0.20 WHY IS IT THAT, AS YOU SAY, MOST ACCIDENTS ARE CAUSED BY HUMANS AND MOST HUMANS ARE STILL CAUSED BY ACCIDENTS? WHAT CAN I AS A PRESCRIBER DO ABOUT THIS?

It is no good just blaming the method-users. Prescribers can fail them in a number of ways, both by errors but more commonly by omissions: for example, simply not allowing enough time for basic instructions and for them to ask questions. 'You cannot make the horse drink' ... but in the first place have we *properly* 'taken the horse to the water?' More on this follows in Chapter 8 (see Qs 8.3–8.16): we need first to be fully informed about the methods available.

Table 0.3 shows current usage of the methods in Great Britain.

TABLE 0.3 PERCENTAGE OF WOMEN AGED 16–49 USING THE PILL, STERILIZATION AND THE CONDOM AS MAIN METHOD, BY AGE (GREAT BRITAIN, 1995)

Method of contraception	Age								
	All Ages	16–17	18–19	20–24	25–29	30–34	35–39	40–44	45–49
Sterilization	24	0	0	1	7	18	32	45	46
Female	12					9	15	24	26
Male	12					9	17	21	20
Pill (COC + POP)	25	25	37	49	41	29	20	9	3
Condom (male)	18	13	26	21	20	20	16	16	14
IUD	4	0	0	1	4	5	5	4	5
Other birth control, possibly infertile, or sterile after hysterectomy	6	0	2	3	8	9	12	16	23
Pregnant or wanting pregnancy	8	1	4	8	13	14	6	1	0
Abstinence/no partner	14	64	38	21	10	9	10	10	10

*General Household Survey. 1995, OPCS 1996.
Percentages may add to more than 100 because of use of more than one method (and rounding of numbers).

Aspects of human fertility and fertility awareness: Natural birth control

Apparently, after God created Adam, He said to him: 'I have some NEWS for you: two bits of good news and one bit of bad news. Which would you like to hear first?' And Adam said, 'The good news first please, God.'
So God said to Adam: 'The first good news is that I am going to create for you an Organ. This Organ is called the Brain. With this gift of mine you will be able to think, and to learn, and to feel – and if you use it well you will be a good steward of all the other creatures I have made.'

'Thank you very much', said Adam. 'What's the other good news?'

'Well', said God, 'I am going to create for you another Organ. This Organ is called the Penis. With it you will be able to give to your wife and receive back from her, much pleasure – and with my help, create children to follow you, and so you will be fruitful and multiply.' 'Thank you again', said Adam. 'So, what's the bad news?' 'YOU WILL NEVER BE ABLE TO USE BOTH AT THE SAME TIME', said God.

BACKGROUND CONSIDERATIONS

1.1 HOW FERTILE ARE HUMAN BEINGS?

Given that disjunction between brain and genitalia (in both sexes, though men are undoubtedly the worse affected ...): both the devising and the practising of effective contraception are difficult!

We break no records in the animal kingdom, but we are fertile enough to become numerically by far and away the most successful vertebrate that this planet has ever known. The first half of this chapter deals with physiological factors which promote conception. We have first to consider aspects relating to intercourse, then the sperm, the ova, fertilization and implantation.

We can at least be grateful that the fertility of average couples is not as great as the human maximum, which must have been approached by the couple described in the Guinness Book of Records:

> *The greatest officially recorded number of children produced by a mother is 69 by the first of the two wives of Feodor Vasilyev (b. 1707), a peasant from Shuya, 241 km east of Moscow. In 27 confinements, she gave birth to 16 pairs of twins, 7 sets of triplets and 14 sets of quadruplets. ... Almost all survived to their majority.*

1.2 WHAT FEATURES OF HUMAN INTERCOURSE ARE PARTICULARLY FAVOURABLE TO FERTILITY?

1 Obviously the attraction is frequently powerful and mutual, and the human female is exceptional in having no breeding season and in being potentially receptive on most days of the cycle.

2 Some indication of the power of the human sex instinct is provided by the calculation (never mind the assumptions) by WHO in the early 1990s, that intercourse takes place about 42 000 million times per year. This worked out, somewhere in the world, to over 1300 ejaculations per second ... and even more by now.

3 The drive towards copulation in both sexes is in 'real-time', now, and feels irresistible. This frustrates forward planning and the successful use of intercourse-related methods. And men are the worst culprits – they omit to tell their partners important nuisance details (e.g. that the condom split!) and tell the most flagrant lies (whether about their undying love or their HIV status).

4 In many women maximum desire concides with the most fertile phase, when there is an abundance of oestrogenic mucus, very favourable to sperm survival; whereas minimum desire is in the premenstrual 'safe' phase.

5 The outpouring of vaginal transudate described by Masters and Johnson raises the pH of the vagina so that it becomes favourable to sperm.

6 There is evidence that, at least in some women, there is a negative pressure in the uterus at orgasm which may promote physical aspiration of sperm into the cervix and uterus. Sperm are found in the cervix within 90 seconds of ejaculation.

1.3 HOW DO THE MECHANICS OF INTERCOURSE INTERFERE WITH THE EFFICACY OF VAGINAL METHODS?

1 The ballooning of the whole upper two-thirds of the vagina, also described by Masters and Johnson, leads to:
   (a) an increased risk of sperm passing over the rim of a diaphragm or other cervical cap, and
   (b) the risk of displacement of any cervical device into a fornix.

2 The penile thrusts themselves lead to:
   (a) the potential to dislodge all forms of female barrier, particularly in certain positions of intercourse, and
   (b) if a vaginal spermicide is used, it is probable that the spreading effect of intercourse means that there is ultimately too little spermicide around the external os of the cervix at ejaculation. This may in part explain how spermicides have usually appeared far more effective in vitro than in vivo (see Q 3.63).

1.4 WHAT ARE THE RELEVANT FACTS ABOUT CERVICAL MUCUS?

Cervical mucus is only the most obvious component of the genital tract mucus and fluid, which extend right through the cavity of the uterus and both tubes. Under the influence of unopposed oestrogen in the follicular phase it becomes increasingly fluid and receptive to sperm, with a marked Spinnbarkeit. It helps to capacitate sperm and provides an optimum environment for them to proceed to the upper tract. The ability to promote sperm survival for prolonged durations varies from women to woman and from cycle to cycle, as does the length of time within the cycle that ovulatory mucus is present.

The characteristics of mucus change abruptly under the influence of progesterone, even though the corpus luteum continues to secrete oestrogens. It rapidly becomes impenetrable and hostile to sperm. Women can be taught to feel the change from the earlier slippery 'ovulatory' mucus to the sticky mucus of the luteal phase. But before ovulation WHO found (1983) 'a substantial' probability of pregnancy if intercourse occurs (even) in the presence of sticky mucus (see Q 1.25).

1.5 WHAT OTHER CHANGES OCCUR AT THE CERVIX DURING THE CYCLE?

Continuing research into birth planning by methods of fertility awareness has shown that women can be taught to detect the changes occurring in the size of the external cervical os, and also in its position relative to the introitus. The cervix starts low and rises appreciably during the follicular phase, until around ovulation it reaches peak height from the introitus with maximum softness and sufficient dilation to admit a finger tip. The cervix then descends and narrows rapidly early in the luteal phase, becoming once more closed, firm and close to the vulva. It is reported that daily autopalpation of these cervical changes can be of particular value in the detection of the return of fertility towards the end of lactation (see Q 1.35).

1.6 WHICH ARE THE MOST IMPORTANT PHYSIOLOGICAL FACTS ABOUT SPERM WHICH PROMOTE CONCEPTION?

All of us whose work involves family planning rapidly develop an enormous respect for these little swimmers! There is great individual variation between men, and between individual sperm within the same man's ejaculate. Sperm counts and quality have fallen in some areas, attributed to oestrogenic chemical pollutants in the environment: is Nature biting back, against the species that is multiplying like there were no tomorrow? (Q 0.1ff).

Yet there is still an overkill of numbers produced by most men. From the point of view of preventing pregnancy we have to consider the very best sperm with regard to motility, survival and fertilizing ability, rather than those exhibiting average or lesser qualities.

1.7 HOW MANY SPERM ARE PRESENT, AND WHAT ARE THE IMPLICATIONS?

Spermatogenesis proceeds in normal men at rates of the order of 1000 per second from each testicle! With a count of say 80 million/ml being not unrepresentative, it would not be unusual for there to be 350 million sperm in the 3–5 ml of a typical ejaculate. If each sperm could find an egg this would be enough to populate most of North America! One per cent of this number (enough to people Costa Rica or New Zealand) might very well cause a pregnancy (see Q 1.9). Yet this would be contained in the hardly visible volume of less than 0.05 ml.

This has obvious implications for coitus interruptus (see Q 2.7) and also for any lack of care when using the condom (see Q 2.20). In contraceptive terms, semen is a dangerous fluid!

1.8 WHAT IS THE EXTREME LIMIT OF SPERM SURVIVAL IN GENITAL TRACT MUCUS, AND WHAT ARE THE IMPLICATIONS?

This has proved very difficult to study directly, since the studies themselves are liable to alter what is being observed. It seems clear that sperm *normally* survive no more than about 6 hours in the vagina, as its pH reverts to its normal low value subsequent to intercourse. Motile sperm have been found even in the vagina up to 16 hours after intercourse, however, and survival in the cervical, uterine and tubal fluid appears very variable. Survival depends on features of the sperm themselves, the seminal fluid, and to what degree the oestrogenic mucus approaches the ideal – in that woman or in that particular cycle.

In the past most authorities have talked in terms of average survival times of about 3–4 days. However, with so many millions ejaculated one must be concerned not with average sperm survival but lunatic fringe sperm survival! It is the duration of the ability to fertilize of the first centile of the sperm (i.e. the most vigorous 3 million or so) which is the relevant figure. This is not known; but both direct studies and indirect studies suggest that this can certainly exceed 5 days. On some rare occasions in some rare couples, particularly where the woman produces good mucus for an unusually long time, it might even reach 7 days. Mucus assessment (see Qs 1.4 and 1.24) should theoretically give more advance warning of ovulation than usual in those very cases, but it can fail to do so.

The main implication is the likely ineffectiveness, in long-term use by most couples, of the *first* phase of the so-called 'safe period' (see Q 1.16).

1.9 HOW CAN IT BE THAT 1% OF A MAN'S EJACULATE (I.E. ABOUT 3 MILLION SPERM) COULD CAUSE A PREGNANCY, WHEN MEN WITH THAT NUMBER OF SPERM/ML ARE COMMONLY INFERTILE?

This question implies a common misunderstanding of the nature of semen analysis in an infertility clinic. For a start, an excessively high count can actually be associated with male subfertility. And when a low count is present, it is mainly acting as a marker for other much more important features of the sperm which are causing the subfertility, such as poor motility, frequent abnormal forms, or the presence of antibodies. The paucity of sperm goes along with them being pretty poor individuals. This does not apply when 3 million good sperm from a fertile man are deposited at the cervix, for example because of too late use of a condom.

Evidence for the above comes from routine sperm counts in men having vasectomies who have fathered children. Counts less than 2 million/ml are not uncommon; and in a study of late recanalization reported from Oxford, it appeared that one man with counts of only 500 000 and 750 000/ml (with motility demonstrated) was responsible for his wife's pregnancy.

1.10 WHAT ARE THE RELEVANT PHYSIOLOGICAL FACTS ABOUT OVA?

1 More often than expected by many couples, ovulation occurs early. Many women claiming 28-day menstrual cycles really sometimes have 26-day cycles, and some can feature fertile cycles as short as 21 or 22 days in length (see Q 1.15 for the implications).
2 Ovum fertilizability is short – practically the only physiological fact so far discussed which helps contraception. From in vitro fertilization research, maximum ovum survival is believed to be 24 hours but successful fertilization appears to be unlikely beyond 12 hours. This means that if a pregnancy is desired, the best chance of successful fertilization is when that fragile ovum arrives at a tube which is already populated with adequate numbers of vigorous, motile sperm.

1.11 CAN HUMAN FEMALES BE LIKE RABBITS, OVULATING ON INTERCOURSE?

I think the answer to this question which is often asked can (fortunately) be a fairly definite 'no'. First there is no need to postulate any such mechanism, when one adds together the data mentioned above concerning sperm survival and the frequent occurrence of ovulation earlier than usual. Intercourse can be fertile almost any time, not excluding during the menses, if sperm may survive for up to 7 days and ovulation can be unexpectedly early or late.

A more important reason for rejecting this hypothesis is the fact that, were it to be true, newly married women would have shorter menstrual cycles than women who were abstaining from intercourse (such as nuns). Such a shortening of the mean duration of menstrual cycles has not been observed.

1.12 AFTER FERTILIZATION HOW MUCH PREIMPLANTATION WASTAGE OCCURS?

Here we have another fact which, fortunately, reduces the size of the contraceptive task. Assessments of postfertilization wastage vary considerably, but a good modern estimate would be around 30–40%. Frequently there are chromosomal abnormalities, but local factors affecting the receptivity of the endometrium to the blastocyst are also important. These can be enhanced by contraceptive methods (see Qs 5.4 and 7.6).

FERTILITY AWARENESS AND NATURAL FAMILY PLANNING

BACKGROUND AND MECHANISMS

1.13 PUTTING THE ABOVE PHYSIOLOGICAL FACTS TOGETHER, HOW LONG IS THE POTENTIALLY FERTILE PHASE IN THE HUMAN FEMALE?

This had traditionally been termed 'midcycle', or say days 10–17 of a 28-day cycle; but recent in vivo and in vitro studies, which form the basis of the physiology described in the last ten questions, clearly indicate that the fertile phase both starts and finishes earlier. The latest work would imply that under optimal conditions for sperm survival the potentially fertile phase is not less than days 7–14 (i.e. the whole of the second week of a 4-week cycle). If ovulation takes place on day 14–15 a further 1-plus days needs to be added to allow for maximum ovum survival, i.e. in all from *day 7 to day 15–16*, all adjusted as appropriate of course, if the cycle is longer

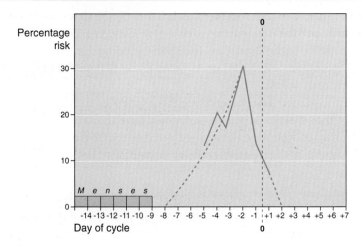

Figure 1.1 The risk of conception on different days of the menstrual cycle (Barrett JC and Marshall J 1969) (See text Q 1.14–1.16). (Redrawn from Table 2 in *Population Studies* 1969; 23: 455–461)

or shorter than 28 days. It is fascinating that recent studies with biochemical markers of ovulation, and the artificial reproduction work on sperm and ovum survival, reflect so accurately the 1969 findings of Barrett and Marshall (Fig. 1.1).

1.14 HOW WAS THE BARRETT AND MARSHALL STUDY DESIGNED? WHAT IS THE RISK OF CONCEPTION ON EACH DAY OF THE CYCLE (FIG. 1.1)

In brief, 241 previously fertile women who had been fully trained to keep basal body temperature (BBT) charts also kept a careful record of every act of intercourse. Whether conception took place in a given cycle was also known. Some were attempting to conceive; others to avoid pregnancy. All the data on 1898 cycles and 6015 acts of coitus were fed into a computer, and for each woman the day of BBT shift, and hence presumed ovulation, was identified in a standard way for that cycle.

The analysis gave figures for the percentage risk of conception for intercourse on each day of the cycle relative to the BBT shift, and these have been charted to produce Figure 1.1 (0 represents the BBT shift). The continuous line joins the points for which the data were sufficient for an estimate of percentage risk of conception to be made; the dotted lines are no more than approximate projections down to the horizontal axis.

1.15 WHAT ARE THE MAIN OBSERVATIONS FROM FIGURE 1.1?

1 The percentage risk of conception exceeds zero between days 7 and 16 of a 28-day cycle, as predicted from sperm and ovum survival studies (see Q 1.13).
2 Peak fecundability occurs well before ovum release, again congruent with the notion that it is best for the sperm to be waiting in the tubes in advance of ovulation.
3 The first 'infertile' phase of the cycle is shown to be short, even in a woman who never ovulates earlier than day 14. Since it is well known that very many women do occasionally ovulate earlier in the cycle, in a 24-day cycle intercourse any later than day 3 might, on the basis of these data, sometimes result in conception!
4 The good news from Figure 1.1, however is that the second phase is potentially a very 'safe period', dependent only on the reliability of ovulation detection. There is, normally, only one ovum, and it is fertilizable for a predictable, short time.

This is quite unlike the first phase which is beset by problems: the millions of sperm, the capriciousness with which enough of them may just survive on occasion for as much as a week, coupled with the possibility of a random, early ovulation. So far no means have been devised of *predicting* ovulation accurately, far enough ahead, to eliminate the risk of sperm survival up to the point of fertilization.

1.16 WHAT ARE THE IMPLICATIONS OF THE FECUNDABILITY CURVE (FIG. 1.1) FOR FAMILY PLANNING?

In my view, with any combination of present technologies, only the second infertile phase should be relied on by a woman who feels that she must avoid pregnancy. The first phase is only suitable for those who are delaying a wanted pregnancy ('spacing'). The one exception to this recommendation might be a woman with very regular longish menstrual cycles (never less than 28 days) who is good at detecting mucus and cervical changes. She should abstain in each cycle from the first day of detection of mucus or from 20 days before her shortest cycle would end, whichever comes earlier, to identify the first potentially fertile day (Q 1.18).

But the capriciousness of sperm survival under occasional optimal conditions in the female reproductive tract still means that, whatever methodology based on fertility awareness is used, the preovulatory phase will always be 'in a different ball-park' of potential efficacy, as compared with the postovulatory phase.

1.17 WHY HAVE FAMILY PLANNING SPECIALISTS TRADITIONALLY DECRIED NATURAL FAMILY PLANNING METHODS? WHAT SHOULD BE THEIR ATTITUDE NOW?

The bad reputation of these methods followed from the high failure rate of the old calendar/rhythm approach (see Q 1.18), coupled with a lack of awareness of the fundamental difference in effectiveness potential between the first and the second infertile phases, however they might be determined. That lack of awareness is still common today among both the opponents and the proponents of the methods.

The correct attitude today should be a very positive one to this *choice* for couples, with accurate information and appropriate advice about the appropriateness of the choice in each case.

1.18 THOUGH NOT RECOMMENDED AS THE SOLE METHOD, WHAT CALCULATIONS ARE REQUIRED FOR THE CALENDAR/RHYTHM METHOD?

1 First the woman should define the shortest and longest menstrual cycle over the previous six (preferably 12) cycles.
2 Second she should subtract 20 days from the length of the shortest cycle to derive the first day of the fertile phase. This allows 14, 15 or 16 days for the length of the luteal phase plus 6, 5 or 4 days for maximum sperm survival. Sadly both these durations may sometimes be longer! But in the identification of the start of the fertile phase, this particular calculation is an important additional safeguard (to the first appearance of any mucus, Q 1.24). Third, subtract 11 from the longest cycle observed to derive the last day of the fertile phase, so allowing 12–14 days for minimum length of a fertile luteal phase and 1 day for the duration of ovum fertilizability. This is not a reliable guide to the end of the fertile phase (and better indicators exist).

Even with good compliance this method has a high failure rate. Compliance is also difficult, because few women have regular menstrual cycles so the amount of abstinence required becomes intolerable to many couples.

1.19 HOW ARE THE PHASES OF THE FERTILITY CYCLE DEFINED? SEE FIGURE 1.2.

1 The first infertile phase starts on day 1 of the menses and ends with the earliest time that any sperm could survive to cause a pregnancy. It varies very much in length depending on the rapidity of the follicular response to the pituitary hormones.

2 The *true* fertile phase extends from the end of phase 1 until that time following ovulation when the ovum is incapable of being fertilized. Its duration is therefore the sum of the maximum number of days of sperm survival (say 7 days) and the maximum duration of fertilizability of the

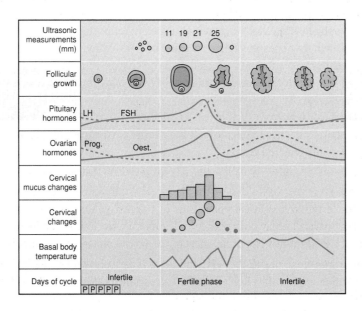

Figure 1.2 The relationship during the cycle of serial ultrasound measurements, hormonal control and clinical indicators of fertility. Q 1.19. (Reproduced courtesy of the late Dr A. Flynn, Birmingham Maternity Hospital, Queen Elizabeth Medical Centre, Birmingham)

ovum (say 24 hours). In practice the identified fertile phase tends to be longer than this, because the clinical indicators of fertility are not 100% accurate.

3   The second infertile phase extends from the end of the fertile phase until the onset of the next menstruation. This phase has a mean duration of 13 days with a range, in likely fertile cycles, of about 11–15 days. It is often called the 'absolute' infertile phase as significantly delayed superovulation never occurs in the human. (If two or more eggs are released this is believed to be always on the same day.) Provided ovulation is accurately determined and sufficient time is allowed for the ovum to succumb, conception really is impossible in this phase.

1.20 HOW MAY THE PHASES BE DETERMINED, IN PRACTICE?

We must distinguish carefully between:

1   The biological events themselves which delineate the phases – these are clearcut and defined in Q 1.19. But they are not the same as:
2   The biological indicators of the events. These can be further classified into:
   (a) biophysical methods (e.g. serial ultrasonic monitoring of follicular growth, changes in vaginal, ovarian or hand blood flow, etc.);
   (b) biochemical methods which detect the change in concentration of the sex steroids or their metabolities in body fluids such as urine or saliva;
   (c) clinical indicators such as BBT, mucus and cervical changes. The accuracy of these indicators of the events at (1) varies, and must also be distinguished from:
3   The ability of the woman and her partner accurately to detect the indicator. And finally after detection and recording of the indicator we have to consider:
4   The compliance of the woman and of her partner, which is a different matter again.

The importance of numbers (3) and (4) was well shown in a celebrated study, which apparently showed that the pregnancy rate was higher when charts of clinical indicators were interpreted by the woman's husband than when the woman decided when it was safe to have intercourse!

1.21 WHAT ARE THE MAJOR CLINICAL (PATIENT-IDENTIFIABLE) INDICATORS OF FERTILITY?

1   Changes in the cervical mucus (see Qs 1.4 and 1.24).
2   Changes involving the cervix itself (see Q 1.5).
3   Changes in the BBT (see Q 1.22).

1.22 HOW ARE THE CHANGES IN THE BBT USED?

The biphasic nature of the temperature cycle is caused by metabolites of progesterone, hence this can only be used to detect the onset of the second infertile phase. A woman must measure her temperature under basal conditions after a period of sleep, without getting out of bed, having a drink or smoking a cigarette. The shift of temperature is small (0.2–0.4°C), hence a special expanded-scale mercury thermometer should be used, or better still a modern, direct-reading, electronic version. The temperature should be taken orally or vaginally for an absolute minimum of 3 minutes, sticking to the same orifice for any given cycle.

The results are plotted daily on a special chart. To detect the shift a cover line is drawn 0.05°C over the lower phase temperatures of which there should be a minimum of six. The second infertile phase is held to begin on the morning of the third consecutive high temperature after the temperature shift; each being a minimum of 0.2°C higher than those six earlier temperatures, covered by the line drawn as just described.

1.23 WHAT ARE THE DIFFICULTIES OF BBT ASSESSMENT?

Some women have problems with using and reading thermometers, and with keeping interpretable charts. But the main danger is of a mild infection occurring prematurely say around day 10, so raising the temperature before ovulation in what is actually going to be a relatively long cycle. A false signal (rise in temperature, back to normal) could also follow use of a prostaglandin synthetase inhibitor in the early follicular phase.

1.24 HOW ARE THE MUCUS CHANGES USED TO DETECT THE FERTILE AND INFERTILE PHASES?

At every micturition the woman is instructed to observe the quantity, colour, fluidity, glossiness, transparency and stretchiness of the mucus.

The most fertile characteristics of the mucus over the entire day are charted each night. The client fills in either a colour (green for dry, yellow for mucus, and red for bleeding) or writes in a description of the mucus seen.

The peak mucus day can only be identified retrospectively, and corresponds closely with the peak secretion of oestrogen in the blood. This is the last day during which the mucus is clear, wet, slippery with an elastic quality allowing it to be stretched for several centimetres before it breaks, like raw egg-white. After ovulation, the rise in progesterone causes within a day a profound change in the amount and characteristics of the mucus. If present at all it resembles the opaque, sticky and tacky postmenstrual type. The peak mucus day can hence be identified. Allowing 2–3 days for ovulation to be completed and 1 day for ovum fertilizability, the second infertile phase is defined as beginning on the evening of the fourth day after the peak mucus symptom.

Changes in the cervix itself (see Q 1.5) can be used to check on the other indicators, though this is not essential.

1.25 WHAT PRACTICAL PROBLEMS CAN CONFUSE MUCUS ASSESSMENT?

1   The most serious is the effect of intercourse, and of sexual excitement without intercourse. Both the fluid of sexual arousal and semen can mimic the sensations and the features of ovulatory mucus. This is another problem if use of the *first infertile phase* is attempted. Unprotected intercourse is then only allowed on alternate days to allow mucus assessment. To identify the first potentially fertile day, *the calculation at Q 1.18 (shortest cycle less 20) must have priority* over mucus observations: since WHO (1983) has reported that in almost 20% of cycles no mucus at all was observed at the vulva until 3 days or less before the peak day. Therefore mucus of any type must equate to potential fertility: sticky mucus is not reliably 'infertile'.
2   Spermicidal jellies and lubricants can similarly cause confusion, particularly if the diaphragm is used in the fertile phase.
3   Mucus assessment is impossible during bleeding – a problem in some short menstrual cycles.
4   Vaginal infections and discharges: these can cause difficulty, notably thrush and its treatments which tend to 'dry' the mucus.

1.26 WHAT ARE THE MINOR CLINICAL INDICATORS OF FERTILITY?

These tend to be specific to individual women, or only occur in some ovulatory cycles. When present they can be helpful in *confirming* the major signals. Among them are:

1 Ovulation pain (Mittelschmerz). Ultrasound scan studies show that this regular unilateral (rarely bilateral) pain occurs 24–48 hours preovulation, not at the event itself. It is probably caused through stretching of the ovarian tissue by the rapidly growing follicle.
2 A midcycle 'show' of blood.
3 The onset of breast symptoms, acne and other skin changes, and variations in mood and sexual desire.

The second infertile phase may be held to commence 5 days after Mittelschmerz ends, provided this matches the findings on a woman's temperature/mucus chart (see Q 1.27).

1.27 COMBINING INDICATORS IS OBVIOUSLY SAFER, BUT WHAT SHOULD BE DONE IF DIFFERENT CLINICAL INDICATORS BEING USED BY THE WOMAN GIVE VARIABLE RESULTS?

In identifying the second phase, for example, the woman should be instructed to act only on the latest of the signals being used. For example, if peak mucus plus 4 days would suggest that intercourse was safe on a Thursday evening, but only two higher temperatures had been recorded, intercourse would be deferred until the third higher temperature was recorded the following (Friday) morning.

For those who are 'spacing' rather than limiting pregnancy, and therefore wish to rely on both infertile phases, the following summary rule is helpful:

- **The fertile time starts 20 days before the woman's shortest cycle would end or earlier when any secretions are detected**
- **It ends after at least three higher temperature have been recorded all *after* the peak mucus day.**

1.28 WHAT ABOUT 'PERSONA®' – THE UNIPATH PERSONAL CONTRACEPTIVE SYSTEM? SEE FIGURE 1.3.

Charting mucus and temperatures and other symptoms is obviously rather a 'hassle'. This innovative product, first marketed in 1996, consists of a

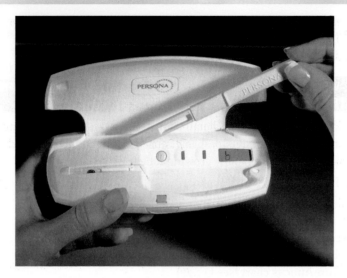

Figure 1.3 'Persona®' (Unipath Personal Contraceptive System). From: Kubba A, Sanfilippo J, Hampton N (1999) *Contraception and Office Gynecology: Choices in Reproductive Healthcare* p. 45. London: WB Saunders. With permission.

series of disposable test sticks and a hand-held computerized monitor. As instructed by a yellow light on the monitor the test sticks are dipped in the user's early morning urine samples and transferred to a slot in the device. There the levels of both estrone-3-glucuronide (E-3-G) and luteinizing hormone (LH) are measured by a patented immunochromatographic assay, utilizing an optical monitor (see Fig. 1.3). As soon as the first significant rise in the E-3-G level is detected the fertility status is changed to 'unsafe', i.e. a red light replaces the green one on the monitor. After subsequent detection of the first significant rise of LH, the end of the fertile period is not signalled by a green light until four further days have elapsed: to allow for the time to ovulation and then demise of the ovum.

The system initially requests 16 tests in the first cycle, dropping to eight thereafter. Utilizing data on the individual's previous six menstrual cycles as well as the current one, it is sensitive to cyclical changes so that the number of 'red' days varies. In the first few months there are typically 12–15 red days, falling later according to the manufacturer's brochure to as low as 6 to 10 days among those with the most regular cycles; but rising if urine tests are missed out, or subsequent to an unusually long or short cycle.

Given the facts about potential sperm survival, above, the group given only 6 infertile days must include those at a higher risk of follicular-phase method failures. See also Q 1.30 and 1.31.

1.29 WHO CAN USE PERSONA®? THE SHORT- AND LONG-TERM CONTRAINDICATIONS

PERSONA® is usable if cycle lengths are between 23 and 35 days, and can accommodate variations of up to 10 days within this range. It should not be used:

1   if the woman has experienced menopausal (vasomotor) symptoms;
2   while breastfeeding, or after recent childbirth;
3   after recent use of any hormonal contraception, including all pills and injectables;

If numbers 2 and 3 apply (including a single use of *hormonal emergency contraception*) the user is advised to wait for two natural consecutive cycles, each of 23–35 days, and *only* initiate use of PERSONA® when the third menses start.

4   during a cycle in which tetracycline is used (itself, *not* any of its relatives such as doxycycline). This can lead to an enhancement of the LH signal from the urine.

The main contraindication, of course, relates to suitability of the method to the lifestyle of the couple, and often too little thought is given to the man's views. If he is going to come home drunk on a Saturday night and (maybe only metaphorically) kick the PERSONA® across the bedroom whatever light it shows, this is hardly the right method! Much attention also needs to be paid to explaining its known failure rate even with correct use (Q 1.30).

1.30 WHAT IS THE FAILURE RATE OF PERSONA® AS CURRENTLY MARKETED (1998)?

Preliminary efficacy information from European trials by the manufacturer suggests a first-year failure rate in consistent users of around 6 per 100 woman-years. This is a *derived* rate from the pre-marketing trials in which a higher rate was actually observed, particularly among women with short cycles and/or put on 'red alert' for too few days. The algorithm of the device as marketed was subsequently altered, increasing the number of 'red' days appropriately. However it is important to note that this quoted failure rate of

PERSONA® has *not* yet been substantiated: I understand that a new trial with the marketed PERSONA® devices (as modified to utilize the new algorithm) is underway in the US. Until that is published we have to work on the basis of the manufacturers' claim of 94% effectiveness if it is used according to the instructions. (The 'perfect use' rate (Q0.18) would be even lower).

This is comparable to the best previous results using fertility awareness – but it is lower than would be acceptable to those accustomed to the efficacy of the COC. The device is certainly more convenient and usually signals a shorter fertile period than the 10–12 days' abstinence typically demanded by the multiple index methods.

Couples should be reminded that they might well themselves be among the 6% in whom the method fails, and that this equates to a 1 in 17 chance of pregnancy in the next year.

1.31 WHAT IF THAT 1 IN 17 RISK OF CONCEPTION IS NOT ACCEPTABLE?

If so, they should be given another option. Indeed, in my opinion this should always have been on offer, it should have been described in the instructions with this product. Given the higher inbuilt risk of intercourse before ovulation (due to those capricious sperm! – see Qs 1.8 and 1.16), I recommend the following combination method, for a monogamous couple wanting high efficacy:

- From Day 1 until the red light first appears: *use condoms*
- Throughout the 'red' phase: *abstain*
- After the second 'green' phase starts: *unprotected sex*

I would confidently give a low failure rate of 1–3% if this advice were accurately followed; and the scientists involved in the testing of PERSONA® confirm that this was achieved in the trials by those who relied solely on the second 'green' phase.

EFFECTIVENESS

1.28 WHAT IS THE EFFICACY OF MULTIPLE-INDEX NATURAL FAMILY PLANNING (NFP)?

If the second infertile phase only is relied on, highly acceptable method-failure rates of 1–3/100 woman-years are obtainable. Higher rates should not necessarily be blamed on the NFP approach, if the couple have used a barrier method during part of the fertile phase, it may well be the latter that has failed.

In fairness, it should be reported that similar excellent method-failure rates have sometimes been reported for the use of multiple-index methods even where intercourse has been permitted in the first, preovulatory, phase. This is partly because the most highly fertile couples tend to drop out of, or never enter, the studied population. And as Trussell (see Q 0.18) has also pointed out, rates as low as 1–3/100 woman-years are not relevant for *average* potential users of natural family planning; there is no doubt that it is extremely unforgiving of less-than-perfect use, which let us face it, is *normal* use of any method for most normal people. (Contrast the pill: most people forget pills from time to time, but the difference is that they are much more likely to get away with it.)

See Q 1.30 above for a discussion of the effectiveness of PERSONA®.

ADVANTAGES AND INDICATIONS

1.33 WHAT ARE THE ADVANTAGES OF METHODS BASED ON FERTILITY AWARENESS?

1 First and foremost, they are completely free from any known physical side-effects for the user (but see Q 1.34).
2 They are acceptable to many with certain religious and cultural views, not only Roman Catholics. According to strict interpretations, they are used rightly when the intention is family spacing, with the possibility of conceiving retained.
3 The methods are under the couple's personal control (abstinence is always available!)
4 The methods readily lend themselves, if the couple's scruples permit, to the additional use of an artificial method such as a barrier at the potentially fertile times.
5 Once established as efficient users, after proper teaching, no further expensive follow-up of the couple is necessary.
6 Understanding of the methods can help subfertile couples to achieve a pregnancy.

PROBLEMS AND DISADVANTAGES

2

1.34 WHAT ARE THE PROBLEMS OF NATURAL FAMILY PLANNING METHODS?

1 Interestingly enough, the majority of *established* users believe the method to be helpful to their marriage/relationship rather than causing stress – but conflicts and frustrations are also reported.

2 A worrying potential hazard is fetal abnormalities due to conceptions resulting from fertilization involving ageing gametes. Animal work and a couple of retrospective human studies have suggested this. However, several others including the WHO study mentioned above have shown no hint of an increase in the incidence of birth defects. The risk, if real, must clearly be very small.

1.35 CAN FERTILITY AWARENESS PREDICT THE RETURN OF FERTILITY AFTER LACTATION?

Full breastfeeding, in which the baby takes no fluids other than from its mother, is a highly efficient natural contraceptive. The most important factor is the frequency and duration of suckling. In practice therefore the return of fertility is a prolonged process, during which many spurious attempts at follicular growth and ovulation occur over weeks or months before actual ovulation. Moreover the first ovulation often antedates the first vaginal bleed. The cervical mucus pattern at this time is not sufficient to help the woman distinguish false alarms from genuine ovulation. If artificial contraception is acceptable to her, she will simply have to play safe and begin to use it from the very first mucus sign of ovarian follicular activity.

For those who wish to continue the natural methods, workers in Birmingham have found that marked changes in the cervix (i.e. softening in consistency, widening of the external os and elevation of position) occur only in the days immediately preceding the first true ovulation. The reliability of the cervix as an indicator at this time requires further testing (see Q 1.5.)

See Q 8.53 for the problems of identifying the infrequent ovulations of women approaching the menopause.

BREASTFEEDING AS NATURAL BIRTH CONTROL

1.36 CAN BREASTFEEDING BE A SATISFACTORY METHOD?

Very much so, and no method could be more natural. A consensus statement from a conference in Bellagio, Italy, is summarized in the algorithm of Figure 1.4. If all three facts apply – amenorrhoea since the lochia ceased, baby not yet 6 months old, and breastfeeding total or very nearly so – the risk of conception by 6 months is only 2%. This compares favourably with other accepted methods of birth control. Hence it may be presented just like any other method to a woman – provided there is the usual caveat, that she is not promised that she will not be one of those 2% for whom the method fails.

However for even greater efficacy and peace of mind many women will prefer to use the progestagen-only pill in addition to their breastfeeding – see Qs 5.55 and 5.56.

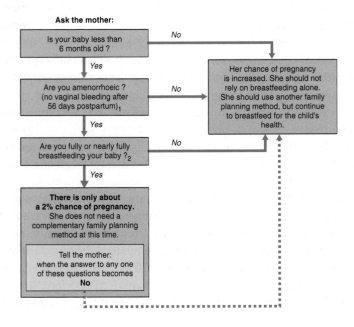

Figure 1.4   Use of the lactational amenorrhoea method during the first 6 postpartum months. Q 1.36. *Notes*: 1. Spotting that occurs during the first 56 days is not considered to be menses. 2. 'Nearly full' breastfeeding means that very occasional non-breastfeeds are given.

THE (NEAR) FUTURE

1.37 WHAT OF THE FUTURE? ARE THERE ANY DEVELOPMENTS WHICH MAY MAKE FERTILITY AWARENESS METHODS MORE ACCEPTABLE?

Some of these are suggested in Figure 1.2. One (PERSONA®) has already arrived in the UK.

1   Ultimately, the relative price of **ultrasound** machines may fall so low, and their user-friendliness may increase to such a degree, that women could simply plug them in to their television sets. Follicular growth, rupture and corpus luteum formation could then be monitored by the woman and her partner themselves!

2   More realistically, a number of new **home kits** are being devised based on the cyclic changes in the hormones of the menstrual cycle, or their metabolites and other substances in body fluids. The most useful fluids are urine, saliva and breast milk; but biochemical changes in the mucus are also being studied.

3   Other approaches include:

(a) The **Rovumeter**. This is a device which simply measures the daily amount of cervicovaginal fluid aspirated from the posterior vaginal fornix by the woman into a sterile, disposable, calibrated, plastic aspirator. Volume changes are more objective than the usual mucus awareness approach, and can apparently be used for family planning purposes.

(b) New possibilities may arise by serendipity, such as some research at King's College Medical School in London into Raynaud's phenomenon. In normal women (as well as those with Raynaud's phenomenon) the findings are different at different phases of the menstrual cycle. It appears that oestrogen tends to increase the reactivity of the arteries of the hand. Progesterone tends to relax the vessels producing an overall increase in blood volume. Appropriate daily measurements in the hand could in theory therefore be used both to predict and to detect the woman's fertile period. No device for possible home use has yet appeared, however.

2 Male methods

COITUS INTERRUPTUS

2.1 WHAT IS COITUS INTERRUPTUS?

This is well described by its commonest euphemism, 'withdrawal' (in time, before ejaculation, ensuring that all sperms are deposited outside the vagina). There are many other terms, notably 'being careful' and also local idioms such as 'getting off at Fratton instead of going through to Portsmouth' (used in Hampshire, but having many regional equivalents!). These have often misled interviewers into thinking that no contraceptive method is being used.

2.2 WHAT IS THE HISTORY OF THE METHOD?

It is doubtless the earliest form of birth control. It is mentioned in Genesis, the only explicit mention of contraception in the Bible:

> *Then Judah said to Er's brother Onan, 'Go and sleep with your brother's widow. Fulfil your obligation to her as her husband's brother, so that your brother may have descendants.' But Onan knew that the children would not belong to him, so whenever he had intercourse with his brother's widow he let the semen spill on the ground, so that there would be no children for his brother. What he did displeased the Lord and the Lord killed him also.*

Although this text is widely quoted as implying that withdrawal is itself sinful, and by extension that other 'artificial' methods that prevent the sperm meeting the egg are wrong: according to most commentators the sin was not in the method at all. It was Onan's failure to comply with the Levirate Law and perform his family duty.

Though Islamic societies and numerous Imams are basically pronatalist, the Koran describes a more liberal attitude to withdrawal and by inference to other methods of contraception. In the Tradition of the Prophet we find:

> *A man said, O Prophet of God! I have a slave girl and I practise coitus interruptus with her. I dislike her becoming pregnant, yet I have the desires of men. The Jews believe that coitus interruptus constitutes killing a life in miniature form.*

The Prophet (Mohammed) replied,

> *The Jews are liars. If God wishes to create it, you can never change it.*

Right up to the second half of the twentieth century, withdrawal remained a major and often the primary method of contraception. As late as 1947 the Royal Commission on Population in England found that amongst recently married couples with contraceptive experience, 43% used withdrawal as the sole method of birth control, the proportion rising to 65% in social class V. Studies in developing countries have shown its use, at least on some occasions, by more than half of all couples in Jamaica, Puerto Rico, and Hungary in the 1960s.

2.3 WHAT IS THE EFFECTIVENESS OF COITUS INTERRUPTUS?

High failure rates alleged by the early family planners have been quoted and requoted by subsequent generations of writers. Yet the evidence contradicts that view. In 1949 the Royal Commission (see above) reported that 'no difference has been found between users of appliance and users of non-appliance methods as regards the average number of children'.

Withdrawal was by far the most popular of the non-appliance methods, and the pregnancy rate was found to be a creditable 8/100 woman-years of exposure. A study in Indianapolis revealed a failure rate of only 10, compared with an average rate of 12 for all other methods, and amongst high-income couples the rate was precisely the same as for the diaphragm.

2.4 WHAT ARE THE ADVANTAGES OF COITUS INTERRUPTUS?

Chiefly that the method is free of charge, requires no prescription, and cannot be left at home when the couple go on holiday. Moreover it does not cause nausea or weight gain! Its use has been associated with some of the lowest birth rates in history, for example in eastern Europe after the Second World War. It is obviously acceptable to many users.

2.5 WHAT ARE THE DISADVANTAGES?

Obviously intercourse is incomplete, and many find the method very unsatisfying to both partners. Yet no significant adverse effects have ever been demonstrated among those who do choose to use it. It seems to be assumed without discussion that there would be an inevitable lack of satisfaction of the woman, compounded by anxiety that her partner would not withdraw 'in time'. Psychological problems are assumed to follow. Yet in a survey of nearly 2000 British women questioned in 1967–68 by Cartwright, only 31% of 311 who had discontinued use of the method did so because they found it unpleasant, and only 4% because they believed it harmful to health. In contrast, 54% of 381 former condom users gave up the method because they found it unpleasant to use.

Even among those professionally engaged in family planning, this method is unjustifiably overlooked, condemned or ridiculed. Marie Stopes stated that it was 'harmful to the nerves as well as unsafe'.

2.6 WHY HAS THE METHOD BEEN SO NEGLECTED, EXCEPT PERHAPS BY GERMAINE GREER?

One reason perhaps is that it has no manufacturers to advertise its virtues. It has the reputation of being unsatisfying and ineffective. It should certainly not be *promoted*. But it is unfortunate that many unplanned pregnancies among young people having intercourse unexpectedly are probably caused by the conventional teaching of doctors and nurses. Withdrawal is often not attempted when it might have been, because the message that it is 'ineffective' has been so well conveyed. We must remember the old slogan:

Any method of family planning is better than no method, though some methods are better than others.

While encouraging the use of more modern methods, we should remember that for many this one works; and that 'in an emergency' it is a very great deal better than nothing.

2.7 AREN'T THERE SPERM IN THE PRE-EJACULATE?

Yes there are, sometimes. Abraham Stone in 1931 asked several medical friends to examine preorgasmic secretions for sperm. He finally collected 24 slides from 18 individuals. Two showed many sperm, two contained few, and one an occasional sperm. Stone correctly reported that the figures were 'insignificant for a definite conclusion'. The chances of such sperm causing fertilization must be low, though not negligible (see Q 1.9).

A much more probable cause of failure results from partial ejaculation of a larger quantity of semen sometimes occurring a short while before the final male orgasm; or withdrawal during the latter rather than before it starts. Hence the suggestion for those who want to continue using the method that they might use a spermicide as well (see Q 2.9).

2.8 SHOULD A COUPLE ALWAYS BE DISCOURAGED FROM USING COITUS INTERRUPTUS?

The answer has to be no. We must remember the basic teaching of psychosexual medicine, that there are innumerable methods of giving and receiving sexual pleasure, which the couple should feel free to devise for themselves. Why should they not be able to have a sexually satisfying life and choose to use coitus interruptus, if that is their mutually agreed choice?

2.9 HOW DO YOU COUNSEL A COUPLE WHO VOLUNTEER THAT COITUS INTERRUPTUS IS THEIR USUAL METHOD?

Clearly, other options should always be discussed. If, however, they find the alternatives unacceptable, then I always suggest the additional use of spermicide (a pessary, or perhaps Delfen foam). This should cope satisfactorily with any small deposit of sperm before withdrawal.

2.10 YOUR CONCLUSION?

Malcolm Potts, to whom I am indebted for much of this section, concludes in his 1983 book with Peter Diggory, *Textbook of Contraception Practice*:

> *Coitus interruptus is like a bicycle or a buffalo cart; there are better methods of transport and better methods of contraception, but for a great many people it represents a practical solution to an every day problem.*

THE CONDOM

BACKGROUND AND MECHANISM

2.11 WHAT IS THE DEFINITION OF A MALE SHEATH/CONDOM?

This is a closed-ended, expansile, tubular device designed to cover the erect penis and physically prevent the transmission of semen into the vagina. It is traditionally made of vulcanized latex rubber which is as thin as possible while maintaining adequate strength and often lubricated – to minimize 'loss of sensitivity' during intercourse, which is perhaps the method's chief disadvantage. It is also a method for use by (often) the least well-motivated of the partners: hence the renewed interest in female-controlled condoms, as well as more effective spermicide/virucides (see Qs 3.55–3.58 and 3.61)

2.12 WHAT IS THE METHOD'S HISTORY?

This apparently dates back to Roman times, when animal bladders were used chiefly to prevent the spread of sexually transmitted disease. In folklore, the invention was much later, by Dr Condom, reputedly a physician at the court of Charles II. It is doubtful whether Dr C. even existed. Much more probably, the word condom was derived from the Latin (*condus*: a receptacle), as a euphemism for an item already well known. The earliest published description is that of the Italian anatomist Gabriel Fallopio, who in 1564 recommended a linen sheath moistened with lotion – again in order to protect against veneral infection. Only in the 18th century do we find described the use of condoms specifically to prevent pregnancy. Condoms were then made from the caeca of sheep or other animals. Similar 'skin condoms' are still available but they have always been expensive and hence beyond the means of ordinary couples. They are also not recommended for safer sex – to prevent virus transmission.

It was the process of vulcanization of rubber, first carried out by Hancock and Goodyear in 1844, which revolutionized the world's contraception as well as its transport.

2.13 HOW ACCEPTABLE AND HOW FREQUENTLY USED IS THE CONDOM METHOD?

An estimated 40 million couples use the condom worldwide, but with striking geographical differences. Japan accounts for more than a quarter of all condom users in the world. Seventy-five percent of couples who use any contraceptive in that country use this method, generally purchased by the woman. This may change if the pill should ever become a realistic option in Japan. By contrast, and despite the massive problem of the acquired immune deficiency syndrome (AIDS), condom use remains low in Africa, the Middle East and Latin America, which together account for less than 10% of worldwide use.

2.14 WHAT IS THE ACCEPTABILITY AND USAGE OF THE CONDOM IN THE UK?

For many, 'spoilt' by modern non-intercourse-related alternatives, it must be admitted the method remains completely unacceptable for sustained use. There is an undeniable change of sensations reported especially by men, though this sometimes has the benefit of prolonging intercourse.

In most recent surveys, approaching 20% of all couples use the condom. Estimates are always approximate as many couples use the sheath as an occasional alternative if not addition to other methods; but it continues to be the second most prevalent method within each 10-year cohort, during the reproductive years. In the 1996 National Opinion Poll (Schering) 13% of pill-takers claimed to use it in combination with the condom for protection against infection: a definite increase.

2.15 HOW CAN THE IMAGE OF THE CONDOM AS A METHOD BE IMPROVED?

In the past condoms had a very poor image. AIDS has changed all that – or has it? There are still widespread misconceptions about efficacy and reduced sensitivity. For centuries, condoms were associated with prostitution and extramarital intercourse. Even today as he purchases his condoms a married man may sense that the retailer assumes they surely cannot be for intercourse with his wife. Removal of this unfortunate image is unlikely so long as the media maintains double standards: there is widespread portrayal of intercourse on television, for example, yet it is perceived as against morality or good taste to mention the condom in the storyline.

EFFECTIVENESS

2.16 HOW EFFECTIVE IS THE CONDOM METHOD?

Method-failure rates can be less than 1 pregnancy/100 couple-years. These are based on selected populations where there has been no sexual contact whatever without the rubber intervening, the only failures being caused by condoms bursting due to a manufacturing defect (some bursts and most cases of condoms slipping off are user errors, see Q 2.20 below). Since successful use depends so very much on the motivation and care taken by the couple, failure rates do vary widely: from a low of 0.4/100 woman-years in the north of England, 1973, to a high of no less than 32/100 woman-years in Puerto Rico in 1961. A large population-based US study of the 1980s documented between eight and 11 failures at 1 year for single women. In four UK studies the range was more relevant to the *careful user*, from 3.1 to 4.8/100 woman-years.

As usual, failures are more frequent with the young and inexperienced, and among couples who wish to delay rather than prevent pregnancy. Among such, *average* use leads to at least 10% conceptions in the course of 1 year, a one in ten chance (and we do such couples a disservice if this information is withheld from them). Older couples use the method better, perhaps because of diminished fertility and a lower frequency of intercourse, as well as more careful use. For example, in the Oxford/Family Planning Association (FPA) study a pregnancy rate of only 0.7/100 couple-years was reported among women aged 35 and older, as compared with a rate of 3.6/100 couple-years for women aged 25–34 (in both cases the husband having been before recruitment a condom-user for more than 4 years).

2.17 WHY ARE MEN SO BAD AT USING CONDOMS (AT ALL, OR WELL)?

Clearly, it has a lot to do with themselves not getting pregnant! A report from two university campuses in Georgia, USA, just about says it all:

Among 98 male students aged 18–29 (mean age 22.4 years) who participated in a standardized interview about their use of condoms, 50% reported ever experiencing condom breakage.

Among these 49 men, 15 (30%) had at some time failed to disclose knowledge of a broken condom to their female sex partner, nine of them many times! Overall, 13.2% of condom breakage episodes were never revealed to the partners! The reasons given were (N = number of individuals out of the 15):

- *unwillingness to interrupt intercourse because orgasm was approaching (N = 6);*
- *wanting to avoid being blamed for the break (N = 5);*
- *desire to minimize anxiety of the partner about the break (N = 4).*

I was rendered quite speechless when I first learnt of this little study (*JAMA* 1997;278:291–292). Its implications, for example for emergency contraception, are devastating!

2.18 HOW IMPORTANT IS ADDITIONAL SPERMICIDE USE TO CONDOM EFFECTIVENESS?

This theoretically should increase contraceptive protection. However:

1. Since the pregnancy rate among consistent users is already very low, it would be difficult to prove the extra degree of protection.
2. Spermicides alone tend to be rather inefficient at preventing pregnancy when the whole ejaculate is spilled, though they may be more effective if there are leaks of small amounts of semen.
3. The requirement to use a separate spermicide may be perceived as a messy additional intrusion during intercourse, and so might actually cause more pregnancies because of irregular use of the condom (or occasional reliance on the spermicidal pessary alone).

> **NOTE:** There is also now a possible problem that the commonest spermicide (nonoxynol-9 or -11) causes apparent damage to the vaginal epithelium in very frequent use. This affects recommendations about virus transmission prevention but not those about routine contraception, see Q 3.67.

2.19 ARE SPERMICIDALLY LUBRICATED CONDOMS THEREFORE PREFERRED?

Because of doubts about interference with regular use (see Q 2.18) and some other anxieties (see Qs 3.67 and 3.68), the UK FPA has not for some years considered spermicides mandatory. All the same, the best protection in the event of spillage is probably provided by separate pessaries or foam; followed by a brand with an adequate additional spermicidal dose within the teat of the condom; and then by brands which are simply spermicidally lubricated. This would be almost impossible to prove because controlled trials are so difficult to mount and would necessarily involve a vast number of volunteers.

The highest priority should be given to making things as easy as possible for the variably motivated couples who choose to use this method.

2.20 WHAT ARE THE COMMON ERRORS IN CONDOM USE THAT MAY LEAD TO PREGNANCY?

Particularly when the combined oral contraceptive (COC) has to be stopped on medical grounds after many years, most couples have no idea just how 'dangerous' a fluid semen will now become. It is important to stress that the 4–5 ml of an average man's ejaculate can easily contain 3–400 million sperm, and hence a minute proportion of this volume in a fertile man might cause a pregnancy. Common unrecognized errors include:

1 Genital contact, with the condom put on just before ejaculation – but often not in time to catch the first fraction of sperm.
2 Loss of erection, perhaps due to overexcitement or anxiety, so condom slips off unnoticed before ejaculation. Another cause of slippage is mentioned at Q 2.22.
3 Leakage on withdrawal, when the penis is flaccid.
4 Later genital contact with sperm already on glans and in urethra of the penis (from earlier intercourse) before a new condom is applied.
5 Damage to the sheath – see Q 2.21.

2.21 WHAT MAY CAUSE CONDOM BREAKAGE, ASIDE FROM MANUFACTURING DEFECTS?

1 *Mechanical damage*, e.g. by sharp fingernails, especially during attempts to force it on the wrong way, rolling it up tighter rather than unrolling it (an easy mistake while excited!).

TABLE 2.1 VAGINAL AND RECTAL PREPARATIONS WHICH SHOULD BE REGARDED AS UNSAFE TO USE WITH CONDOMS OR DIAPHRAGMS	
Arachis oil enema	Monistat
Baby oil	Nizoral
Cyclogest	Nystan cream (pessaries OK)
Dalacin cream	Ortho Dienoestrol
E45 (and similar)	Ortho-Gynest (Ovestin OK)
Ecostatin	Petroleum jelly (Vaseline)
Fungilin	Premarin cream
Gyno-Daktarin	Sultrin
Gyno-Pevaryl (Pevaryl OK)	Witepsol-based products

Note: Some suntan oils and creams are similarly not 'condom-friendly'. But water-based products such as 'KY jelly', also ethylene glycol, glycerol and silicones are not suspect.

2 *Chemical action.* It is still not widely enough known that vegetable and mineral oil-based lubricants, and the bases for many prescribable vaginal products, can seriously damage and lead to rupture of rubber. Baby oil for example, often suggested as part of sex play, destroys over 90% of a condom's strength after only 15 minutes contact! The Durex Information Service (1991) has produced a useful leaflet listing 20 common vaginal preparations which should be regarded as unsafe to use with condoms and diaphragms, and there may be others. See Table 2.1. Here lies a definite advantage of plastic condoms!

2.22 WHAT INSTRUCTIONS SHOULD BE GIVEN TO COUPLES PLANNING TO USE RUBBER MALE CONDOMS?

1 Use only good-quality condoms: the voluntary UK kitemark means more than the mandatory European CE mark.
2 Avoid any chemical or physical damage: do not use oil-based lubricants such as Vaseline or baby oil. Use jelly such as KY, or a spermicidal product. See Qs 2.20 and 2.21.
3 Put the condom on the penis before any genital contact whatever. If there is no teat, make room for the semen by pinching the end of the sheath as it is applied. (Otherwise there is the risk of semen tracking up the shaft of the penis and either escaping or causing the condom to slip off.)

4 After intercourse, withdraw the penis before it becomes too soft, holding the base of the condom during withdrawal and taking care not to spill any semen.

5 Use each condom once only. Inspect it for damage/possible leaks before disposal.

6 For maximum effectiveness, your partner should use a spermicide (e.g. foam or pessary).

7 *Most importantly, if the condom ruptures or slips off, on any potentially fertile day, obtain **emergency (postcoital) contraception** (see Q 7.5) within 72 hours.*

ADVANTAGES AND INDICATIONS

2.23 WHAT ARE THE ADVANTAGES OF THE CONDOM METHOD?

The advantages are many:

1 easily obtainable, relatively cheap or free from NHS clinics;
2 free from medical risks;
3 highly effective if used consistently and correctly;
4 no medical supervision required;
5 protection against most sexually transmitted diseases including viruses;
6 possible protection against cervical neoplasia and invasive carcinoma;
7 offers visible evidence of use (particularly to the woman, who has the greatest motivation to avoid pregnancy);
8 involves the male in sharing contraceptive responsibility, though with some men this can be a definite disadvantage;
9 may sometimes increase the woman's pleasure by prolonging intercourse;
10 minimizes post-intercourse odour and the messiness of semen, for those who perceive these as problems.

2.24 IN WHAT SITUATIONS MAY THE CONDOM BE PARTICULARLY INDICATED?

1 Where couples are unable or unwilling to make use of formal family planning services.
2 During short-term contraception (e.g. while waiting to start oral contraceptives).
3 Where intercourse takes place only infrequently and unpredictably.

4 For protection against sexually transmitted infections, notably HIV.
5 With the agreement of the man (not always obtainable), for the prevention of cervical neoplasia, particularly when that has already been treated (Q2.26).

Items 4 and 5 are indications which might apply even if the main birth control method being used is an IUD, a hormone or sterilization (either sex).

2.25 AGAINST WHICH SEXUALLY TRANSMITTED DISEASES DOES THE CONDOM PROVIDE PROTECTION?

A major benefit from the woman's point of view is the reduced risk of upper genital tract disease (pelvic infection with its serious threat to her future fertility). Consistent condom use is protective against gonorrhoea and *Trichomonas vaginitis*, the spirochaete of syphilis, chlamydia, and similar bacterial and protozoal organisms. It obviously provides little or no protection against infestations such as scabies and lice.

Most importantly, the rubber or plastic of which male or female condoms are made is an effective barrier when intact to viruses, including HIV, the far more infectious hepatitis viruses, herpes simplex types I and II and the wart viruses.

Whereas fertilization is possible only during about 8 days per cycle, viruses can be transfered at any time. As we have seen, condom conceptions are not uncommon. So the method can only provide relative protection ('safer sex'). Bilateral (two-sided) monogamy has much going for it! (see pp. 23–31 of my handbook for women, *The Pill*).

2.26 WHAT EVIDENCE IS THERE THAT THE CONDOM MAY BE PROTECTIVE OR EVEN THERAPEUTIC AGAINST CERVICAL CELL ABNORMALITIES?

In a UK case-control study, for example, the relative risk of developing severe cervical dysplasia decreased with duration of condom or diaphragm use while it increased with duration of oral contraceptive (OC) use. After 10 years the relative risk for women using any barrier method was 0.2 compared to 4.0 for the pill-users.

In an American study, as many as 136 out of 139 women with cervical cell abnormalities who received no treatment apart from their partners adopting use of the condom showed complete reversal of the condition. Unfortunately there was no control group, and the findings need confirmation.

PROBLEMS AND DISADVANTAGES

2.27 WHAT ARE THE POSSIBLE DISADVANTAGES OF THE METHOD?

There are few, but enough to put many people off:

1 coitus-related and interrupts spontaneity of intercourse;
2 decreased 'sensitivity', especially for the male (much less with modern products);
3 perceived as acting as a barrier in psychological as well as physical terms;
4 perceived to be messy, rubber has a distinctive odour which is hard to mask;
5 they may slip off or rupture;
6 few users appreciate how very small leaks of semen may yet cause a pregnancy (see Q 1.7);
7 hence a very high degree of motivation and extremely meticulous use are required for long-term avoidance of pregnancy; these characteristics are regrettably possessed by relatively few men!

2.28 WHAT ARE THE POSSIBLE UNWANTED EFFECTS OF THE CONDOM?

Very few, it is difficult to imagine how death might occur – perhaps by inhalation?

1 *Allergy.* Most 'allergies' are excuses (especially by men). But irritation is not uncommon and true allergy to residues left in the rubber after the manufacturing processes does exist. The solution now is generally found by transferring to use of a plastic condom (see Q 2.32).
2 Of course the method fails to protect against disorders linked to the normal/abnormal menstrual cycle, such as menorrhagia, premenstrual syndrome, functional ovarian cysts, endometriosis, and carcinoma of the ovary and endometrium. These can therefore be described as side-effects of the condom, but even more as 'side-effects of not using the pill' (see Q 4.55).

2.29 HOW CAN THE DISADVANTAGES BE MINIMIZED?

By using ultra-thin and lubricated condoms, innovative materials and shapes, and perhaps by involving the female more in the selection of specific brands and in their actual use. For example, if a condom (perhaps brightly coloured or ribbed) is applied by the woman as part of foreplay, this can counter the first and foremost disadvantage in Q2.27 above, and even heighten eroticism. Or a female condom may be tried, for variety.

PRESENT AND FUTURE DESIGNS

2.30 ARE THERE ANY CONDOMS WHICH ARE NOT RECOMMENDED?

So-called American Tips which are designed to fit only over the glans penis, have a bad reputation for slipping off during use. Also not approved are some 'fun' condoms available from sex shops which do not conform to BSI kitemark specifications.

2.31 HOW ARE RUBBER CONDOMS MANUFACTURED?

In a highly automated process, condom-shaped metal or glass moulds are dipped into latex solution, from where they pass to a drying oven. After a second immersion in latex, the moulds pass into another heated air chamber for drying and vulcanization. The finished product is usually rolled off the mould by nylon brushes and then subjected to quality control testing. Each of the millions produced is tested electronically for pin-holes; and samples are put through a water test for holes and also now an air inflation test to bursting point. The international standard (ISO 4074) permits only seven samples out of 200 to rupture after inflation with 15 litres of air.

2.32 DOES THE FUTURE PERHAPS LIE WITH PLASTIC CONDOMS?

Very likely, in my view. They have no smell and are good heat conductors, non-allergenic and unaffected by any chemicals in common use. One version, Avanti®, has been on the UK market since 1966. It is well lubricated and ultrathin, which many men find preferable. But despite using polyurethane, a material with good intrinsic strength, its thin-ness means it is at least as likely as (in one US study more likely than) a good rubber condom to rupture in use.

An exciting new product is now CE-marked and on the market since 1998 in the Netherlands: **ez.on**^{tm} **condooms**. It is the first baggy or loose-fit male condom. Each has a patented soft flange at the open end, with which it is 'pulled on like a sock' (either way, it is 'bidirectional' unlike all rubber condoms) over the erect penis – which it then firmly but comfortably grasps at its base. Importantly, loose-fit ensures that the major part of the shaft and all the glans of the penis feel free within the well-lubricated sac. Unlike all other condoms it is completely bi-directional – there is no wrong way to put it on. It has good tensile strength since there is no need for its walls to be especially thin. Quotes from preliminary acceptability trials suggest that it allows more 'normal' sensations during penetrative intercourse for the male partner and has 'no disadvantages compared with rubber condoms' for the female. It is a little 'noisier' than they are, although less so than the female condom – see Q 3.68!

Let us hope that its 'feel-good' features usefully improve male acceptance of the condom method, and that it soon becomes available in other countries.

See Qs 3.55–58 for the female condom.

QUESTIONS ASKED BY USERS ABOUT THE CONDOM/SHEATH

2.33 THE CONDOMS KEEP BREAKING – WHY IS THIS?

There are several possible explanations (see Q 2.21). Are you allowing any oily chemicals to come into contact with them? Sometimes you or your partner may be causing damage with fingernails while it is being put on. Waiting until she is more aroused and lubricated before penetration may help, or the use of KY jelly. Otherwise you could try a different brand – discuss with your chemist.

2.34 DO I HAVE TO USE A SPERMICIDE WITH THE CONDOM?

This is no longer an absolute requirement. However, if you have ever had a sheath slip off or break it is more secure if your partner inserts a dose of spermicide first. And certainly if you ever 'cheat' a little – meaning there is some penetration before you actually put the condom on – additional spermicide could be important in case of an early leak of sperm. Spermicidally-lubricated sheaths will not help there, but may otherwise be slightly more effective.

2.35 SOME CONDOMS HAVE RIBS AND BUMPS ETC. – ARE THESE CONTRACEPTIVES SAFE?

If they are kite-marked (BSI tested), the answer is yes. Beware of those that are not so approved.

2.36 IF A CONDOM BREAKS OR SLIPS OFF, IS THERE ANYTHING YOU CAN DO TO AVOID A POSSIBLE PREGNANCY?

Yes, preferably in the next 24 hours, make sure you obtain *emergency contraception* (Ch. 7).

2.37 I SEEM TO BE DEVELOPING AN ALLERGIC RASH FROM THE CONDOM – IS THERE ONE SPECIALLY MADE WHICH OVERCOMES THIS PROBLEM?

It is best for a doctor to examine your penis in case for example your 'allergy' is caused by something else such as thrush. If you are using a spermicidally lubricated condom, you could try one without the spermicide. Otherwise the best bet now would be plastic condoms such as Avanti® or **ez.on**tm (2.32). You could also try natural skin condoms which are available by mail order.

2.38 DO CONDOMS HAVE A SHELF-LIFE?

Yes: It is usually stated to be a long one of about 5 years, but it is important to realize that rubber ones can deteriorate more rapidly in abnormal conditions, such as in the tropics – and anywhere if exposed to strong ultraviolet light. See also Q 2.21.

2.39 CAN I USE THE CONDOM MORE THAN ONCE?

This is not recommended – it was feasible with the old-style reusable types.

2.40 WHY CAN'T YOU EASILY GET CONDOMS FREE FROM YOUR FAMILY DOCTOR?

Why indeed? This is an excellent method which in my view should certainly be available from GPs, as it is from clinics.

2.41 CAN YOU THROW A CONDOM AWAY DOWN THE TOILET?

From the environmental point of view it is better to use a dustbin.

2.42 MY PARTNER FEELS VERY DRY, IS THERE A LUBRICANT YOU CAN SAFELY USE WITH THE CONDOM?

Some of this dryness may be removable by better sex technique – particularly by more foreplay so increasing arousal fluid. If she has any soreness or itching she should be checked for thrush or allergy. Otherwise use a water-based lubricant (Qs 2.21, 2.22) sparingly, or better still a jelly which is also contraceptive. See also Qs 3.52 and 3.53.

3 Vaginal methods of contraception

OCCLUSIVE CAPS

3.1 WHY SHOULD WE TRY TO AVOID THE TERMS 'FEMALE OR VAGINAL BARRIERS'?

Although these are convenient, ideally I wish we could find better terms to use. They should preferably be avoided in discussions with prospective users, since sexual intercourse has to do with closeness, and one can reinforce wrong feelings and fantasies about the method being a 'barrier'

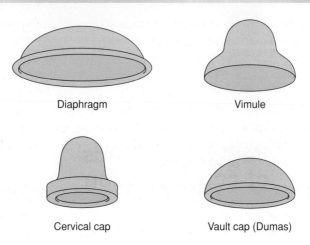

| Diaphragm | Vimule |
| Cervical cap | Vault cap (Dumas) |

Figure 3.1 Diaphragm and cervical vault caps. Q 3.2.

3.2 WHAT TERMINOLOGY WILL YOU BE USING? WHAT TYPES ARE AVAILABLE?

See Figure 3.1. To avoid confusion, I shall use the term occlusive caps for all the standard female barriers. This has two subgroups, namely the diaphragm and the cervical/vault caps, with the vimule being here considered as a modified vault cap.

3.3 WHAT IS THE METHOD'S HISTORY?

It is a very ancient method, with descriptions dating back to 1850 BC; the Petri papyrus describes a spermicidal pessary made partly of crocodile dung. A section of the Talmud from the second century AD recommended a moistened sponge in the vagina before coitus. Rubber occlusive pessaries did not appear until the 19th century, in Germany, and the first diaphragm was popularized by Mensinga, the pseudonym of a German physician Dr C. Hasse. The development of vulcanized rubber enabled him to produce a thinner and more pliable device incorporating a flat watch spring in the rim. It became known as the Dutch cap through publicity given to it by the Dutch neo-Malthusians.

The occlusive pessary was referred to in the famous manual *The Wife's Handbook*, published in 1887; for this action its author, Arthur Allbutt, was struck off the British Medical Register. Because of this kind of opposition, occlusive pessaries became readily available only in the 1920s. Then, to quote Malcolm Potts, 'diaphragms and caps were to Family Planning what the steam locomotive was to transportation; they were the first in the field, brought emancipation to millions, and for a long time had no rivals'. Ultimately they were overtaken by a new technology; yet the methods only have two major problems: some lack of independence from intercourse and relative lack of effectiveness. If these could be overcome, there could be a large-scale return to vaginal methods.

3.4 HOW POPULAR ARE VAGINAL METHODS WORLDWIDE?

The diaphragm reached the peak of its popularity around 1959, when it was reported that the method was used by about 12% of British couples practising contraception. Usage declined rapidly with the advent of the pill, and now less than 1% of contracepting women used the method in the UK. In most developing countries prevalence of use is too low to measure; and is likely to remain so until vaginal barriers are devised that do not require medical fitting or special training in use, and do not pose storage and supply problems.

3.5 HOW IMPORTANT IS MEDICAL ATTITUDE AND TRAINING TO THE ACCEPTABILITY OF VAGINAL METHODS?

Crucially: it has been well said that often the biggest 'barrier to the barriers' is the medical profession, and sometimes (though less so) the nursing profession. Many women introduced for the first time to the diaphragm at the age of 35–40 express surprise at its ease and convenience. Often they complain that doctors and nurses had earlier damned the method with exceedingly faint praise.

This is a highly practical subject. The right attitude and skills can only be acquired by observing and being taught by unhurried and experienced professionals: in my experience family planning trained nurses are usually best! (see Qs 3.33–3.40).

3.6 WHAT IS THE MODE OF ACTION OF THE DIAPHRAGM AND CERVICAL/VAULT CAPS?

The *diaphragm* lies diagonally across the cervix, the vaginal vault and much of the anterior vaginal wall. Since the vagina is known to 'balloon' during intercourse (see Q 1.3), a sperm-tight fit between the diaphragm and the vaginal wall is impossible. On a theoretical basis, the main functions of the diaphragm are:

1 to act as a carrier of the spermicide to the most important site, namely the external os, and prevent the spreading effect of intercourse (see Q 1.3);
2 holding sperm away as a barrier from the receptive alkaline cervical mucus, long enough for them to die in the acid vagina;
3 preventing this mucus from entering the acid vagina and thereby providing a film within which the sperm can swim to the external os, and possibly:
4 preventing physical aspiration of sperm into the cervix and uterus.

Some authorities question the importance of the spermicide (see Q. 3.7).

Cervical/vault caps are meant to stay in place by suction, which makes it possible that the barrier effect is more important to their contraceptive action than is the case with the diaphragm.

3.7 HOW IMPORTANT IS THE USE OF SPERMICIDE WITH OCCLUSIVE CAPS?

This is questioned, particularly by the Australian Family Planning Association, and especially for the cervical/vault caps which act by suction. It is a fact that with no type of occlusive cap has there ever been a proper controlled trial. This should compare (preferably by random allocation) women who follow the full routine of instructions concerning the use of spermicide (see Q 3.44), in every detail, with women who use exactly the same method carefully and after the same fitting routine but without any spermicide at all. Such a study has been performed at the Margaret Pyke Centre, and although the power of our study was not great enough to show statistical significance, the spermicide-using group did achieve better results.

EFFECTIVENESS

3.8 HOW EFFECTIVE IS THE DIAPHRAGM?

Table 0.2 (see Q 0.19) quotes an overall failure rate for the diaphragm of 4–20 per 100 woman years, a surprisingly wide range, perhaps. As usual the lower failure rate relates to the older woman. Her conscientiousness in regularly using the method efficiently is of greatest importance.

Professor Trussell of Princeton has made a special study of contraceptive failure rates. The first year pregnancy rates were much higher in parous

TABLE 3.1 DIAPHRAGM FAILURE RATES PER 100 WOMAN-YEARS ACCORDING TO AGE, DURATION OF USE AND COMPLETENESS OF FAMILY

Duration of use	Age 25–34			Age 35+		
	≤2 years	2–4 years	4 years+	≤2 years	2–4 years	4 years+
Family complete	6.1	3.5	2.3	2.1	1.6	0.7
Family not complete	5.3	4.3	2.4	4.5	2.0	1.3

Source: Oxford/FPA Study, 1982

women if they used the cervical cap (ranging up to over 25%, even with 'perfect use'!). Parous diaphragm 'perfect users' had similar rates to nulliparae, however, though still in the range of 4–8% in the first year. This, it should be noted, is an order of magnitude higher than the best rates obtainable by conscientious COC use.

Table 3.1 relates the failure rates to an indicator of motivation recorded in the Oxford/FPA study, namely whether or not the woman considered her family to be complete. As clearly shown, the failure rate tended to be higher when the family was not felt to be complete, implying less careful use of the diaphragm when another baby would be acceptable (i.e. 'spacers').

3.9 ARE THE DIAPHRAGM FAILURE RATES OF THE OXFORD/FPA STUDY A GOOD INDICATION OF THE RATES TO BE EXPECTED IN ROUTINE FAMILY PLANNING PRACTICE?

No.

1 At recruitment, every woman was aged 25–39 years, married, a white British subject, and had to be already a current user of the diaphragm of at least 5 months standing.

2 The women were basically 'middle class' and were probably unusually well motivated and careful.

3 Younger and more fertile women having intercourse more frequently must be expected to have a higher failure rate, even if the method were properly fitted and always used.

The most important factor is the recruitment in the Oxford/FPA study only of established users. By 5 months the most fertile and least careful women, along with those with anatomical problems interfering with the effectiveness of the method, would not have been available for recruitment – by virtue of already becoming pregnant! All studies show the highest failure rates in the first few months of use. Even using the data of Table 3.1, faced with an 'Oxford/FPA type' woman under 35 one can only quote a failure rate of around 5–6/100 woman-years for the first year of use. This is about the best to be expected, with a rate of around 10 for most young unmarried women of average motivation. (All these rates include user failures.)

3.10 WHAT FAILURE RATES CAN BE GIVEN FOR CERVICAL CAPS?

These are considered later (Qs 3.27–3.32). Available effectiveness data are sparse, but Trussell's review in the book *Contraceptive Technology* (17th Edition, 1998) gives a best estimate of 9% at 1 year of use for nulliparous 'perfect users': possibly acceptable for 'spacers'. His quoted rate of 26% for parous women suggests to me that this is no longer a method to be recommended for most in that group of potential users.

3.11 IN SUMMARY, WHAT FACTORS PROMOTE THE EFFECTIVENESS OF THE DIAPHRAGM AND SIMILAR VAGINAL METHODS?

The following questions need to be asked:

1 Is she an established user or starting the method from scratch?
2 What is her age?
3 What is her frequency of intercourse?
4 What is her motivation for obsessionally careful and regular use? In particular is she really trying to avoid a pregnancy or just to delay one?
5 Is she at all uncomfortable about handling her own genitalia? This important factor is not at all linked with intelligence.
6 Are there any anatomical problems on examination? (see Qs 3.22, 3.30, 3.31 and 3.35).
7 During initial training, is she good at inserting the device and particularly at checking that the cervix is covered?

3.12 WHAT COMMON ERRORS IN THE USE OF OCCLUSIVE CAPS MAY LEAD TO PREGNANCY?

The commonest clearly is failure to use, at intercourse on one or more occasions in the cycle of conception. Women often report minor errors in use of the spermicide. It is not at all clear how important these are, especially as they are frequently reported also in non-conception cycles.

During use, the most important error is failure to make a secondary check after insertion that the cervix is correctly covered.

Clinicians' errors include: wrong selection of users, poor fitting (with regard to size, choice of flat spring, coil or arcing diaphragm or other cap) and poor teaching.

ADVANTAGES AND BENEFICIAL EFFECTS

3.13 WHAT ARE THE ADVANTAGES OF OCCLUSIVE CAPS?

1 Effective if used with care.
2 Much more independent of intercourse than the sheath (see Q 3.14).
3 In general, neither partner suffers any loss of feeling.
4 The method is under a woman's control and needs only to be used when required.
5 Aesthetically useful for intercourse during uterine bleeding.
6 No proven systemic effects.
7 Some definite non-contraceptive benefits (see Q 3.15).

3.14 ARE OCCLUSIVE CAPS NECESSARILY INTERCOURSE-RELATED METHODS?

No. In counselling, this is a most important point to explain. It is perfectly in order to insert a diaphragm several hours ahead of intercourse. Opinions differ as to how soon it becomes necessary to add extra spermicide just before intercourse (see Qs 3.44 and 3.49). But certainly removal of the requirement to put the cap itself in just before is beneficial to compliance. Since keeping the cervical mucus out of the vagina may be one of the most important mechanisms (see Q 3.6), it could even be that insertion well ahead of intercourse actually increases effectiveness, though this has not been established.

3.15 WHAT ARE THE BENEFICIAL MEDICAL EFFECTS?

1 Protection against most sexually transmitted infections (STIs), including the agents causing pelvic inflammatory disease. (However the method is

not believed to give adequate protection against HIV and other sexually transmitted *viruses*.)

2 Reduction in the risk of cervical neoplasia.

These are most important benefits in the modern world.

3.16 HOW ARE OCCLUSIVE CAPS PROTECTIVE AGAINST STIS?

In two ways:

1 Partly by providing a mechanical barrier which reduces the chance of organisms reaching the cervix and upper genital tract. This will not be enough protection against the viruses including herpes; or non-viral diseases like syphilis which can form lesions of the vagina, vulva and elsewhere.

2 The associated spermicide is also relevant. Spermicides tend also to be 'germicides' (see Qs 3.66 and 3.67).

3.17 WHAT IS THE EVIDENCE FOR AT LEAST SOME PROTECTIVE EFFECT AGAINST CERVICAL NEOPLASIA?

In the Oxford/FPA study, the rate per 100 woman-years for oral contraceptive (OC) users was 0.95 and for intrauterine device (IUD) users 0.87. For diaphragm users, however, the rate was 0.23 after adjustment for age at first coitus, number of partners and smoking patterns. Another Oxford study showed a steady decline in the relative risk of severe cervical neoplasia for users of all types of barrier method from 1 down to 0.2 after 10 years. However diaphragm users may also be protected from this condition by their own sexual lifestyle and that of their partners.

MAIN PROBLEMS AND DISADVANTAGES

3.18 WHAT ARE THE DISADVANTAGES OF OCCLUSIVE CAPS?

1 Though not necessarily coitus-related, they involve a woman handling her genitalia, some forward planning, and a slight loss of spontaneity.

2 Loss of cervical and some vaginal sensation (unnoticed by most).

3 May rarely be felt in use by the woman's partner, though not by her if properly fitted.

4 Require fitting by trained personnel and a period of training in use, usually 1 week, during which another method must be used.
5 In practice less effective than hormonal contraception, or the IUD.
6 Perceived as being 'messy' due to the spermicide.
7 Capable of producing some local adverse effects (see Q 3.19).

3.19 WHAT ARE THE POSSIBLE ADVERSE MEDICAL EFFECTS?

1 Increased risk of urinary tract infections and symptoms. This problem seems to apply only to the diaphragm. See Q 3.51.
2 A small minority of women develop vaginal irritation and allergy due either to the rubber or more commonly to the spermicide.
3 Pressure effects due to the rim of the occlusive cap itself, leading rarely to vaginal abrasions or ulcers (see Q 3.54).
4 A significant increase in hospital referrals for the treatment of haemorrhoids was found in the Oxford/FPA study – no other researchers appear to have studied this possible effect.

There are also a few unresolved safety issues, considered later (see Qs 3.67–3.74).

> **NOTE:** An excipient used in Cyclogest (progesterone) pessaries can damage rubber. If a cap-user is given this unproven form of treatment for the premenstrual syndrome, she should therefore be advised to use the rectal route of administration. (See also Q 2.21 for other substances which may damage rubber.)

SELECTION OF USERS AND DEVICES

3.20 WHAT ARE THE CONDITIONS FOR THE SUCCESSFUL USE OF OCCLUSIVE CAPS?

In the main, the answer depends on favourable answers to the questions about the woman herself, listed at Q 3.11 above. In addition, experience plus a positive attitude by the providers, ideally both a doctor and a nurse, are of paramount importance. Skilful fitting, knowledge of when to suggest a cervical/vault cap instead, and above all really satisfactory teaching of the woman, are vital factors. The diaphragm is the first-choice medically fitted vaginal method for most women.

1 The woman's choice.
2 As an alternative to medical methods (hormones, IUDs) for a woman who can accept reduced efficacy in return for getting rid of the side-effects of the medical method.
3 The need for contraception on an intermittent yet predictable basis.
4 For protection against pelvic infection or recurrence of cervical neoplasia. This can be worth suggesting even if another method is in use as the main contraceptive.

3.22 WHAT ARE THE CONTRAINDICATIONS TO THE DIAPHRAGM?

These include:

1 aversion to touching the genital area;
2 congenital abnormalities such as a septate vagina;
3 most forms of uterovaginal prolapse;
4 inadequate retropubic ledge on examination;
5 poor vagina or perineal muscle tone;
6 inability to learn the insertion technique;
7 lack of hygiene or privacy for insertion, removal and care of the cap;
8 acute vaginitis – treat first;
9 recurrent urinary infections – indication for vault or cervical cap;
10 past history of cap-induced vaginal trauma;
11 true allergy to rubber;
12 past history of toxic shock syndrome – though this not proved related to occlusive caps;
13 *virgo intacta* – sheath use is commonly advised first, until the vagina is 'ready'. But well-motivated tampon-users can receive a small diaphragm, with refitting planned to follow 1 month's regular use. Items 3, 4, 5 and 9 do not always contraindicate cervical/vault caps (see Q 3.32), and an arcing diaphragm may solve 6.

3.23 WHAT IS THE STRUCTURE OF A DIAPHRAGM?

See Figure 3.2. This is the most commonly used occlusive cap. It consists of a thin latex rubber hemisphere, the rim of which is reinforced by a flexible

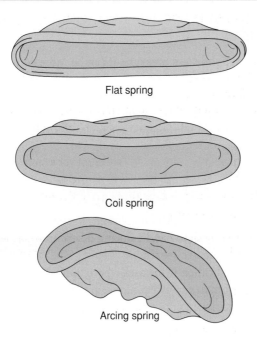

Figure 3.2 Types of diaphragm. Q 3.23 and following. *Note:* flat and coil spring diaphragms may also be fitted dome down instead of up (Q3.27).

flat or coiled metal spring. The sizes, measuring the external diameter, range from 50 to 100 mm in steps of 5 mm.

3.24 WHAT TYPES OF DIAPHRAGM ARE AVAILABLE?

1 *The flat-spring diaphragm.* This has a firm watch spring and is easily fitted, remaining in the horizontal plane on compression. It is suitable for the normal vagina, and is often tried first.
2 *The coil-spring diaphragm* has a spiral coiled spring. This makes it softer than the flat-spring.
3 *The arcing-spring diaphragm* combines features of both the above and consists of a rubber dome with a firm double metal spring. It exerts strong pressure on the vaginal walls, but its main characteristic is that when compressed it forms an arc, directing the posterior part of the diaphragm downwards and away from the cervix during insertion. This can be an advantage, see Q 3.26.

65

3.25 WHAT ARE THE INDICATIONS FOR THE COIL-SPRING DIAPHRAGM?

1 Because it exerts slightly less pressure, it can be more comfortable for some women than the flat-spring.
2 The reduced pressure makes it seem to the woman like a half-size smaller than the equivalent flat-spring diaphragm. This can be useful since half-sizes (2.5 mm increments) are no longer available for any diaphragm.

3.26 FOR WHOM MIGHT THE ARCING-SPRING DIAPHRAGM BE INDICATED?

This is the most widely used type of diaphragm in some countries. Some women find it more difficult to handle during insertion because of its non-horizontal shape when squeezed.

Its main positive indication is in cases where the length or direction of the cervix, or the woman's own technique, are leading to a tendency to squeeze the diaphragm into the anterior fornix. See Q 3.40 (7).

3.27 WHAT TYPES OF CERVICAL/VAULT CAPS ARE AVAILABLE?

1 *The cervical cap*. This is shaped like a thimble (Fig. 3.1) and is designed to fit snugly over the cervix. The commonest variety is the cavity rim cap with an integral thickened rim incorporating a small groove. This is intended to increase suction to the sides of the cervix. The available internal diameters of the upper rim are: 22, 25, 28 and 31 mm. Other varieties are available abroad.
2 *The vault cap*. This rubber cap is shaped like a bowl with a thinner dome through which the cervix can be palpated. It covers but does not fit closely to the cervix. Five sizes are available ranging from 55 to 75 mm in 5 mm steps.
3 *The vimule*. This is a variation of the vault cap with a hat-shaped prolongation of the dome to accommodate longer cervices. There are three sizes: small (45 mm), medium (48 mm) and large (51 mm).

3.28 WHAT IS THE MODE OF ACTION OF CERVICAL/VAULT CAPS?

1 They all operate by suction, not by spring tension as the diaphragm. Otherwise the mode of action – and the uncertainties about the importance of spermicides – are the same as for the diaphragm, see Qs 3.6 and 3.7.

3.29 WHAT INDICATIONS AND ADVANTAGES DO THE CERVICAL/VAULT CAPS SHARE?

1. They share the advantages of the diaphragm but are suitable for patients with poorer muscle tone and some cases of uterovaginal prolapse.
2. They are generally not felt by the male partner.
3. There is no reduction of vaginal sensation.
4. They are unlikely to produce urinary symptoms.
5. Fitting is unaffected by the changes in the size of the vagina, either during intercourse or as a result of changes in body weight.

3.30 WHAT ARE THE CONDITIONS NECESSARY TO FIT A CERVICAL CAP?

1. The cervix must be easily felt.
2. The cervix must be healthy, not torn.
3. The cervix must not point backwards, and ideally should point down the axis of the vagina.
4. The cervix must be straight sided.

3.31 WHAT CONDITIONS ARE NECESSARY FOR FITTING A VAULT CAP?

1. The cervix must be easily felt.
2. The cervix must be fairly short, but it may be quite bulky if it does not protrude too much into the vaginal vault.

3.32 IN WHAT CIRCUMSTANCES WOULD YOU RECOMMEND A TRIAL OF THE VAULT OR VIMULE CAPS?

The vault cap is under-used. It can be very useful where there are contraindications to the diaphragm (see Q 3.22), particularly absence of the retropubic ledge, poor muscle tone and a history of recurrent cystitis. It is a little easier for the woman to fit and remove than the cervical cap, and the precise contour and direction of the cervix are much less important.

Where there is a choice I would recommend a trial of the vault cap before the cervical cap. The vimule is rarely used – its sole indication is to accommodate a cervix which is so long that it prevents suction being exerted in a woman for whom a vault cap would otherwise be selected.

INITIAL FITTING, TRAINING AND FOLLOW-UP ARRANGEMENTS

The factors in Qs 3.9 and 3.11 above should be very carefully explored with the woman, particularly determining that the method is socially and psychologically acceptable to her and in particular that she will be a regular conscientious user. She must also in fairness be told that the method has a moderately high failure rate *despite* ideal fitting, and compliance with every detail of the instructions as to use.

In a sensitive and unhurried way.

The practical aspects cannot be learnt from books. Apprenticeship is necessary in two aspects: fitting technique, and instruction of the woman.

1 The apparent health and direction of the uterus and cervix. Tenderness must be absent.
2 The type of retropubic ledge. This can be more fully assessed with a practice diaphragm in position.
3 Assessment of the vaginal musculature and tone, including the perineal muscles.
4 If the diaphragm is chosen the distance from the posterior fornix to the posterior aspect of the symphysis is measured as shown in Figure 3.3.

Cervical cytology and other screening procedures are performed according to local practice.

1 The woman should have emptied her bladder and an initial choice of practice diaphragm is made based on the distance measured at the first examination (Fig. 3.3). A fitting ring can be used at this stage.
2 With the index inside the rim, compress the practice diaphragm between thumb and the remaining fingers. The labia are separated and

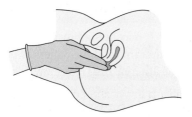

To measure for diaphragm size
Hold index and middle fingers together and insert into vagina up
to the posterior fornix. Raise hand to bring surface of index finger to
contact with pubic arch. Use tip of thumb to mark the point directly
beneath the inferior margin of the pubic bone and withdraw
fingers in this position.

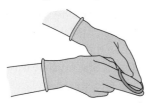

To determine diaphragm size
Place one end of rim of fitting diaphragm or ring on tip of middle finger.
The opposite end should lie just in front of the thumb tip.
This is the approximate diameter of the diaphragm needed.

Figure 3.3 Diaphragm – procedure for estimating the size of practice diaphragm to be tried.
Q 3.36. (Reproduced courtesy of Janssen Cilag Pharmaceutical Ltd, Diaphragm Teaching Aid)

the diaphragm inserted downwards and backwards to the posterior
fornix, tucking the anterior rim behind the symphysis pubis.
3 Check that the cervix is covered.
4 Insert a *finger tip* between the anterior rim of the cap and the symphysis:
   (a) if the cap is too small, a wider gap will be felt or it may be found that
       the whole diaphragm is in the anterior fornix;
   (b) if the cap is too large it projects anteriorly/inferiorly and may cause
       immediate discomfort (or become uncomfortable or distorted later,
       after wearing).
5 The woman should be asked to stand and walk a few steps. On
   re-examination anterior protrusion may be due to a small cystocele
   or a poor retropubic ledge. In this event a vault or possibly a cervical
   cap should be tried.

3.37 WHICH WAY UP SHOULD DIAPHRAGMS BE FITTED?

This really does not matter. It may be slightly easier to remove a flat-spring type if it is inserted dome upwards and the patient is instructed to hook her index finger under the anterior rim. However, this is a non-problem anyway if she simply uses both index and middle fingers to grasp the rim. The arcing diaphragm forms the correct shape (with its leading edge pointing downwards) more readily if it is initially held dome upwards. This requires careful demonstration.

3.38 WHAT ARE THE IMPORTANT POINTS WHEN TEACHING THE PROSPECTIVE USER?

Thorough teaching which generates confidence in the user is essential for success. A three-dimensional plastic model helps but a short video is better still. Unless the doctor is a woman the nurse usually takes over at this stage (if she did not do the initial fitting). She must be very encouraging and able, without embarrassment on either side, and in secure privacy, to supervise closely all aspects of the learning process.

3.39 SUCCESSFUL TEACHING – HOW IMPORTANT IS THE POSITION THE WOMAN SHOULD ADOPT?

This important aspect is often overlooked by the trainer. Unless instructed to the contrary, many women automatically adopt a half- standing, half-squatting position when inserting the diaphragm or when checking that it is correctly located over the cervix. This should be discouraged, as it makes it almost impossible for the fingers to reach the cervix. It may explain some so-called 'cap failures', caused solely because the woman was unable to check that the device was correctly positioned. The two best positions are:

1   Standing with one foot resting on a chair – a right-handed woman should raise her left leg and vice versa (Fig. 3.4).
2   Squatting right down on the ground.

Other positions are possible according to the woman's choice.

3.40 SUCCESSFUL TEACHING (DIAPHRAGM) – WHAT ARE THE STEPS?

1   In her own preferred position as just described, teach the woman to locate her cervix. Most women prefer to use one finger, but it is an error

to insist on this. Even 'short-fingered' women can learn to feel their cervix if taught to use both index and middle fingers.

2 The instructor then inserts the cap for the patient, allowing her to feel her cervix covered with thin rubber.

3 The patient then removes the diaphragm for herself, either by hooking it out or (and this needs stressing) the use of two fingers each side of the anterior rim. If this is found difficult, practising with a slightly too large diaphragm may be all that is necessary to boost confidence.

4 She should feel again for the cervix to emphasize the different feel when it is uncovered.

5 She should then be taught to insert the diaphragm as described above and shown in steps 6–8 of Figure 3.4. Emphasis is placed on the fact that the direction of insertion is similar to that for a tampon – primarily backwards.

6 *She should then examine herself to check that the cervix is covered by the soft rubber dome.* It is absolutely vital to explain that the fact that a diaphragm fits snugly behind the symphysis and feels comfortable is no guarantee of correct insertion.

7 If the woman repeatedly inserts the diaphragm into her anterior fornix, the following may be tried:

(a) two useful tips from the Sister-in-Charge at the Margaret Pyke Centre (MPC). First, the woman lies on her back and holds the diaphragm in her left hand (if right-handed). She then uses her right hand to separate the labia and guide insertion, vertically. Alternatively, and in any convenient position (see Q 3.39), she inserts the diaphragm halfway only, then the half which is still outside is pressed towards the symphysis while completing the insertion.

(b) the use of an *arcing diaphragm*. When held dome down, compression between middle finger and thumb, with the index finger between to steady it, produces a downward bend (Fig. 3.2 and Q 3.26). This helps the posterior rim to pass below the cervix and so into the posterior rather than the anterior fornix. Occasionally:

(c) with either diaphragm design, the woman's partner may be able to learn to insert it for her.

The use of an introducer is rarely much help, in our experience at MPC.

71

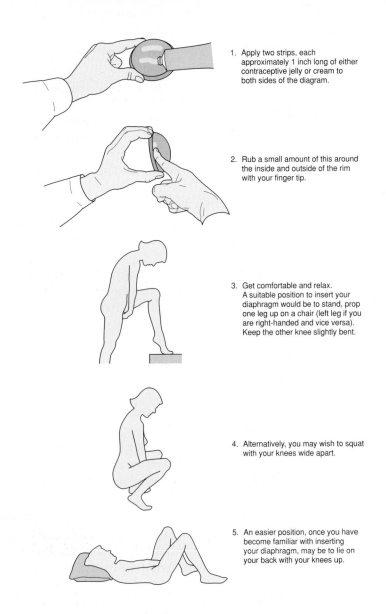

1. Apply two strips, each approximately 1 inch long of either contraceptive jelly or cream to both sides of the diagram.

2. Rub a small amount of this around the inside and outside of the rim with your finger tip.

3. Get comfortable and relax. A suitable position to insert your diaphragm would be to stand, prop one leg up on a chair (left leg if you are right-handed and vice versa). Keep the other knee slightly bent.

4. Alternatively, you may wish to squat with your knees wide apart.

5. An easier position, once you have become familiar with inserting your diaphragm, may be to lie on your back with your knees up.

Figure 3.4 Instructions for prospective user of the diaphragm. Q 3.39. (Reproduced courtesy of Janssen-Cilag Pharmaceutical Ltd, Diaphragm Patient Teaching Aid)

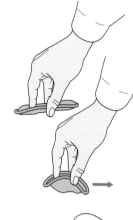

6. To insert your diaphragm fold it in half by pressing the middle of the opposite sides together between the thumb and forefinger of one hand. You may find it helpful to place your index finger in the dome between your thumb and fingers to help prevent it springing away.

If you have been given an arcing spring diaphragm hold it with the arc pointing downwards to ensure that the cervix will be covered.

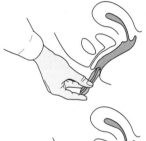

7. Hold the lips of your vagina apart with your other hand. Gently slide the folded diaphragm into your vagina, placing your index finger on the rim to guide it. Aim towards the small of the back as if inserting a tampon. You may feel the rim pass over the cervix.

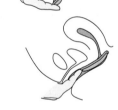

8. Use the index finger to push the front rim up behind the pubic bone.

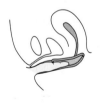

9. To check if the diaphragm is in place insert your index finger into your vagina and touch the dome. You should feel the cervix underneath. Move your index finger to the front of the diaphragm and make sure it is firmly in place behind the pubic bone. Finally check that the back rim is behind the cervix.

10. Do not remove your diaphragm for 6 hours after intercourse. Put your index finger in your vagina and hook it behind the rim of the diaphragm under your pubic bone. Gently pull the diaphragm down and out. You may find it useful to bear down slightly especially if it is well tucked up behind the pubic bone. The diaphragm should not be left in place for more than 24 hours.

3.41 HOW ARE CERVICAL AND VAULT CAPS FITTED?

1 The correct size allows the rim of the chosen cap to touch the fornices with no gap, comfortably to accommodate the cervix (the cervical cap being the only one that truly fits it), and to show evidence of a suction effect.

2 To insert the chosen cap, the rim is compressed between thumb and first two fingers and guided along the posterior vaginal wall towards the cervix. The cap is allowed to open by removing the thumb, and then is pushed over the cervix with the fingertips. A final check is made to ensure that the cervix is palpable through the cap and that there is no gap above the rim.

3 Cervical and vault caps are removed by inserting a fingertip above the rim and then easing the cap downwards, before removal with the index and middle fingers.

3.42 SUCCESSFUL TEACHING – WHAT INSTRUCTIONS FOR VAULT AND CERVICAL CAPS?

Feeling for the cervix, insertion and removal are taught as just described for the fitting. The important point is that if the right sort of woman has been chosen for these caps (which are a little more tricky to use than the diaphragm), she rapidly develops her own technique both for insertion and removal. Provided this is shown to lead to correct location, she should be encouraged to continue.

The correct size for vault and vimule caps is that which fits snugly into the vaginal vault and covers the cervix without exerting pressure upon it.

Further practical details about fitting these smaller suction caps are best learnt in the practical, clinical situation.

3.43 SUCCESSFUL TEACHING – WHAT IS THE TRAINING 'TIMETABLE' FOR ANY TYPE OF OCCLUSIVE CAP?

It is usual and preferable to provide the woman with a practice cap for the first week, during which she should use an alternative contraceptive. This enables her to increase her confidence in the techniques of insertion and removal, and to test whether the method is comfortable during all normal activities. She should be informed with the aid of the most recent edition of the Family Planning Association's leaflet of all the 'rules' as below before she leaves after the first visit. The same points should again be run through at the return visit, before she starts to rely on the method.

3.44 SUCCESSFUL TEACHING – WHAT ACTUAL INSTRUCTIONS ARE GIVEN AT THE FIRST VISIT? SEE FIGURE 3.4.

The wording that follows is addressed to a particular woman and relates specifically to the diaphragm (see also Q 3.49):

1   Always use the recommended spermicidal cream or jelly. Apply two strips, each of 1 inch (2.5 cm), to each side. It is unnecessary to smear the surfaces too much, but you may want to put some on the leading part of the rim.

2   Put your cap in place, using the position and technique you found most comfortable when you were fitted. This could be at any convenient time before lovemaking.

3   If you are having a bath, you should put your diaphragm in after rather than before it. (See also Q 3.86).

4   Most important: check the position of your diaphragm with either your index finger, or with index and middle finger as you prefer. The important thing is that you check that the diaphragm covers your cervix. This feels a bit like a rounded nose with a single nostril, upwards and backwards somewhere near the top of your vagina. You should get used to the particular way your cervix points, which may be forwards, backwards or straight downwards. Check that the rubber on your diaphragm actually covers the cervix – do not rely just on it feeling comfortable.

5   Should lovemaking take place more than 3 hours after you put the cap in, either insert more cream or jelly or foam with an applicator, or use a spermicidal pessary or film pushed well up with the finger. You need to allow about 10 minutes for pessaries to disperse in the vagina before your partner actually deposits semen there.

6   If you have intercourse more than once, more spermicide should be added beforehand, leaving the diaphragm in place.

7   You should leave your cap in place for at least 6 hours after the last intercourse. It can be kept in longer, but should be removed once a day for cleaning.

8   It is no problem if your period starts while the cap is in place. Also it is quite possible to get pregnant during your period. So continue to use your cap for any intercourse, especially towards the end or just after a period, when many people think they can get away without using it.

9   After removal the cap can be washed in warm water with mild toilet soap. It should then be dried and stored in its box in a cool dry place.

Do not use disinfectants, detergents or any mineral or vegetable oil-containing oils or lubricants (see Q 2.21), as these may spoil the rubber.

10 Inspect your cap regularly for holes by holding it up to the light.

> **NOTE:** Although you have been given the cap with spermicide, everything is just for practice during the first week. Wear it during the day to make sure it stays in place. You should not be able to feel it if it is the right size and in the right position. Report any discomfort or other problems when, after 1 week, you return to the clinic or surgery. You should come with it in position so that the doctor or nurse can do a proper check.

3.45 WHAT SHOULD TAKE PLACE AT THE SECOND VISIT?

1 Any discomfort or problems should be identified.
2 If there are problems a change in the size of the cap or use of a different spermicide may be recommended.
3 Repetition of the instructions above is important before the woman actually begins to rely on her method.
4 A final warning about the danger of risk-taking may be useful, coupled with a reminder about *the availability if ever needed of postcoital contraception* (see Ch. 7).

3.46 WHAT EXTRA INSTRUCTIONS ARE GIVEN FOR USERS OF CERVICAL/VAULT CAPS?

1 A usual recommendation is to one-third fill the bowl of either cervical, vault or vimule caps. None is used on the rim for fear of impairing suction.
2 With these caps, an extra measure of spermicidal jelly or a pessary should be added on the vaginal side before the first as well as subsequent acts of intercourse after insertion.

3.47 WHAT ARRANGEMENTS ARE MADE FOR ROUTINE SUBSEQUENT FOLLOW-UP?

1 After the first two visits it is usual to see the patients at 3 months and then at least annually. (Six-monthly visits used to be recommended but this is probably unnecessarily frequent.) The most important thing is:

2 the woman should feel free to return more frequently if difficulties occur.
3 Reassessment of the fitting is particularly required:
   (a) after full-term delivery;
   (b) after any unplanned pregnancy whether ending in a termination or miscarriage (chiefly to assess possible improvements in fitting or the user's technique);
   (c) after having vaginal surgery;
   (d) after the woman loses or gains more than 3 kg in weight.

3.48 WHAT IS THE SCIENTIFIC BASIS FOR THE RULES AND REGULATIONS ABOUT USE OF OCCLUSIVE CAPS, AS IN QS 3.44–3.47 ABOVE?

Rather weak: many assumptions, some of them fundamental ones, have never been tested in proper controlled trials, namely:

1 that spermicides add significantly to the effectiveness of occlusive caps. Actually this has now been tested with a good study design at MPC, but the statistical power was insufficient for a conclusive result (Q 3.7);
2 that fitting the largest diaphragm that the woman finds comfortable will improve its effectiveness;
3 that extra spermicide should be used at each intercourse;
4 that extra spermicide should be used if intercourse is delayed for more than 3 hours after placement of the cap;
5 that the spermicide should be applied both to the top and under surface of the diaphragm;
6 that the shortest safe time after intercourse that any occlusive cap can be removed is 6 hours (based on assumptions about the spermicidal effects of the acid vagina);
7 that gain or loss of as little as 3 kg in weight would influence the effectiveness of occlusive caps.

3.49 WHAT VARIATIONS IN THE INSTRUCTIONS GIVEN TO PATIENTS ARE WORTH CONSIDERING?

Numerous variations are accepted practice in different countries around the world. In Australia use of spermicide at all with occlusive caps is often left to the patient's choice. The rationale for this is the high rate of user-failure in that country and the belief that increased compliance is likely when 'messy' spermicides are avoided. This Australian view, however, is a minority view. Pending more data most authorities feel that spermicides should be used; but all possible efforts should be made to reduce the problems of non-compliance with which they are associated. For example, newer spermicidal jellies with a far better appearance, texture and smell are being marketed. In addition two variants seem reasonable:

1 Application of spermicide to the superior surface only of the diaphragm. This is the norm in America, and is becoming more usual also in this country (about an 8 cm (3 in) strip of cream or jelly from the tube being applied).
2 Increasing to 6 hours the interval after placement of the diaphragm and before intercourse after which further spermicide is advised.

Other minor variations are also permitted by various family planning authorities.

MANAGEMENT OF SIDE-EFFECTS AND COMPLICATIONS

3.50 WHAT SHOULD BE DONE IF THE PARTNER CAN FEEL THE DIAPHRAGM DURING INTERCOURSE?

1 Check the size – a bigger or smaller variety may be needed.
2 Re-teach the patient. The couple may have already decided not to use certain positions (e.g. for rear entry vaginal intercourse they might use the condom instead).
3 Change from a flat- to a coiled-spring diaphragm.
4 Change to a vault or perhaps a cervical cap.
5 Change the method.

3.51 WHY ARE URINARY TRACT INFECTIONS COMMONER IN DIAPHRAGM USERS, AND HOW SHOULD THEY BE MANAGED?

1 The fact that urinary tract infections develop more frequently is believed to be caused mainly by the pressure of the rim on the urethra and bladder base, predisposing to urethritis and cystitis.
2 Some work has also suggested that use of the diaphragm and other occlusive caps with spermicide alters the vaginal flora so as to promote infections. Vaginal cultures from cap-users grow *Escherichia coli* more often than those from relevant controls.

It would appear that the first explanation is the more important, since the following actions usually help (especially item 2):

1 change to a smaller size of diaphragm;
2 change to a vault cap (or cervical cap).

The woman is also advised to empty her bladder both before and just after intercourse.

3.52 WHAT ARE THE POSSIBLE CAUSES OF THE COMPLAINT OF 'VAGINAL SORENESS'?

1 There may be an incidental infection such as trichomoniasis or thrush (or urethritis, see above).
2 Inflammatory reactions, abrasions or even frank ulcers can also be caused by local pressure.
3 Allergy is possible, either to the spermicide or to chemicals in the rubber of the occlusive cap.

3.53 HOW SHOULD VAGINAL SORENESS BE MANAGED?

1 First examine the patient: particularly her vulva and the whole vaginal surface. If there is widespread erythema and multiple vesicles or scaling, suspect allergy. Allergy can be treated by change of spermicide (see Table 3.2), but in this country plastic caps are no longer sold.

TABLE 3.2 SPERMICIDES AVAILABLE IN THE UK

Name	Manufacturer	Active ingredients
Foams		
Delfen Foam	Janssen-Cilag Pharmaceutical Ltd	Nonoxynol-9 12.5%
Creams		
Ortho-creme	Janssen-Cilag Pharmaceutical Ltd	Nonoxynol-9 2%
Jellies		
Duragel	LRC Products Ltd	Nonoxynol-11 2%
Gynol II	Janssen-Cilag Pharmaceutical Ltd	Nonoxynol-9 2%
Pessaries		
Double Check	FP Sales Ltd	Nonoxynol-9 6%
Ortho-Forms	Janssen-Cilag Pharmaceutical Ltd	Nonoxynol-9 5%

All these products have vehicles which do not have adverse effects on rubber (see Q 2.21).

2 Swabs should be taken for possible infections. If there is a discharge with a slightly fishy odour a useful test is the pH using test paper whose range is pH 4–6. A result which is >4.5 suggests either bacterial vaginosis (BV) or trichomoniasis, both treatable with metronidazole. For BV, clindamycin (Dalacin) 2% cream can also be used – but beware its possible adverse effects on rubber (Q 2.21).

3.54 WHAT SHOULD BE DONE IF ACTUAL ABRASIONS OR ULCERS ARE SEEN?

I have personally only seen one severe case, in an arcing diaphragm user, but they have been described in users of other diaphragms, vimules and cervical caps.

In our case the ulcers were posterolateral on each side, 2–3 cm long and about 0.5 cm wide and deep, and very indurated. At first a carcinoma of the vagina was suspected! However, complete recovery followed non-use of the diaphragm (which was size 85 and fitted correctly) and abstinence from intercourse for 3 weeks. No other treatment was required.

The woman concerned had met a new partner, and intercourse had been unusually vigorous and frequent with the diaphragm left in place for long periods of time. Cases reported from the USA had similarly worn the diaphragm or vimule cap for 3 or more days in succession. This rare complication is also said to be more likely if the diaphragm is too large, and may be related to variations in individual anatomy (see also Q. 3.85).

NOTE: The 'Today®' collatex contraceptive sponge
Regrettably, this product, which was actually very user-friendly, and popular among women whose fertility could be expected to be low, has been removed from the market for commercial reasons. Its place has now been taken to some extent by Delfen foam (see Q 3.64).

FEMALE CONDOMS

3.55 WHAT IS THE NEW FEMALE CONDOM, FIRST MARKETED DURING 1992?

Various designs have been proposed, including the *bikini condom* with its integral latex pouch, from America, and more recently the Janesway

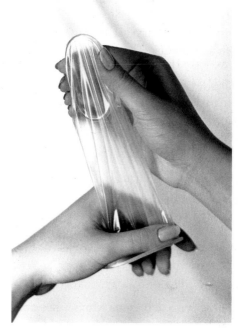

Figure 3.5   Femidom. Q 3.55.

panty-condom, with a latex pouch attached to frilly knickers! Neither of these have reached the market to date.

The most successful product is *Femidom* (*Reality* in the USA), first devised in Denmark. Made of polyurethane and preloaded with an efficient silicone lubricant, it is shown in Figure 3.5. The currently marketed version is 17 cm long. Both have a large (70-mm) diameter outer ring attached at the opening, designed to prevent it advancing beyond the vulva. A 60 mm diameter loose ring at the inner closed end aids its retention within the vagina and is also squeezed like a diaphragm for insertion. The whole device thus forms a well lubricated secondary vagina.

3.56 WHAT ADVANTAGES ARE CLAIMED?

Advantages:

1 over-the-counter method not requiring fitting by any outsider;
2 under the woman's control;

3 insertable pre-intercourse, like the diaphragm;
4 does not require erect penis at outset;
5 male sensations: usually reported as feeling more normal than intercourse with a male rubber condom;
6 odour free;
7 very complete barrier against STIs including viruses;
8 worth suggesting if local soreness makes sex uncomfortable or during menses or postpartum lochia.
9 shown to be less likely than the male condom to rupture in use;
10 not damaged by any common chemicals.

Its use-effectiveness (up to 95% effective to one year with perfect use) is broadly similar to the male condom.

3.57 ARE THERE ANY PROBLEMS?

Users report several in-use problems:

1 Prominence during foreplay
2 The potential for the penis to become wrongly positioned (between the sac and the vaginal wall). Users should be warned about this risk.
3 It is rather noisy in use: prompting the suggestion to 'have the music on!'

3.58 WHAT IS THE PLACE OF FEMIDOM IN THE RANGE OF METHODS?

Reports about its acceptability are mixed. It was given qualified approval as a method by about half the users in the first MPC study, who tried it up to 10 times but used a different method for contraception. Among 106 volunteers in MPC's trial of Femidom as sole contraceptive more than half found it unacceptable. However, nine of the 11 users who continued for 1 year, and most of 20 who had to stop using it solely because supplies ran out, would have wished to continue long term. As the first female-controlled method with high potential for preventing HIV transmission it must surely be welcomed to the range of contraceptive options. Further development of new variants will hopefully make it even more acceptable and use-effective.

A proportion of users ring the changes along with male condoms according to choice: i.e. having 'his' night followed by 'her' night!

SPERMICIDES

3.59 WHAT ARE SPERMICIDES?

These are a range of substances which chemically immobilize or destroy sperm. They are one of the oldest and simplest forms of fertility control and make a useful contribution, chiefly to increase the efficacy of other methods.

3.60 WHAT IS THE MODE OF ACTION OF SPERMICIDES?

They have two main components: a relatively inert base and an active spermicidal agent. Hence they operate both physically and biochemically, forming a partial barrier and also immobilizing sperm. The base materials vary in their physical characteristics, the best being water soluble. The active ingredients are of five main types:

1 surface-active agents, of which the most widely used worldwide is nonoxynol-9. Indeed, due to commercial pressures this has now become the only spermicide still on the UK market – leading to real difficulties for users of occlusive caps who develop an allergy to it;
2 enzyme inhibitors;
3 bactericides;
4 acids;
5 local anaesthetics and other membrane-active agents.

3.61 WHAT TYPES ARE AVAILABLE?

All the spermicides currently used in the UK are listed in Table 3.2. Regrettably there is very little real choice.

With the arrival of the AIDS problem we are now suffering from neglect of this field by a generation of scientists: far too little research has been done to devise better substances, more effective and safer not only as spermicides but also potentially as *virucides* (see Qs 3.66 and 3.67).

3.62 HOW ARE SPERMICIDES USED?

To be effective, the products should disperse quickly but yet remain in sufficient concentration at the cervix to exert their action at the end of intercourse. Aerosol foams such as Delfen seem to be preferable in this respect. The products listed can be inserted just before intercourse, with the important exception of the pessaries and foaming tablets. These should be inserted at least 10 minutes before ejaculation to allow sufficient time for dispersal.

3.63 HOW EFFECTIVE ARE SPERMICIDES USED ALONE?

Spermicides are far more effective in vitro than they ever prove to be in vivo. This is fully discussed in Q 1.3. There are greater variations in reported effectiveness for spermicides than for almost any other birth control method. The limits range from less than 1 to over 30 pregnancies/100 woman-years! In a study of almost 3000 well-motivated women attending six family planning clinics in the USA with the proper instructions and follow-up, Bernstein documented a pregnancy rate of only 4/100 woman-years. Trussell indicates a 'perfect use' rate of 6% in the first year.

3.64 ARE SPERMICIDES RECOMMENDED FOR USE ALONE AS CONTRACEPTIVES?

General teaching in this country has been that spermicides are not effective enough for use alone. Delfen Foam is believed to be more effective than the other presentations available in this country, and it is very user-friendly, non-greasy and unobtrusive in use. However, they can very useful under certain conditions, mainly where reduced fertility and good compliance are both expected:

1 Women's natural fertility may be less due to:
   (a) *Age*. Fertility declines, most steeply after the age of 45, though less so in those with continued regular cycling (see Qs 8.33 and 8.34). Hence Delfen foam *may* be very appropriate, as well as acceptable from the age of 45 if irregular cycles with some vasomotor symptoms are occurring (and even more so after 50) – through until 1 year after the menopause.
   (b) *Lactation*. The method could be used until uterine bleeding begins to return at weaning.
   (c) *Secondary amenorrhoea* (see Q 4.64), though if the woman is hypo-oestrogenic the COC or HRT may be preferable.
2 Spermicide may also be used as an *adjunct* to other methods of birth control, such as the IUD or *coitus interruptus*.

3 It may also be used for those who are planning their first child fairly soon, or who are *spacing* their family.
4 It would certainly be better than nothing for women who are unable or unwilling to use any other more effective method.

3.65 WHAT ARE THE ADVANTAGES AND DISADVANTAGES OF SPERMICIDES?

These are summarized in Table 3.3.

3.66 DO SPERMICIDES PROTECT AGAINST SEXUALLY TRANSMITTED INFECTIONS?

In vitro studies have shown that most of the common spermicides can kill sexually transmitted pathogens. Nonoxynol has activity against the organisms causing gonorrhoea, *Chlamydia*, *Trichomonas* vaginitis, genital herpes and even AIDS (HIV). In vivo studies have mostly been small and uncontrolled, but in general they confirm a useful protective effect of nonoxynol, with one unwanted exception relating to the risk of virus transmission – see Q 3.67 below.

TABLE 3.3 ADVANTAGES AND DISADVANTAGES OF SPERMICIDES

Advantages	Disadvantages
1. Easy availability.	1. Perceived to be messy.
2. Freedom from major health risks.	2. Not highly effective in general use.
3. No medical intervention/ supervision necessary.	3. Are coitus-dependent and thus inconvenient to use.
4. Need only be used when required.	4. Waiting period of 10 minutes before some products effective.
5. Provide some protection against some sexually transmitted diseases.	5. Not effective if inserted more than 60 minutes ahead.
6. Allow the female to be in control of contraception.	6. Can cause local heat (foaming tablets), irritation or allergy.
7. Provide some genital lubrication.	7. Questions are now being asked about risks of damage to vaginal epithelium. See Q 3.67
8. Are a valuable adjunct to other methods.	

VAGINAL CONTRACEPTION: UNRESOLVED SAFETY ISSUES

3.67 IS IT TRUE THAT NONOXYNOL SEEMS CAPABLE OF SOMETIMES DAMAGING THE VAGINAL EPITHELIUM?

A study in Nairobi prostitutes of nonoxynol-containing spermicides as a possible aid to safer sex reported 'soreness' as a frequent complaint. This was at first thought to be linked in part with trauma from very frequent coitus, but subsequent studies have shown that frequent use of the product itself is the main factor. When used four times a day for 14 days, nonoxynol-9 released from pessaries caused erythema and colposcopic evidence of minor damage to the vaginal skin. This might or might not cause irritation or other symptoms, but it has naturally led to concern that this adverse effect might actually increase the likelihood of transfer of HIV infection, even though nonoxynol does have virucidal activity in vitro. Coupled with the doubts about its effectiveness against intracellular virus, these data mean it should not be promoted as an anti-HIV virucide.

However, pending the development of more alternatives, for the time being it is considered good practice to continue to recommend nonoxynol and the similar surface-active agents listed in Table 3.2 for *normal contraceptive use* (less frequently than four times a day!), whether alone or with diaphragms or condoms. The Margaret Pyke Trust is actively involved with other bodies in urgent and previously neglected research into new and better substances for vaginal use as virucides and spermicides.

3.68 ARE SPERMICIDES ABSORBED, AND IS THERE THEREFORE A RISK OF SYSTEMIC EFFECTS?

Yes, most substances in the vagina can be absorbed into the circulation. Hence it is impossible to say that any method that uses a spermicide is entirely free of the risk of systemic harmful effects. These could be by toxicity to vital organs, idiosyncrasy, or through carcinogenesis or teratogenesis. There have been some reports suggesting an association with unwanted effects (see Qs 3.69 and 3.70) following spermicide absorption, but the overall picture remains a reassuring one.

3.69 WHAT IS THE EVIDENCE THAT STANDARD SPERMICIDES MIGHT HAVE TOXIC EFFECTS AFTER ABSORPTION?

In 1979 it was suggested from animal experiments that nonoxynol-9 might have hepatotoxic effects and cause changes in serum lipids. However, controlled studies of the blood chemistry of women using spermicides have not demonstrated any significant changes, though long-term data are not available. Certainly no obvious harm has ever been reported among long-term users of vaginal contraceptives.

3.70 WHAT IS THE EVIDENCE ABOUT TERATOGENESIS?

Exposure to the spermicide early in pregnancy, or fertilization of an ovum by a sperm damaged by the spermicide, might in theory increase the rate of malformations. In 1981, one study reported an increase in various unrelated fetal abnormalities among the children of women who may have used spermicides around the time they became pregnant. This study has been criticized because of flaws in the study design. More recent studies have completely failed to show the risk. Present opinion is that spermicides do not have any detectable teratogenic effect in ordinary use.

3.71 ARE THERE REPORTS OF AN INCREASE OF NEOPLASIA IN WOMEN USING VAGINAL CONTRACEPTION?

No – neither as a consequence of systemic absorption, nor because of any effect of spermicide or rubber on the vaginal or cervical epithelium. A few women who are sensitive to spermicides may develop hyperkeratosis of the cervix or vagina. This has not been shown to result in neoplasia. Indeed, it is very likely that barrier methods are protective against cervical neoplasia (see Q 3.17).

3.72 CAN VAGINAL CONTRACEPTION PROMOTE INFECTION?

This may seem improbable, in view of the fact that both the barrier effect and the spermicide seem to protect against many STIs. Concern arises from evidence that *Staphylococcus aureus* and some streptococci, and *E. coli* can tend to proliferate in the presence of a diaphragm or a cervical cap at the expense of the usual protective *Lactobacilli*. This has already been mentioned as a possible factor in the increased risk of urinary infections. It may also be relevant to toxic shock syndrome (TSS).

3.73 CAN THE DIAPHRAGM OR OTHER CAPS CAUSE TOXIC SHOCK SYNDROME?

Sporadic cases have been reported in the USA. However, the rate is so low that the risk is unlikely to be greater than that already existing from use of tampons by those diaphragm-users.

3.74 WHAT IS THE OVERALL SAFETY OF VAGINAL CONTRACEPTIVES?

Even allowing for the unresolved safety issues above, potential users may be told that all these methods are still believed to be medically safer than the hormonal methods. However, honesty is necessary, and it would be wrong to say that any method that uses an absorbable spermicide is completely free from systemic effect.

In assessing safety it is also important to remember that unwanted pregnancies are overall more frequent among users of any of these methods. One then has to consider the potential health hazard of the resulting unwanted pregnancies.

THE (NEAR) FUTURE IN VAGINAL CONTRACEPTION

3.75 WHAT INNOVATIVE SPERMICIDES ARE BEING STUDIED?

Inhibitors of the sperm's own enzymes, principally acrosin, show promise: and several surprising drugs (like propranolol), normally used for non-contraceptive indications, have aroused interest because of their effect on the sperm membrane and motility. Derivatives of natural products such as gossypol are also being screened. Another approach is to develop agents that directly alter cervical mucus both chemically and physically. Disinfectants/antibiotics are important because of their particular potential also as microbicides. Among these are chlorhexidine and gramicidin. Procept 2000 and Dextrin sulphate are substances showing promise as agents to block virus entry through the epithelium, and are particularly harmless to it (unlike nonoxynol itself, see Q 3.67 above).

More research is also urgently required into better carrier (base) materials and systems.

3.76 WHAT IS THE STATE OF RESEARCH INTO OCCLUSIVE CAPS?

1 *Disposable spermicide-coated diaphragms.* These have been studied, designed to overcome the perceived 'messiness' of any vaginal contraceptive that requires separate application of the spermicide.

2 *New sponges* with different spermicides, or combinations of spermicide, or microbicides should be useful, judging by the high acceptability of the sponge method in the MPC trial.

3 *New cervical caps.* There was great interest in the mid-80s in the so-called custom-fitted cervical cap, made from a mould of the user's cervix. Trials of this *Contracap* gave a quite unacceptable failure rate. However the objective remains attractive – of a non-coitally related appliance designed to be left in the place in the upper vagina for long periods of time. *Lea's Shield* and *Femcap* are American inventions: preliminary results with the latter, which does not require fitting like a diaphragm, but must still be used with a spermicide, are reasonably promising. See Figure 3.6.

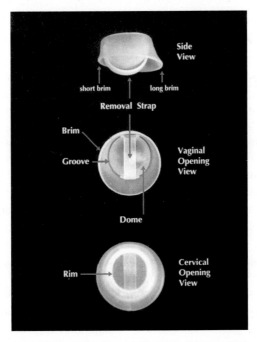

Figure 3.6 Femcap. From: Kubba A, Sanfilippo J, Hampton N (1999) *Contraception and Office Gynecology: Choices in Reproductive Healthcare* p. 124. London: WB Saunders. With permission.

The *Oves cap*, also an over-the-counter product used with spermicide, has (disturbingly) actually arrived on the UK market with almost no efficacy data! The *Gynaeseal diaphragm-tampon* devised by an Australian and mentioned in my last edition, seems to have sunk without trace.

4 *Intracervical devices*. Both medicated and non-medicated devices with some kind of flange or protruding arms to anchor them in the lower part of the uterus are possibilities which have been studied.

5 *Vaginal rings*. WHO did some preliminary work on a silicone rubber ring that releases nonoxynol-9 at a constant rate for at least 30 days. This seems a very promising approach, preferably using a more advanced spermicide or better still a virucide.

QUESTIONS ASKED BY USERS ABOUT VAGINAL CONTRACEPTION

3.77 CAN I USE SOME KIND OF CAP IF MY WOMB TILTS BACKWARDS?

It is a myth that this makes it impossible to use the method. Some positions of your cervix (entrance to the womb) may make it preferable for you to be given an arcing diaphragm, and could lead to rejection of a cervical cap; but the method is not ruled out if you wish to use it.

3.78 IN AMERICA THEY HAVE INSERTERS FOR DIAPHRAGMS – ARE THEY AVAILABLE HERE?

Yes they are, but you need to ask yourself whether your wish to use one might be connected with some reluctance to touch yourself in the genital area. It may be that can be overcome by counselling, or perhaps you should think about using another method.

3.79 HOW DO I KNOW WHERE MY CERVIX IS?

It is absolutely essential that you feel confident that you can find your cervix, whatever the kind of occlusive cap you are going to use. It is often helpful to ask your doctor or the nurse to tell you in which direction its little opening points. You may also find it much easier to feel if you use two fingers rather than one.

3.80 HOW MUCH CREAM OR JELLY SHOULD I USE WITH MY DIAPHRAGM?

A common error is to use too much. See Q 3.44 for the standard instructions. If you find messiness a particular problem but still wish to use the method, ask your doctor or nurse about the possibility of following the American teaching, of putting spermicide only on the top of the cap when it is first inserted. (Continue to follow all the other rules you were taught.) Delfen foam may be preferred.

3.81 CAN THE CAP FALL OUT WHEN YOU GO TO THE TOILET?

Normally, this will not happen. If it does, soon after intercourse, consider postcoital contraception (see Ch. 7). Moreover, if your diaphragm or other cap comes out, it may be that you have a prolapse, or the wrong size, or are not inserting it correctly. So you should make an early appointment to discuss things with the doctor or nurse.

3.82 CAN CAPS AND DIAPHRAGMS BE FITTED WITH STRINGS TO HELP REMOVAL? I HAVE DIFFICULTY IN GETTING MINE OUT.

There are no longer any marketed with strings. You may have been taught to use just one finger to hook out the diaphragm but the solution to your problem may well be just to use two fingers, one each side of the front rim.

3.83 HOW DO I CHECK THE DIAPHRAGM IS IN GOOD CONDITION? ITS DOME HAS BECOME MUCH SOFTER AND FLOPPIER AND IT HAS LOST ITS NEW WHITENESS – DO THESE CHANGES MATTER?

You should hold your diaphragm up to the light and stretch it, being careful not to damage the rubber with your fingernails. If no holes are seen, and if the rim can readily be restored to a reasonable shape, then all is well. The change in colour and texture of the rubber is quite normal.

3.84 CAN I LEAVE THE CAP IN DURING MY PERIODS?

The US FDA advises against this because of an unproven extra risk of the rare TSS. To reduce messiness if you fancy lovemaking during any bleeding a better solution might be Femidom (see Q 3.55).

3.85 I HAVE HEARD YOU CAN LEAVE THE CAP IN ALL THE TIME – IS THIS RIGHT?

If you follow the rules, yes – almost! It can be in position most of the time if your love life is unpredictable and frequent. The important thing is to remove it at least once in 24 hours, 6 hours after the last intercourse, wash it in mild soap, rinse it thoroughly and then it can be reinserted. Continuous use without giving your vaginal wall an occasional rest seems a bad thing, however (see Q 3.54).

3.86 CAN I HAVE A BATH OR GO SWIMMING WHILST THE CAP IS IN PLACE?

Yes. However, it is ideally best if this is not until at least 2 hours after intercourse, in case it helps the sperm to escape the action of the spermicide. And if you make love after bathing with the diaphragm in, put in some extra spermicide first.

3.87 I HAVE A BABY – CAN I GO BACK TO USING MY OLD DIAPHRAGM OR CAP?

Quite possibly not. It is certainly important to get the fitting rechecked and have a full retraining in correct use (see also Q 3.47).

3.88 HOW OFTEN SHOULD I CHANGE THE DIAPHRAGM OR CAP FOR A NEW ONE?

Only when your inspection at Q 3.83 shows damage, or as recommended by your clinic. Occlusive caps are quite expensive on the NHS and successful regular use of the same one for 2 years is very common. Remember too that if you lose your cap you can buy the right size over the counter at any chemist.

3.89 IS FEMIDOM A RECOMMENDED METHOD?

Yes. Follow the instructions which come with it most carefully, every time. If you are careful to avoid wrong positioning of the penis (see Q 3.57), and the sperm are caught completely within the Femidom, it is as good as a male condom both as a contraceptive and for safer sex.

3.90 CAN I USE A HOME-MADE BARRIER, 'IN AN EMERGENCY'?

Improvised barriers can be made. Probably the best is a suitable piece of sponge or plug of cloth, soaked either in vinegar solution diluted 1 in 20 with water, or in a soap solution.

3.91 DO YOU RECOMMEND THE 'HONEYCAP', WHICH MY FRIEND USES?

Definitely not. Available from some doctors in private practice in London, this is really only a size 60 arcing-spring diaphragm which is first soaked in honey for 7 days; and then used without spermicide for up to a week at a time. The honey is meant to reduce the risk of vaginal infection or odour, but even this is unproven: and its effectiveness has also not been properly tested.

All in all it is highly likely to have the same failure rate as in a Marie Stopes Centre study of the 'non-spermicide, fit-free diaphragm' (same 60 mm size) – which amounted to a risk, in the first year, that one woman would get pregnant out of every four users!

4

Oral contraception – the combined oral contraceptive (COC)

BACKGROUND: EFFICACY AND MECHANISMS

4.1 WHAT IS THE DEFINITION OF ORAL CONTRACEPTION?

An orally administered substance or combination which prevents pregnancy. Specifically at the present time such substances are only for use by women. Steroids and other potential systemic contraceptives may also be given by non-oral routes (see Chs 5 and 8). In this chapter I shall consider only the combined oral contraceptive (COC), which is a combination of oestrogen and progestagen. Unless qualified, the word 'pill' refers to the COC. The progestagen-only pill (POP) is considered in Chapter 5.

4.2 WHAT IS THE HISTORY OF ORAL CONTRACEPTION?

This is discussed in more detail elsewhere (see my book *The Pill*, Further Reading). In brief, it was shown by the early 1900s that the corpus luteum of pregnancy stops further ovulation. In 1921 Haberlandt transplanted ovaries into female rabbits, and rendered them infertile for several months. He suggested that extracts from ovaries might be used as oral contraceptives. In 1941 Marker used diosgenin from the Mexican yam as the raw material for sex steroids. This led to the synthesis of norethisterone (known as norethindrone in the USA) by Djerassi and his colleagues in 1950. Frank Colton independently produced norethynodrel, which with mestranol was the first marketed oral contraceptive. Margaret Sanger, supported by her wealthy friend Catherine McCormack, financed the studies of the biologist Gregory Pincus and M. C. Chang together with the obstetrician John Rock. After systematic experiments in animals the first human trials in North America were reported in 1956. In the Puerto Rico field trial which followed the intention appears to have been to use progestagen alone, but there was contamination with mestranol. Thus the invention of the 'combined pill' – which was shown later to give much better cycle control than any progestagen-only method – owes a definite debt to chance.

The combined pill became available in the USA in June 1960 and in the UK during 1961. In 1963 the Wyeth Company achieved the total synthesis of norgestrel.

The first case report of venous thromboembolism was reported in *The Lancet* in 1961 by an astute British GP. Subsequently there have been numerous case-control studies, and three main prospective (cohort) studies, researching both the adverse and beneficial effects. Much more money has been spent on testing than on originally developing the method.

4.3 WHAT IS THE USAGE OF THE PILL, WORLDWIDE AND IN THE UK?

There is enormous variation between countries, and within countries according to age groups. The differences have more to do with medical politics, religion, and the inertia of institutions, than with the acceptability or otherwise of the method to potential consumers. Estimated overall usage varies between less than 2% of married women in Japan through to about 40% in the Netherlands. According to the UK General Household Survey (1995), the COC is used by about 25% of the 13 million women aged 16–49, of which the POP accounts for one tenth i.e. 2.5%. A more recent (1998) estimate from pill-cycles sold is 23% (i.e. 3 million users). In the peak age group 20–24, 49% of all women (which is about 70% of all contraception-users) use pills, mainly the COC. See Table 0.3, page 15.

In several surveys over the last 15 years, for the RCGP and other bodies, up to 95% of sexually active UK women under the age of 30 reported use of oral contraceptives at some time.

4.4 WHAT ARE THE MAIN MECHANISMS OF CONTRACEPTIVE ACTION OF THE COMBINED PILL?

These are summarized in Table 4.1. Without exception all steroidal methods operate by some combination of the mechanisms there described. The COC has a very similar primary action in most women, namely the prevention of ovulation: both by lack of follicular maturation and by abolition of oestrogen-mediated positive feedback which leads to the luteinizing hormone (LH) surge. The other mechanisms shown – reduction in sperm penetrability of cervical mucus (see Q 5.16) and of the receptivity to the blastocyst of the endometrium (see Q 5.17) – are primarily back-up mechanisms for the COC. They have greater relevance to the mechanisms of some of the oestrogen-free methods of Chapter 5. See also Q 5.34 for tubal effects.

4.5 WHAT ARE THE TYPES OF COC?

Current COCs are either fixed-dose or phasic. The latter are like the former in containing both oestrogen and progestagen. The ratio of the two is not fixed, however, but changed in a stepwise fashion, either once (biphasic pills) or twice (triphasic pills) in each 21-day course. They are discussed in more detail below (see Qs 4.174–4.179). We should note here, however, that like all COCs the phasic types remove the menstrual cycle; but they attempt to replace it with cyclical variations, chiefly in the progestagen dose. There is as yet no proof that this has important health benefits (aside, that is, from the giving of a low dose of each hormone).

TABLE 4.1 VARIOUS PROGESTAGEN DELIVERY SYSTEMS (ALL EXCEPT COC ARE OESTROGEN-FREE)

	Oral		Injectable		Implant
	COC	POP	NET-EN	DMPA	Implanon
Administration					
Frequency	Daily	Daily	2-monthly	3-monthly	3-yearly
Progestagen dose	Low	Ultra-low	High	High	Ultra-low
Blood levels	Rapidly fluctuating		Initial peak then decline		Constant
First pass through liver	Yes	Yes	No	No	No
Major mechanisms					
Ovary: ↓ Ovulation*	+++	+	++	+++	++
Cervical mucus: ↓ sperm penetrability	Yes	Yes	Yes	Yes	Yes
Endometrium: ↓ receptivity to blastocyst	Yes	Yes	Yes	Yes	Yes
Use effectiveness	0.2–3	0.5–4	<2	0–1	0–0.1
Menstrual pattern	Regular	Often irregular	Irregular	Very irregular	Irregular
Amenorrhoea during use	Rare	Occasional	Common	Very common	Common
Reversibility					
Immediate termination possible?	Yes	Yes	No	No	Yes
By woman herself at anytime?	Yes	Yes	No	No	No
Median time to conception *from first omitted dose/removal*	c. 3 months	c. 2 months	c. 3 months	c. 6 months	c. 2 months

*By two mechanisms – no pre-ovulatory follicles formed, plus no LH surges occur.

4.6 WHAT ARE 'EVERYDAY' (ED) VARIETIES OF COC? DO THEY HAVE ADVANTAGES?

These are regimens which include, usually, 7 days of placebo tablets. They have the advantage of a reduction in the risk that the user will forget to restart her next packet on time – a potent cause of pill failure (see Q 4.18). This system is also one way of removing the necessity for numbering, as opposed to putting the day of the week, against the pill blisters in phasic packets (compare Logynon ED with Logynon). A simpler solution, as in Trinovum, is the use of 7-day phases. 'Sunday start' schemes, with instructions for extra contraception in the first packet, are common in the USA.

4.7 WHAT ARE THE DISADVANTAGES OF ED PACKAGING?

This is often complicated by a starting routine involving a variable number of placebos, so extra contraception has to be advised for 14 days. Some women dislike the implication that they are too unintelligent to remember when to stop and restart treatment. It has even been suggested, thirdly, that some women think that the dummy lactose (sugar) pills might be bad for them!

For these reasons ED packaging has never been popular in the UK. However, in other countries well over half of all pill cycles are of this type – which I personally favour as an aid to compliance. There are ways of simplifying the starting routine so as always to start with an *active* tablet; and the placebos should perhaps be made of bran, as everyone knows that bran is good for you!

4.8 WHAT MODIFIED REGIMENS WOULD YOU LIKE TO SEE MARKETED?

Since as will be described fully below the pill-free interval (PFI) is 'the Achilles' heel' of the COC's efficacy, there would be particular merit in returning to an earlier scheme of 22 active pills with six placebos. Indeed even without placebos this is good for compliance, since the 'finishing day' is then the same day of the week as the 'starting day'.

ED packets of monophasic brands with four placebo tablets would also be useful. Instead of or as well as tricycling (see Q. 4.31) these regimens with a much shortened pill-free time could be used by women with a history of past conception while taking the COC (Q 4.27). Moreover if the PFI were shortened, new products for general use could safely offer even lower doses of both hormones than are currently viable. These are already marketed in some countries.

4.9 WHAT ABOUT OTHER OESTROGEN-PROGESTAGEN AGENTS (ESPECIALLY SEQUENTIAL PILLS AND REGIMENS OF HORMONE REPLACEMENT THERAPY)?

High-oestrogen sequential pills were shown to double the risk of endometrial carcinoma and have rightly been consigned to history.

Older women are now frequently given a similar regimen of oestrogen alone, typically for 16 days, followed by oestrogen plus progestagen for 12 days. The oestrogen is, of course, a natural oestrogen, in doses which have a far smaller effect on the endometrium; and there is good evidence that these regimens do not increase (they may even reduce) the risk of endometrial cancer. But they are not safely contraceptive. For most fertile women a modified (usually non-cyclical, no-bleed) regimen which would be definitely contraceptive as well treating any oestrogen deficiency would be preferable. This whole matter is discussed further in Chapter 8.

4.10 WHAT LINK IS THERE BETWEEN THE COC CYCLE AND THE MENSTRUAL CYCLE?

Very little, but endless confusion is caused by the fact that women consider their hormone withdrawal bleeds as the same thing as 'periods'. In reality of course the normal menstrual cycle is removed during use of the COC. The ovaries show no follicular activity *during pill-taking* (contrast the situation between packets, see Q 4.15) and hence produce minimal endogenous oestrogen. Withdrawal bleeding (WTB) is an end-organ response to withdrawal of the artificial hormones, and is irrelevant to events elsewhere in the body and specifically at the pituitary and the ovaries. In physiological terms, everywhere except at the endometrium, the pill causes secondary amenorrhoea for as long as the woman takes it.

Absence of WTB is totally irrelevant to future fertility, though a pregnancy test is indicated after two WTBs have been missed: sooner if there are good reasons to suspect pill-failure. Aside from pregnancy-testing, it is pointless to investigate this.

Breakthrough bleeding (BTB) is likewise a purely endometrial response, but it may be heavy enough to simulate a 'period' to the woman. This also needs explaining in advance as a reason to continue taking her daily pills with extra diligence (until an early appointment), rather than stopping.

Lack of adequate instruction about WTB and BTB commonly causes avoidable 'iatrogenic' pregnancies (see Q 8.12, 8.17).

Enormous – yet it is still not explained in most pill leaflets or by many prescribers. It influences all the following issues:

1 the *efficacy* of the COC, in that lengthening of the PFI risks ovulation whereas mid-packet pill omissions are unimportant;
2 the improved *recommendations* once pills are omitted or vomited;
3 short- or long-term use of *interacting drugs* or use of the pill if past 'breakthrough pregnancies' have occurred;
4 the minimizing of *health-risks*;
5 and, possibly, even the *reversibility* of the pill method.

All these points will be expanded in the next group of questions.

EFFECTIVENESS OF THE COC – CIRCUMSTANCES IN WHICH IT MAY BE REDUCED

There is no simple answer to this question, since efficacy is so user-dependant. According to Trussell, during 'perfect use' only 0.1% of women in the US will experience a pregnancy during the first year of use, but in 'typical' use he gives a figure of 5% – a fiftyfold range! The UK FPA settles for 'over 99%' for consistent users.

The theoretical effectiveness approaches 100% partly because of the adjunctive mechanisms mentioned above (see Q 4.4). However it appears that for some women the modern (less than 50 µg oestrogen) pills are only just sufficient for efficacy, particularly if omitted tablets lead to the slightest lengthening of the pill-free week. I argue below that in a few susceptible women this time cannot be lengthened by even a few hours with impunity. Minor errors of compliance are extremely common, and most pill-takers (through provider failure) are uninformed about the critical importance of not lengthening the pill-free time.

The slightly higher pregnancy rate with modern pills is thus explained chiefly in terms of 'reduced margin for error'. But, regrettably, this problem is often amplified by insufficient pill teaching by hurried health care professionals: who regularly omit any explanation of the implications of the pill-free interval (Qs 4.15–4.28) and fail to back this with the user-friendly FPA leaflet 'Choosing and Using the Combined Pill.'

4.13 WHAT IS THE EFFECT OF INCREASING AGE ON EFFICACY?

The Oxford/Family Planning Association (FPA) study shows the (slight) expected decline in pregnancy rate with increasing age, due mainly to declining fertility and also some reduction in the frequency of intercourse (see Table 0.2 columns 3 and 4, and Q 0.19).

4.14 ARE OVERWEIGHT WOMEN MORE LIKELY TO CONCEIVE WHILE TAKING MODERN ULTRA-LOW-DOSE COCS?

No. This has not been demonstrated, although it might be expected pharmacologically, since a 75-kg woman receives exactly the same dose in normal pill-taking as her 50-kg friend. Moreover *there is a definite weight influence on the efficacy of some progestagen-only methods* (see Q 5.13).

My own theory is that the combined pill is contraceptively so very strong, along with its back-up actions, that it has sufficient margin to cope with women of any weight. Other factors like compliance will affect efficacy far more (relatively) than body mass, which is perhaps more detectable as a factor if a systemic method has a method-failure rate above 1/100 woman-years.

4.15 SINCE IT IS THE CONTRACEPTIVE-FREE PART OF THE PILL-TAKING CYCLE, DOES NOT THE PILL-FREE INTERVAL (PFI) HAVE EFFICACY IMPLICATIONS?

Precisely. When you think about it we have here a bizarre contraceptive: one that we providers actually instruct the users *not* to use – for 25% of the time. Any systemic contraceptive must be at its lowest ebb when it is longest since it was actually ingested (Fig. 4.1). Hardly surprisingly, biochemical and ultrasound data demonstrate varying degrees of return of pituitary and ovarian follicular activity during the pill-free time.

Figure 4.2 displays the findings from a 1979 study based on patients attending the Margaret Pyke Centre (MPC). It is the rapid and sustained decline in the artificial hormones at the start of the pill-free interval (top half of Fig. 4.2) which leads to the withdrawal bleed (WTB). More importantly in this context, the figure shows the resulting slight average

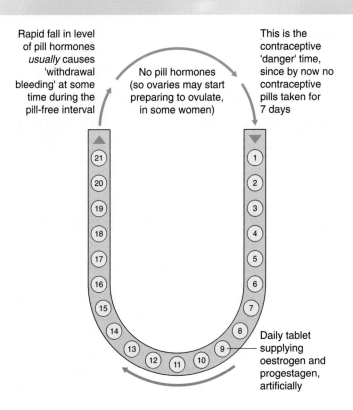

Figure 4.1 The pill cycle displayed as a horseshoe. Q 4.15. *Note*: a horseshoe is a symmetrical object. Hence the pill-free interval can be lengthened, leading to the risk of conception, either side of the horseshoe, by forgetting pills either at the beginning or at the end of the packet.

increase in (natural) oestradiol, implying regular return of ovarian follicular activity during the pill-free week. Wide standard deviations are also shown, meaning that in a subgroup the levels are high – indeed as high as has been observed well into the follicular phase of spontaneous menstrual cycles.

In a more recent MPC study, apparently preovulatory-type follicles of diameter 10 mm or more were present on the seventh pill-free day in 23% of 120 pill-takers; in three women the follicle was 16–19 mm in diameter (i.e. potentially only about 2 days from fertile ovulation). In the other women there was no important change, suggesting continuing quiescence of their ovaries.

The pill-free week

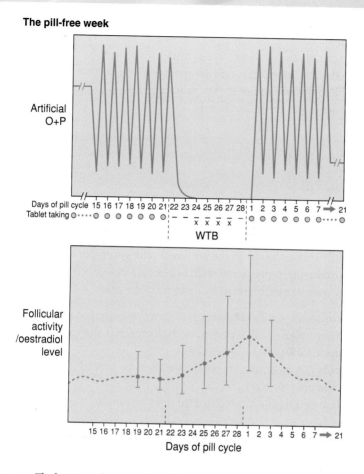

Figure 4.2 The hormone changes of the pill-free week. Q 4.15 and following. Changes through the pill-taking cycle in the blood levels of both the ingested artificial hormones (oestrogen (O) and progestagen (P)), and in follicular activity as demonstrated by growth of the dominant follicle by ultrasound. WTB, withdrawal bleeding. Note the rapid return to low ovarian activity during the first 7 days of pill-taking. (Bottom half of the figure is from a study of patients attending the Margaret Pyke Centre).

However, for the purpose of maintaining contraception all we have to be concerned about is the extreme cases. Among them, breakthrough ovulation is most likely to follow any lengthening of the PFI. Most important, such lengthening may result from omissions, malabsorption due to vomiting, and drug interaction involving pills *either at the start or at the end of a packet*. See the legend to Figure 4.1: pill-taking is depicted as a horseshoe because a horseshoe is a symmetrical object.

Clearly the advice which is still sometimes given, to take extra precautions to the end of her packet, is wrong: it fails to allow for ovarian activity returning in the pill-free time.

4.16 SO WHAT IS THE SCIENTIFIC BASIS OF THE ADVICE WE SHOULD GIVE A WOMAN WHO HAS MISSED PILLS FOR ANY REASON?

In a fascinating study of previously regular pill-takers, it was shown by Smith *et al.* in 1986 that even if only 14 or even as few as seven pills had been taken since the last PFI, no women ovulated after seven pills were subsequently missed! (One in the 7-missed-pills group got mighty close, however, producing progesterone: albeit at non-fertile levels). This and other work may be summarized by three propositions:

1 Seven consecutive pills are enough to 'put the ovaries to sleep'. (Thereafter pills 8–21 in a packet, or many more if she tricycles, simply maintain the ovaries in quiescence).
2 Seven pills can be omitted without ovulation, as indeed is regularly the case in the pill-free week.
3 More than seven pills missed in total risks ovulation.

4.17 SO WHAT IS ACTUALLY NOW RECOMMENDED FOR MISSED COCs?

The 7-day 'Rule' is used by the UK FPA and is also now agreed by the UK manufacturers. It is based on the above pharmacology and can be conveyed in a simple algorithm (Fig. 4.3).

Note that the seven days of added contraception are logical in view of point 1 in Q 4.16 above. If there is already some follicular activity – which applies (almost) only at *the start of the packet after the PFI* and then only to just around 1/5 to 1/4 (23%) of a pill-taking population – seven tablets seem to be capable of putting any ovary back into a quiescent state. Moreover, if it has been too late to stop ovulation, this is likely to occur (and the egg will cease to be fertilizable) during the same seven days of condom use. For added safety, emergency contraception is recommended additionally if the PFI has been lengthened to 9 days or more – actually, *or if in the*

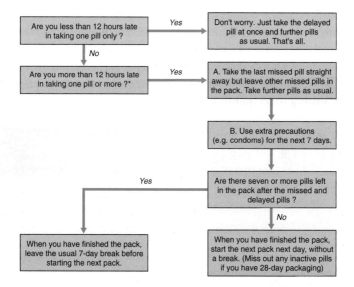

Figure 4.3   Advice for missed pills (21-day packaging). *NB If two or more pills missed *and* if they were all from the first seven in your pack, and if you have had unprotected intercourse since the end of your last pack, talk promptly to your doctor.** You may need emergency pills *as well as* continuing with instructions A and B above. See Qs 4.24 and 7.23(5).
From: Guillebaud J (1998) *Contraception Today* (3rd ed) p. 41, London: Martin Dunitz

prescriber's opinion the net effect of any combination of pill-omissions in the first week equates to a 9-day PFI (Q 4.24).

If 28-day packaging is used the woman must be carefully taught which are the dummy 'reminder' tablets, for omission if she misses any of the last seven active pills. All women should be asked to return for the exclusion of pregnancy if they have no bleeding in the *next* PFI.

How does the advice conveyed in Figure 4.3 apply in various categories of pill omissions? (Qs 4.18–4.20)

4.18 IT IS EASY TO SEE FROM FIGURES 4.1 AND 4.2 THAT MISSING PILLS AT THE START OF A PACKET, LENGTHENING THE CONTRACEPTION-FREE TIME TO MORE THAN 7 DAYS, COULD WELL BE 'BAD NEWS!' BUT WHAT ABOUT OMITTED PILLS IN THE MIDDLE OF A PACKET?

Tablets *omitted following on prior tablet-taking for 7 or more days*, and not followed by a PFI, are very low risk omissions for breakthrough ovulation.

If we allow for the one woman who nearly ovulated and the small numbers in the study just quoted in Q 4.16: once seven tablets have been taken, at the very least up to four pills may be missed mid-packet with impunity!

Yet because of a wrong analogy with the normal menstrual cycle, *unless we prescribers re-educate them*, patients worry most about missed pills when it matters least, in mid-packet. Unless they have been taught (as in the new millennium they must surely be taught! – see Q 4.21) they will rarely even seek advice when pill omissions or a stomach upset *have* led to a lengthening of the pill-free time, or (at the end of a pack) *will now* be leading to a *similar* lengthening. This is the most serious situation of all, but not seen as such e.g.: '*I just started my pack a bit late!*'

4.19 WHAT ARE THE IMPLICATIONS OF LATE-PACKET PILL OMISSIONS?

If a woman omits two or three tablets at the end of her preceding packet and is allowed to recommence the next packet on her usual starting day (something she is sure to do, unless otherwise instructed), there will be an ovulation risk at the end of the thereby lengthened pill-free time, after what is a *falsely reassuring withdrawal bleed*. (One consequence: any questioning later on about missed pills, perhaps in the antenatal clinic, must include asking about missed pills *before* the *last menstrual period* (LMP)!)

If she is properly taught, however, and follows the scheme in Figure 4.3, going straight on to the next packet, she will actually be more protected due to having a shorter PFI than usual. ...

4.20 SHOULD THIS ADVICE FOR LATE TABLET OMISSIONS (Q 4.19) BE DIFFERENT IF THE WOMAN IS ON A TRIPHASIC PILL BRAND?

No, at the end of the packet she should start immediately with the first (lower dose) phase tablets (see 4.174–4.179). She will probably have a 'withdrawal-type' bleed, but contraceptive efficacy will still be increased. This is a different situation from postponing 'periods' as described at Q 4.179.

4.21 CLEARLY IT WOULD BE BETTER IF THERE EMERGED A NEW GENERATION OF PILL-TAKERS WHO UNDERSTOOD THIS PHYSIOLOGY AHEAD OF TIME!

And it could happen, with our help as providers. In my opinion every new pill-taker has the right to know the basics of the 'contraception-free' interval, which are *not* that complicated to explain in lay terms:

- that it is a time when the ovary is 'let off the hook';
- that she could be one of the 23% with extra ovarian activity (Q 4.15);
- that her contraceptive safety in and after the PFI depends crucially on starting her *next* packet on time – so if she switches methods there are *not* seven 'safe' carryover days ... (Q8.17(16));
- that missing pills at the end of a packet is like making her pill-free break early by mistake, which is why it would be a bit silly to add on the regular break on top.

Straightaway when this is done, the advice of Figure 4.3 becomes understandable and compliance much more probable. The *time* for this basic pill-teaching (nurse-time often being better than doctor-time) needs to be found, backed by the FPA's leaflet (Q 4.12).

4.22 HOW MIGHT THE ADVICE IN FIGURE 4.3 BE SIMPLIFIED WHEN FACED WITH INDIVIDUAL WOMEN WHO HAVE MISSED THREE PILLS (A) AFTER SEVEN PILLS HAVE BEEN TAKEN MID-PACKET OR (B) NEAR THE END OF A PACKET?

The recommendations of Figure 4.3 above are in my view still preferred for their general applicability and to avoid confusion *in the written word*. However, the recommended seven days of condom use are actually redundant. See Qs 4.18–4.19. Face to face with the pill-takers mentioned: the second woman at (B) must certainly start the next packet without a break, but aside from that *neither* the woman at (A) nor (B) need take extra contraceptive precautions. After all, having had only a 3-day PFI the first woman is actually less likely to conceive than in a normal pill-cycle! Perhaps future pill leaflets should say something like: 'There are some situations in which your doctor may say that 7 days' condom use are not required.' Moreover, if *in these circumstances* she used condoms as instructed in Figure 4.3 and one ruptured: emergency contraception is *not* indicated.

4.23 WHAT OTHER 'RULES' FOR MISSED PILLS ARE THERE WHICH MY PATIENT MAY HAVE READ OR BEEN TAUGHT?

1   The 'take precautions to the end-of-packet rule' is probably commonest and is delightfully *simple*; but sadly (see Q 4.19) it is also 'dangerously' *wrong* for missed pills near the end of a pack!
2   The 'take precautions for the next 14 days, whatever happens' advice is acceptable; since the *second* 7 days of the fortnight does cover the time of

ovulation risk at the end of a PFI that has been lengthened by missed pills just before it (i.e. near the end of a pack). But because it is so counter-intuitive, many men as well as women see use of the unpopular sheath method as pointless just after what they (falsely!) see as a reassuring 'period'!

We however know that the ovary can be ovulating in synchrony with the endometrium bleeding, since that happens only because of exogenous hormone withdrawal. ...

4.24 IF A WOMAN HAS MISSED SEVERAL TABLETS, WHAT ARE THE INDICATIONS FOR EMERGENCY (EC) CONTRACEPTION?

Almost everything depends on *when* they were missed. The advice summarized in Figure 4.3 will be quite sufficient in every situation except *when two or more tablets have been missed from the first seven at the start of packet: in such a manner as to effectively lengthen the PFI to 9 plus days*. Then, postcoital contraception is justified (see Q 7.23), since the woman might happen to be one of the 23% described in Q 4.15.

Beware the *very* late-starter who is continuing to be sexually active. To minimize the chance of intervening (illegally) after implantation, the Faculty of Family Planning and Reproductive Health Care recommends intervention no later than day 15 of a lengthened PFI (with also consideration of copper IUD insertion in such a case).

For almost all mid-packet and late-packet (day 7–21) pill omissions postcoital treatment would be over-treatment. Exceptions: the Faculty states that it might be appropriate (just) if intercourse took place after four or more had been forgotten or vomited. ... And, rarely, one might only *see a woman after her PFI when it had been lengthened through omitted pills at the end of the last packet. She would need EC* – see Q 7.23(5) for suggested regimen.

4.25 WHAT ADVICE FOR VOMITING AND DIARRHOEA?

If the vomiting started less than 2 hours after a pill was swallowed and continues so a replacement tablet will not stay down, extra contraceptive precautions should start from the onset of the illness. They should continue for 7 days after it ends, along with elimination of the subsequent PFI as indicated above and by Figure 4.3. Warn that BTB is now likely.

Diarrhoea alone is not a problem, unless it is of cholera-like severity!

4.26 SURELY THE ABOVE DISCUSSION OF THE PFI TAKES TOO LITTLE ACCOUNT OF THE ADJUNCTIVE CONTRACEPTIVE EFFECTS (SEE Q 4.4)?

Actually, these do not change the argument about the PFI. The most important extra effect is probably the progestagenic reduction in sperm penetrability of cervical mucus. But this too will be at its lowest ebb at the end of any PFI which has been lengthened: obviously, since it is then as long as is possible since progestagen was last ingested.

Once tablet-taking is resumed, however, the pills in the next pack should be able to operate usefully by their anti-implantation effect on the endometrium.

4.27 PENDING THE MARKETING OF PACKETS WITH A SHORTENED PFI, WHAT IS THE BEST REGIMEN FOR WOMEN WHO HAVE HAD A PREVIOUS COMBINED PILL FAILURE?

Some of these may claim perfect compliance, but most will admit to the complete omission of no more than one pill. Most women admit to missing tablets from time to time (in one NOP survey the modal number missed per year was 8!), yet very few conceive. One can therefore argue that the ability to do so after missing only one tablet *selects out those who are likely to have ovaries with above average return to activity in the PFI.*

Therefore all women in this group should in my view be advised to take two or three packets in a row, the so-called bicycle or tricycle regimens (see Q 4.31 and Fig. 4.4), followed by a shortened pill-free interval. Often 6 days is a good choice in these cases since it is easy to remember, with each PFI start day now being identical to the finish-day – but the gap may be shortened even further in a 'high risk' case (see Q 4.36).

Tricycling is surely more logical than the reaction of many doctors after a woman conceives on the pill, a summary of which is 'read her the Riot Act about better pill-taking and give her the same one as before!' Even giving her a stronger formulation may be of less relevance than *eliminating plus shortening the PFIs.*

4.28 AREN'T THERE OTHER DISADVANTAGES TO TAKING A PFI?

Yes: in summary, *the 'cons' of the PFI are:*

1   Makes the COC method *less effective.*
2   The *withdrawal bleeds* can be heavy or perceived as a nuisance.

3 In some women *migraines* or other types of *headache* most often occur in the PFI, triggered by hormone withdrawal.

4 On theoretical grounds, compared with the normal cycle, it is 'unphysiological' to have a whole week with almost no oestrogen circulating (in the majority with quiescent ovaries, that is, not the one-quarter who start producing their own).

4.29 WITH ALL THOSE SNAGS, WHY DO WE CONTINUE TO RECOMMEND THE PFI TO ANYONE?

Because one can list quite a few 'pros' of the PFI as well:

1 Many women like monthly bleeds to reassure 'that all is normal', and that they are not pregnant, more frequently than every 10 weeks as in tricycling. Explaining pill physiology can overcome this objection in cases where tricycling is indicated.

2 Avoids the complaint of bloatedness which some experience through the last weeks of a tricycle.

3 May avoid the breakthrough spotting which sometimes occurs, especially with low-dose pills during the last packet of a tricycle sequence.

4 Tricycle regimens do entail taking more tablets per year: 15–16 packets rather than the 13 when a regular PFI is taken. This increase in the hormone dose taken runs counter to the general philosophy of giving the lowest dose of both hormones for the desired effect of contraception.

5 One has to remember that all data generated from epidemiological studies about the (great) safety and the (remarkable) reversibility of the COC have been gained from women who *were* taking regular monthly breaks. So it might be best to stay with that concept for most pill-takers. In confirmation of that view:

6 In one study HDL-cholesterol suppression (see Q 4.94) by the COC brand in use was restored towards normal by the end of the PFI. In a major randomised controlled trial now being analysed at MPC this phenomenon has been confirmed for other important substances, including coagulation factors. Hence the PFI may prove to have a special value for homeostasis – allowing regularly some degree of recovery from systemic effects of the pill.

4.30 WHAT DO YOU CONCLUDE, GIVEN THE ADVANTAGES OF THE PFI?

A It can be useful to point out to a woman who actually wants to continue with the method but 'someone has suggested' that she ought to 'take a break' from the pill after 10 years' use, that she has already taken 130 breaks. ... Or, put another way, she has really only taken it for $7^1/_2$ years!

B With the above list of 'pros' it would seem wise only to cut out the gap between packets when there are good indications. In the short term this can be done upon request if the woman wishes to avoid a 'period' on special occasions like honeymoons – see Q 4.179 and Figure 4.15 for the procedure if a phasic brand is in use.

There are also longer term special indications for eliminating the PFI as in Table 4.2 and Q 4.31.

TABLE 4.2 INDICATIONS FOR THE TRICYCLE REGIMEN USING A MONOPHASIC PILL OR ITS VARIANTS (Q 4.32)

1 Headaches including migraine with non-focal aura, and other bothersome symptoms occurring regularly in the withdrawal week (see Q 4.28)

2 Unacceptable heavy or painful withdrawal bleeds

3 Paradoxically, to help women who are concerned about absent withdrawal bleeds (this concern and the nuisance of pregnancy testing therefore arising less often!)

4 Premenstrual syndrome – tricycling may help if COCs used to treat PMS

5 Epilepsy: this benefits from relatively more sustained levels of the administered hormones (see also Q 4.36 for reason related to some antiepileptic treatments which are enzyme inducers).

6 Other enzyme-inducer therapy

7 Suspicion of decreased efficacy (see Q 4.27) for any other reason

8 Endometriosis – a progestogen-dominant monophasic pill may be tricycled, for maintenance treatment after primary therapy

9 At the woman's choice.

Note: In view of the possibility that the monthly pill-free interval has health benefits (see Q 4.26), one of these indications should normally apply. See also page 507 'named patient use' since the tricycle regimens are unlicensed.

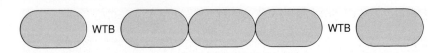

Figure 4.4 Tricycling a monophasic COC. Q 4.31 *Note*: must be monophasic packs. WTB, withdrawal bleeding.

Q 4.31 GIVEN ALL THOSE PROS AND CONS OF THE PFI, WHEN IS THE TRICYCLE PILL REGIMEN (OR ONE OF ITS VARIANTS) INDICATED?

See Figure 4.4. The regimen has nothing to do with triphasic pills. Indeed it necessitates use of *monophasic* pills – which are simply run together, three packets in a row, followed by a PFI of the selected length (either 7 days, or less if the indication is primarily to increase the method's efficacy). Three packets without a break, giving a 10-week cycle, is usually better tolerated than the four in a row which were previously advised. This will produce about five withdrawal bleeds (WTBs) or, if the indication is headaches, only five bad headaches per year – instead of the usual 13!

Bicycling may also be tried as a compromise if cycle control becomes a problem in the third packet (Q 4.32). Table 4.2 summarizes the indications.

4.32 WHAT IS THE SIGNIFICANCE OF BREAKTHROUGH BLEEDING (BTB) OR SPOTTING AFTER THE FIRST PACK DURING 'TRICYCLING'?

If it occurs during the second or third packet in a woman who had no BTB problems with 21-day pill-taking, and *if none of the explanations in Table 4.15 (see Q 4.163) applies*, then it is most likely to be an 'end-organ' effect. In other words, the current formulation is proving to be incapable of maintaining this woman's endometrium beyond a certain duration of continuous pill-taking, i.e. without the 'physiological curettage' of a WTB. Though we lack data, it is my belief that this type of BTB is less likely to be due to low blood levels of the contraceptive steroids than when BTB occurs in the other circumstances discussed at Qs 4.156–4.171.

Therefore the first step, if this is a problem to the woman, is to try 'bicycling' (two packets in a row) rather than to use a stronger pill.

DRUG INTERACTIONS AFFECTING THE COC

4.33 WHAT IS THE ENTEROHEPATIC CYCLE?

See Figure 4.5. After pill ingestion, the progestagens are 80–100%
bioavailable from the upper small bowel, but ethinyloestradiol (EE) is
subject to extensive 'first-pass' metabolism, chiefly by being conjugated
with sulphate in the gut wall. After absorption the artificial oestrogen
and progestagen are carried in the hepatic portal vein to the liver. Liver
metabolism then, or later after the steroids have been transported around
the body, creates metabolites of both steroids. The liver mostly forms
glucuronides. Once these conjugates re-enter the lumen of the bowel,

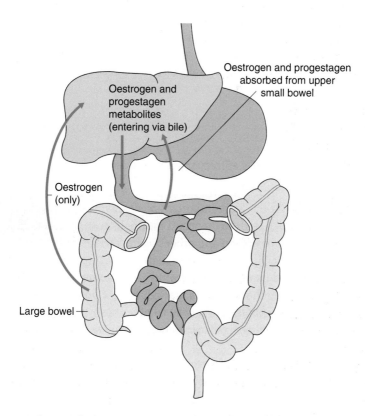

Figure 4.5 The enterohepatic circulation. Q 4.33 and following. *Note*: the progestagen does
not recirculate.

the bowel flora (chiefly *Clostridia* species) are able to remove the sulphate and glucuronide groups. This restores some EE for reabsorption and may help in some women to maintain its level in the circulation.

However in the case of all the artificial progestagens in current use, the progestagenic metabolite which is reabsorbed after the action of the bowel organisms is biologically inactive. This has the important implication that *non-enzyme-inducing antibiotics can have no effect on the efficacy of the progestagen-only pill (POP) or indeed any progestagen-only method.*

Moreover, according to the Liverpool workers, both studies in women with an ileostomy and formal studies with relevant antibiotics suggest that in the vast majority of COC-takers the recycling even of the oestrogen seems to be unimportant for maintaining efficacy. There is some detectable reduction of the AUC (Area Under the (pharmokinetic) Curve for EE) when relevant antibiotics are co-administered, but ovulation has not been shown. It is generally agreed however that, since we do not know which few individuals might be affected by any antibiotics which destroy the relevant bowel flora, it is medicolegally best to play safe as described at Q 4.35.

4.34 WHAT IS THE EFFECT ON PILL EFFICACY OF DRUG INTERACTIONS LINKED WITH THE ENTEROHEPATIC CYCLE?

These may reduce the pill's efficacy mainly in two ways, both related to the pharmacology of Figure 4.3.

1 The first and by far the more important mechanism is by *induction of liver enzymes*, which leads to increased metabolism and thus elimination in the bile of both oestrogen and progestagen. Various drugs are involved, as detailed in Table 4.3. The main ones of importance clinically are rifampicin and its relatives, griseofulvin and some anti-epileptic treatments. Among the latter note that valproate, clonazepam, clobazam and, fortunately (*except for topiramate*) all other newly marketed antiepileptics (including vigabatrin, lamotrigine) *are NOT enzyme inducers.*

2 Alternatively, disturbance by certain *antibiotics* of the gut flora which normally split oestrogen metabolites arriving in the bowel can reduce the reabsorption of reactivated oestrogen, in a very small (but unknown) minority of women. The more relevant ones – as much medicolegally as clinically, see above – are also listed in Table 4.3. Note the following:

(a) This problem does not relate to any of the drugs used to prevent or treat *malaria*, except one, *doxycycline* which has recently acquired that indication; nor (probably) to trimethoprim; nor, certainly, since they somewhat inhibit hepatic metabolism, to co-trimoxazole, sulphonamides and erythromycin (see Table 4.3).

(b) The effect only applies to *short-term antibiotic treatment*; or in long-term therapy *at the time of change to a new antibiotic*. This is because the bowel flora rapidly develop antibiotic resistance, within less than about 2 weeks.

Antibiotic-related diarrhoea is unlikely to be a problem, since any diarrhoea has to be 'cholera-like' before absorption is affected.

4.35 WHAT SHOULD BE ADVISED DURING SHORT-TERM USE OF ANY INTERACTING DRUG?

1 *Enzyme inducers.* If for example *griseofulvin* is to be used (up to say 6 weeks – if longer, see Q 4.40) in the treatment of a cutaneous fungal infection, extra contraceptive precautions are advised for the duration of the treatment. This should be followed by the '7-day rule' as Figure 4.3 above, with omission of the next PFI if the last potentially less effective pill was taken in the last 7 days of the current pack.

   Rifampicin is such a powerful enzyme inducer that even if it be *given only for 2 days* (as for instance to eliminate carriage of the meningococcus), *increased elimination by the liver must be assumed for 4 weeks thereafter*. Extra contraception with elimination of the relevant one or two PFIs should be recommended to cover that time. This advice applies also to its relative, *rifabutin*.

2 *Other antibiotics*: here is the useful fact that the large bowel flora responsible for recycling oestrogens are reconstituted with resistant organisms in about 2 weeks. In practice therefore, if the COC is commenced in a woman who has been taking a tetracycline long term (e.g. for acne), there is no need to advise extra contraceptive precautions. There is a potential – but now believed to be small – problem only in the reverse situation, when the tetracycline product is first introduced to treat a long-term pill-taker. Even then, extra precautions need to be sustained only for the first 2 weeks, but plus the usual 7 days, with elimination of the next PFI if the first 2 weeks' antibiotic use extended into the last 7 days of a pack.

TABLE 4.3 THE MORE IMPORTANT DRUG INTERACTIONS WITH ORAL CONTRACEPTIVES

Class of drug	Approved names	Main action	Clinical implications for COC use
Drug which may reduce COC efficacy			
Anticonvulsants	barbiturates (esp. phenobarbitone) phenytoin primidone carbamazepine topiramate	Induction of liver enzymes, increasing their ability to metabolize *both* COC steroids	Tricycling with shortened PFI preferred, using 50 μg oestrogen COCs, increasing to max 90 μg if BTB occurs. *Sodium valproate, vigabatrin, lamotrigine* and *clonazepam* are among anticonvulsants *without* this effect (Q 4.35)
Other drugs			
(a) Antitubercle	rifamycins (e.g. rifampicin rifabutin)	Marked induction of liver enzymes	Short term, see text. Long term, use of alternative contraception is preferred, e.g. DMPA with 8-week injection intervals (see Q 5.91)
(b) Antifungal	griseofulvin	Enzyme inducer	As for anticonvulsants
(c) Protease inhibitors	ritonavir nelfinavir and probably others	Induction of liver enzymes	Do not use COCs
(d) Miscellaneous	lansoprazole tacrolimus nevirapine modafinil	Induction of liver enzymes	As for anticonvulsants

TABLE 4.3 *(cont'd)*

Class of drug	Approved names	Main action	Clinical implications for COC use
(e) Other antibiotics	penicillins, ampicillin and relatives tetracyclines cephalosporins	Change in bowel flora, reducing enterohepatic recirculation of ethinyloestradiol (EE) only, after hydrolysis of its conjugates	Short courses – wisest to use additional contraception during illness up to 14 days, then follow 7-day rule Long-term low-dose tetracycline for acne – no apparent problem, probably because resistant organisms develop, within about 2 weeks. POP is unaffected by this type of interaction NB doxycycline now in use as anti-malarial prophylaxis
Drugs which may increase COC blood levels			
	paracetamol	Competition in bowel wall for conjugation to sulphate. Therefore, possibly more EE available for absorption	No effect on the progestagen Advise: at least 2 hours separation of the analgesic from the time of pill taking
	co-trimoxazole	Inhibits (weakly) EE metabolism in liver	None, if short course given to low-dose COC-user
	erythromycin ketoconazole	*Potent* inhibitors of EE metabolism	

4.36 GIVEN THAT NO ACTION IS REQUIRED WITH LONG-TERM USE OF 'ORDINARY' (NON-ENZYME-INDUCING) ANTIBIOTICS, WHAT SHOULD BE DONE IF LONG-TERM USE OF AN ENZYME INDUCER IS REQUIRED?

1   *Rifampicin/rifabutin.* These are such potent enzyme inducers that in some women a fivefold increase in the rate of metabolism of the COC was seen by the researchers in Liverpool. So they recommend alternative methods of contraception for long-term users of rifampicin and that the COC be avoided altogether, even in the higher dose tricycling regimen which is described below. Fortunately the main COC hormone affected is EE, so the injectable progestagen Depot medroxyprogesterone acetate (DMPA – see Q 5.82) is a good choice. Even then it is important to compensate for the enzyme induction, logically (as described in Qs 5.85 and 5.91) by shortening the injection interval. If rifampicin (or rifabutin) is the drug, 8 weeks is recommended.

2   *Other long-term enzyme-inducers – mainly anticonvulsant therapies.* Here too an alternative contraceptive option such as an intrauterine method (IUD or IUS) should first be seriously considered. DMPA may be a good choice (see Q 5.91), with a shortened injection interval, usually 10 weeks.

   However, if the combined pill is preferred it is usual to:

   • *prescribe initially a 50 µg oestrogen-containing brand*: specifically this really means Ovran, since the alternative (Norinyl-1; norethisterone-containing – Q 4.124) on the UK market contains mestranol. This is a prodrug for EE and its in vivo conversion is not more than about 75–80% efficient, meaning it effectively provides only 37.5–40 µg of EE.

   • At the MPC *we also advise that the tricycle regimen described at Q 4.31 be used*. This reduces the number of contraceptively 'risky' PFIs. It is particularly appropriate for epileptics since the frequency of attacks is often reduced by the maintenance of steady hormone levels. We recommend that the woman also shortens the PFI at the end of each tricycle to 4 days. A 'diary card' may help her in this, but the main thing is to explain that her 'period' (withdrawal bleed) will tend to continue into the start of the next pack.

4.37 WHAT IF IT SEEMS MORE APPROPRIATE TO USE A GESTODENE, DESOGESTREL, OR NORGESTIMATE-CONTAINING COC FOR A PILL-TAKER NEEDING TREATMENT LONG TERM WITH AN ENZYME-INDUCER?

In selected cases I would prescribe two sub 50 µg pills a day, e.g. one Marvelon plus one Mercilon 20 from the desogestrel 'ladder' (see Q 4.123 and Fig. 4.12). But if so the grounds must be good and record-keeping meticulous ('named patient use' see page 507), since the manufacturer will not accept product liability should a serious problem arise. The same applies if extra pills have to be taken to control BTB (Q 4.38).

4.38 WHAT MAY SIGNAL THE NEED TO CONSIDER AN IMPORTANT DRUG INTERACTION, OR THE NEED FOR A STRONGER PILL?

NB *Having excluded other causes* (see Q 4.163), BTB may be the first clue to a drug interaction in the first place, but may also be used as an indication to *consider* increasing the dose or to advise a change of method. If the user of an enzyme-inducing drug develops BTB on the COC, the first step is to give two or more tablets a day, if necessary to provide a combined oestrogen content of 80 or 90 µg (suggested maximum, and see Q 4.39), titrated against the BTB.

4.39 HOW CAN ONE EXPLAIN THIS INCREASED DOSAGE TO A WOMAN, THAT SHE IS NOT RECEIVING A 'DANGEROUSLY' STRONG PILL REGIMEN?

The risk of this policy, given that BTB is not a fully accurate measure of blood levels (Qs 4.155–163), must be carefully assessed by the prescriber: especially if the woman has any risk factor for arterial or venous disease. Thereafter it can be explained that, as described more fully at Qs 4.157–4.163, one is only attempting to give the minimum dose of both hormones to finish just above the threshold for bleeding. Reassure her that she is metaphorically 'climbing a down escalator'. In other words her increased liver metabolism means that her system is still basically receiving a low-dose regimen while she is taking a 50 µg tablet (or even two per day as may be indicated). She is exposed to more metabolites, but this is not believed to be harmful.

4.40 CAN A WOMAN GO STRAIGHT BACK TO THE NORMAL DOSE AND REGIMEN AS SOON AS THE ENZYME INDUCERS ARE STOPPED?

No: it may be 4 or more weeks before the liver's level of excretory function reverts to normal. Hence if any enzyme inducer has been used for 6 weeks or more (or *at all* in the case of rifampicin) it is therefore recommended by Professors Michael Orme and David Back of Liverpool that there is a delay of about 4 weeks before the woman returns to the standard low-dose pill regimen. This delay should be increased to 8 weeks after more prolonged use of established enzyme inducers. And logically there should then be no gap between the higher- and the low-dose packets (see Q 4.49/Table 4.4).

4.41 WHAT ARE THE IMPLICATIONS OF LONG-TERM AND POSSIBLY CHANGING ANTIBIOTIC TREATMENTS IN WOMEN SUFFERING FROM ACNE OR (FOR EXAMPLE) CYSTIC FIBROSIS?

- On long-term antibiotics and when first starting oral contraception – no problem as discussed above (see Qs 4.34–35).
- On oral contraception, when first starting antibiotics, or *at each switch to a new broad-spectrum antibiotic* – here the counsel of perfection would be to use an additional method such as the condom for the first 3 weeks to permit antibiotic resistance to develop (see Q 4.35).

In practice these precautions are frequently not observed, yet breakthrough pregnancies resulting from this mechanism seem extremely uncommon.

4.42 WHAT ABOUT ANION-EXCHANGE RESINS LIKE CHOLESTYRAMINE, OR ACTIVATED CHARCOAL, OR GUAR GUM WHICH IS SOMETIMES USED TO TREAT POSTPRANDIAL REACTIVE HYPOGLYCAEMIA? MIGHT THEY IMPAIR PILL ABSORPTION?

Any such effect appears to be minimal, but a potential problem could be eliminated by taking them at least 4 hours before or 2 hours after the pill – or indeed any other oral drug.

4.43 WHAT EFFECT DOES A HIGH INTAKE OF VITAMIN C HAVE ON PILL ABSORPTION? AND WHAT ABOUT PARACETAMOL?

- New research on the Vitamin C interaction shows no increase in circulating levels of EE and no rebound on discontinuation – refuting earlier concerns.

- Any effect of paracetamol – in competing for EE conjugation and therefore raising blood levels – is probably clinically unimportant. However in the absence of a definitive (negative) study, it is still best to advise separating pill-taking from the paracetamol by a couple of hours.

4.44 IS THE RUMOUR ABOUT AN INTERACTION OF THE PILL WITH GRAPEFRUIT JUICE FOUNDED ON FACT?

Yes, this one is: though *not* the one that it might make the pill fail, it is the other way round. Grapefruit is a rich source of flavenoids, which compete for the enzymes which metabolize EE: so increasing bioavailability (and blood levels). But even in high grapefruit consumers this is unlikely to cause any significant added prothrombotic risk from the pill. If concerned, the simple solution is to ensure grapefruit juice is always quaffed at least 2 hours after the time of pill-taking. ...

Co-trimoxazole and erythromycin inhibit liver enzymes and so also tend to increase the bioavailability of the COC.

4.45 ARE ANY OF THE INTERACTIONS IN WHICH COCs AFFECT THE METABOLISM OF OTHER DRUGS OF ANY CLINICAL SIGNIFICANCE?

Oral contraceptive (OC) steroids are themselves weak inhibitors of hepatic microsomal enzymes. So they may lower the clearance of diazepam, tricyclic antidepressants, prednisolone, cyclosporin and some other drugs – including according to some reports (but not others) alcohol. Only the enhanced toxicity of *cyclosporin* is important clinically; the others are unlikely to be noticed.

Warfarin. COCs inhibit this drug's metabolism to a variable extent, and also and independently alter clotting factors. Thus the interaction is unpredictable. The combination would need very careful monitoring. In specific individuals it is sometimes appropriate however, since the contraindication to the COC after a venous thrombosis is only absolute *after* anticoagulation ceases.

As COCs tend to impair glucose tolerance, sometimes cause depression and may raise blood pressure, they naturally tend to oppose (pharmacodynamically) the actions of antidiabetic, antidepressant and antihypertensive treatments, respectively. This type of effect is easily compensated by monitoring dose/response of the other drug.

4.46 WHAT ELSE, APART FROM TREATING MY PATIENT, SHOULD I DO IF I SUSPECT A DRUG INTERACTION OF ANY TYPE?

Practitioners who do detect possible drug interactions are asked to continue the practice of completing a yellow card for the Committee on Safety of Medicines.

4.47 SHOULD WOMEN WITH AN ILEOSTOMY OR COLOSTOMY AVOID HORMONAL CONTRACEPTION FOR FEAR OF ABSORPTION PROBLEMS, OR BE GIVEN A STRONGER BRAND THAN USUAL?

Despite the interference in the enterohepatic cycle after an *ileostomy*, the bioavailability of EE as well as the progestogens was not detectably altered in studies by the Liverpool workers. Even when most of the rest of the bowel is absent, the jejunum is highly efficient at absorbing sex steroid hormones.

Yet, because of anecdotes of unexpected conceptions in apparently compliant women with an ileostomy, I would now recommend a regimen with fewer and shorter pill-free intervals in such women (Q 4.31). But I would not advise increasing the dose solely on these grounds.

Colostomy, however, does not (and would not be expected to) have any effect on the enterohepatic circulation of oestrogen.

4.48 DOES COELIAC DISEASE IMPAIR ABSORPTION OF THE COC?

No. Paradoxically, while this disease is active, the diminished function of the gut wall leads to less conjugation of absorbed EE. So more bioactive EE is absorbed than usual! Once coeliac disease is successfully treated absorption is normal.

STARTING ROUTINES WITH THE COC

4.49 WHAT FACTORS NEED CONSIDERATION IN DEVISING STARTING ROUTINES FOR THE COC?

1 First and foremost, women with short cycles may ovulate early in the second week of the menstrual cycle. Hence the value of the Day 1 start, to ensure 7 tablets are taken in time (Q 4.16), and with no need for additional contraception from the outset (Table 4.4).
2 First-timers may usefully be warned that their first 'period' may come on after only about 23 days.

TABLE 4.4 STARTING ROUTINES FOR COMBINED ORAL CONTRACEPTIVES

		Start when?	*Extra precautions for 7 days?*
1	Menstruating	Day 1	No*
		Day 2	No†
		Day 3 or later	Yes†
2	Postpartum		
	(a) No lactation	Day 21 (low risk of thrombosis by then‡, first ovulations reported day 28+)	No
	(b) Lactation	Not normally recommended at all (POP/injectable preferred)	
3	Post-induced early abortion/miscarriage	Same day or next day to avoid postoperative vomiting risk	No
4	Post-trophoblastic tumour	1 month after no hCG detected	As 1
5	Post-higher dose COC	Instant switch§	No
6	Post-lower or same dose COC	After usual 7-day break	No
7	Post-POP	First day of period	No
8	Post-POP with secondary amenorrhoea	Any day (Sunday? see Q 4.50)	No
9	Post-DMPA (risk of pregnancy excluded)	Any day (see text, may overlap the methods)	No‖
10	Other secondary amenorrhoea (risk of pregnancy excluded, see Q 8.22)	Any day (Sunday? see Q 4.50)	YES
11	First cycle after postcoital contraception (see Q 7.39)	1st day/or no later than day 2	No

*14 days' extra precautions if Logynon ED or Femodene ED (see Q 4.7).

† Delay into day 2 may help, to be sure a period is normal. For later starts, up to the old routine day 5, I advise extra precautions for the 7 days which seemingly make any ovary quiescent (Q 4.16). The same can apply beyond day 5 (i.e. not waiting for that elusive next period), IF the prescriber is sure there has been no risk of conception up to the starting day.

‡ Puerperal thrombosis risk lasts longer after severe pregnancy-related hypertension, so delay use until biochemical normality (Q 4.49).

§ This advice is because of reports of rebound ovulation occurring at the time of transfer.

‖ unless overdue most recent injection – if so, see Q 5.133.

3 NB There are studies, especially from Israel, showing that the older routine of a Day 5 start has one advantage: less BTB and spotting in the first cycle. This is well worth considering, since the 1998 Tel Aviv study showed a higher rate of early discontinuations for bleeding in the Day 1 starting group.

If this is preferred, or with even later starts (as is perfectly acceptable if there has been no earlier sexual exposure), extra precautions for 7 days are advisable. In this country this is advised whenever the first tablet of the first pack is taken on Day 3 or later (Table 4.4).

4 After a first trimester pregnancy has ended, the earliest fertile ovulation seems to occur no earlier than about Day 10.

5 After a full-term pregnancy (in the absence of breastfeeding) the earliest possibly fertile ovulation has been shown biochemically at around day 28. However, starting too early has to be avoided because of evidence that the oestrogen in the combined pill can increase the risk of puerperal thromboembolism. The coagulation factor changes of pregnancy are largely reversed by 2 weeks. So for most a start date of Day 21 is appropriate. Starting the COC should be further delayed in those at highest risk of any form of thrombosis, including the obese and after *severe pregnancy-related hypertension* with persistent biochemical abnormalities; with alternative contraception for 7 days if the pill is therefore started beyond Day 21.

6 After injectables such as DMPA the COC can be started immediately. But of more interest is the fact that the COC can also (and often very usefully) be given *concurrently* with it: for example, on restarting after major or leg surgery which has been covered by DMPA (Q 4.195), or to control bleeding problems (Q 5.128). See Q 5.133 for relevant advice if the prospective pill-taker is already overdue her most recent injection.

These and my other recommendations for the COC are summarized in Table 4.4. See Q 5.57 for the progestagen-only pill, which is more suitable than the COC during lactation.

Contraception after pregnancy

This important subject is discussed in much more detail at Qs 8.18–8.33: including, when there is amenorrhoea, how *not* to commence use of a new medical method (IUD, injectable or pill) when an implantation has or may have already occurred (see Q 8.22).

A point to mention here is that, after excluding pregnancy during amenorrhoea, the COC may often best be started on the next Sunday (plus 7 days additional precautions); this avoids future bleeds at weekends. (see Q 4.50.)

4.50 CAN I HELP MY PATIENTS TO AVOID WTB AT WEEKENDS?

Yes, but only if you think to discuss the point! With most starting routines, depending on the weekday their first period happens to start and the length of their WTB, maybe one third of all pill-takers will bleed during part of one weekend in every four. ... This is completely unnecessary!

Starting on the first Sunday of the next period is one option. This is popular in the USA, but must be combined with extra precautions for 7 days. Otherwise, at any time during follow-up you can simply advise additional tablets (one or more as appropriate) from a spare pack to shift the finishing day to a Saturday or Sunday, thereby ensuring that the bleed will be completed during the next Monday–Friday.

MAJOR SYSTEMIC EFFECTS OF THE COC

4.51 WHICH STUDIES HAVE PROVIDED OUR PRESENT INFORMATION ABOUT THE WANTED AND UNWANTED EFFECTS OF THE COC?

There have been many case-control studies, but much of the most useful data has been generated by the cohort studies. Statements made in this book are based wherever possible on congruence of the findings of all the studies, by different investigators in different populations. Three of the most important are:

1   *The Royal College of General Practitioners' (RCGP) Study*. In brief, 23 000 married pill users were recruited from the practices of 1400 GPs and matched (only for age) with a similar number of married control women not using the COC. The GPs informed the study coordinators of all subsequent medical effects, based on every surgery attendance or hospital referral for in- or outpatient care (including for pregnancy). Ex-users have been similarly followed up.

2   In the same year, 1968, Vessey launched the *Oxford/FPA Study*, which has similarly followed a total of over 17 000 clinic attenders since that time. In this study, users of different reversible methods of contraception

act as controls for each other; 56% used oral contraceptives at the outset, compared with 25% who were diaphragm-users and 19% who were fitted with an IUD.

3 *The Nurses' Health Study*. In 1976, 121 700 female registered nurses in the USA completed a mailed questionnaire including items relevant primarily to risk of cancer and circulatory disease. Every 2 years follow-up questionnaires are sent, to update the risk factor data and to ascertain any major medical events.

The completeness of the follow-up in all the above studies is exemplary: e.g. for fatal outcomes, ascertainment in the Nurses' study runs at about 98%.

4.52 WHAT ARE THE STRENGTHS AND DEFICIENCIES OF THE MAIN COHORT STUDIES?

They have the strengths of similar prospective epidemiological studies, particularly with regard to the completeness of data collection over the years, and the possibility of assessment of non-comparability between the groups compared, and of biases. However, they share obvious weaknesses:

1 Random allocation was impossible, so pill-users are different from non-users in many important ways: in the Walnut Creek Study, for example, COC-users tended to be on average taller, more physically active, more likely to smoke or drink in moderation (though not more likely to be heavy smokers or heavy drinkers), to sunbathe more frequently, to have initiated sex earlier and to have had more partners than non-users.

2 All the studies tended to include fewer teenagers than are now normally found amongst a pill-using population, partly because the unmarried are so difficult to follow in long-term prospective studies.

3 In the UK studies, a large number of initially recruited women were lost to follow-up just because they moved house. However, checks on the characteristics of a sample of the latter have not shown them to differ in such a way as to significantly bias the results.

4 By the time the cohort studies report, they are invariably providing information about yesterday's contraceptives. Much of the above data generated by the studies relates to brands containing at least 50 µg of oestrogen and the recently marketed progestagens are under-represented.

4.53 WHAT ARE CASE-CONTROL STUDIES AND WHAT CAN WE LEARN ABOUT THE COC FROM THEM?

1   These are retrospective: Cases are recruited with a condition of interest (e.g. venous thromboembolism, VTE) and attempts are made to match the women with 'controls' (admitted to the same hospital, or from the same community) who are free of the condition but otherwise as similar as possible. The basic idea is that if the frequency of pill-use is greater in cases (relative risk more than 1) the pill may be causing the condition, if it is less (relative risk less than 1) the pill may be protective. Useful studies of this kind are quoted repeatedly in this book, many organised through WHO. Case-control studies never provide absolute rates (attributable cases per 100 000 of population) though these can be roughly calculated if the background prevalence of the condition is known.

2   These studies have a number of problems we cannot discuss in detail here. They are obligatory for very rare events like thrombosis and diseases that take many years of exposure for any causation to become apparent, like arterial wall disease or cancer. But they are notorious for the problems of *bias* and *confounding*. Epidemiologists try very hard to correct for these. But certain confounders (predisposing factors for which pill-use or use of particular brands of pill may be a *marker*, leading to an association which is coincidental *not* causative) may be unknown. In interpreting the observed association of VTE with pills containing desogestrel (DSG) and gestodene (GSD), the confounding effect of duration of use (meaning that use of older brands became associated with being a lower-risk woman through the 'attrition of susceptibles') has been a major bone of contention since that unfortunate CSM letter of October 1995.

3   Epidemiology is particularly weak when it comes to assessing odds ratios which are not much above or below unity (in the ranges 1–2 and 0.5–1). Yet for common conditions these could mean an important attributable risk or benefit.

4   Because of the low prevalence of use, we are unlikely ever to have useful epidemiological data on the side-effects of the POP.

5   It is more difficult to study beneficial than adverse relationships; the death that does not take place as a result of some protective effect is far more difficult to recognize than the one that is linked to COC use. However, good data are available for most of the benefits in Q 4.55.

4.54 CAN WE IDENTIFY THE 'BEST BUY' AMONG THE DIFFERENT PILLS, FOR BENEFITS VERSUS RISKS?

In summary, no. ... We have to say that thus far all the methods of epidemiology, even when backed by 'biological plausibility', have proved too insensitive as research tools. Preoccupation with metabolic minutiae (common among rival drug firms in the 1980s and early 1990s) can also be misleading.

But there are good data to show that we should give formulations with the lowest acceptable dose of both the oestrogen and progestagen. It is also clear that it is essential to have a range of different products for prescribers and users to exercise effective choice – in relation both to the initial prescription, and subsequently when minor side-effects occur.

ADVANTAGES AND BENEFICIAL EFFECTS

4.55 WHAT ARE THE BENEFICIAL EFFECTS OF THE COC?

These can be listed as follows:

Contraceptive

1. Highly effective – and the regular withdrawal bleeds give regular reassurance of that fact.
2. Highly convenient, especially sexually (non-intercourse-related).
3. Reversible – see Qs 4.60 and 4.61.

Non-contraceptive – mainly gynaecological

4. A reduction in the rate of most disorders of the menstrual cycle:
   (a) less heavy bleeding; therefore
   (b) less anaemia;
   (c) less dysmenorrhoea;
   (d) regular bleeding, and timing can be controlled (see Qs 4.256 and 4.257) with tricycling possible as an option (Q 4.31);
   (e) less symptoms of premenstrual tension overall (see Q 4.129), especially if tricycling is tried;
   (f) no ovulation pain, which can be severe in some cycles;
5. Less pelvic inflammatory disease (PID) (see Q 4.58).

6 Less extrauterine pregnancies – since ovulation is inhibited: and as a long-term result of 5.
7 Less benign breast disease (see Q 4.91).
8 Less functional ovarian cysts (see Q 4.59).
9 Less need for hospital treatment due to bleeding from or size of fibroids (see Q 4.91).
10 A beneficial effect on some cancers, notably carcinoma of the endometrium and epithelial cancers of the ovary (see Qs 4.73 and 4.74).

Miscellaneous

11 Less sebaceous disorders (only with selected oestrogen-dominant COCs) (see Q 4.236).
12 No acute toxicity if overdose is taken: only vomiting, and in prepubertal girls the likelihood of WTB a week or so later.
13 Protection from osteoporosis and control of climacteric symptoms in older women up to age 50 (as a valid alternative to natural oestrogen replacement therapy, in risk-factor-free women needing contraception whose ovaries are beginning to function less well – see Q 8.38). The same can apply to younger women with premature ovarian failure, or oligomenorrhoea (see Qs 4.64–4.66). But the COC has been found not to improve bone density when the comparison is with normal cycling women receiving oestrogen from their own ovaries.
14 Beneficial social effects (e.g. postponing childbirth until after tertiary education, as an option)

Other possible benefits have been identified in some studies but have yet to be fully confirmed:

15 Reduction in the rate of endometriosis (see Q 4.227).
16 Less *Trichomonas vaginitis* (see Q 4.228).
17 Less toxic-shock syndrome (TSS) (see Q 4.229).
18 Less thyroid disease (both overactive and underactive syndromes according to RCGP study).
19 Less rheumatoid arthritis. This is now looking more definite, see Q 4.235.
20 ?? Less duodenal ulcers. This apparent effect could well be a good example of confounding (Q 4.53): anxious women prone to ulcers maybe also are more influenced by the media to be afraid of COCs?

4.56 WHAT IS THOUGHT TO BE THE UNIFYING MECHANISM OF THE BENEFITS, ESPECIALLY THE GYNAECOLOGICAL BENEFITS? HOW CAN THIS BE USEFUL IN COUNSELLING PROSPECTIVE PILL-TAKERS?

The removal of the normal menstrual cycle and its replacement by a situation which more closely resembles the physiological state of pregnancy. Women who, due to frequent pregnancies and prolonged lactation, have few menstrual cycles during their reproductive lives (say 50 rather than the 450 plus which would now be typical in developed countries) are less likely to get all the symptoms and conditions listed at items 4, 7, 8, 9, 10, 15 and 19 in Q 4.55. The similarity of the protection that the COC gives against ovarian and endometrial cancers, for example, is probably because there is much less chromosome activity in the endometrium and ovaries than in cycling women. Less chromosome activity means less chance of harmful mutations during frequent epithelial cell divisions.

So taking the pill is in some ways more 'normal' than using a barrier contraceptive and having numerous menstrual cycles, since the latter are in reality 'abnormal' and tend to promote gynaecological pathology: i.e. all the conditions at items 4, 7–10 and 15 above. In a real sense: *any woman who has been on the pill for 10 years has had iatrogenic amenorrhoea for 10 years* – but of a benign pregnancy-mimicking kind since oestrogen and progestagen are still available to the relevant tissues.

Some women find this story reassuring, that in summary the pill can be truly said to tend to 'restore normality'. It reduces the dangers of too many menstrual cycles among those many who now do the 'unnatural' thing, by not having huge families! See also Q 4.129.

4.57 DOES LOWERING DOSES TO REDUCE THE *RISKS* ALSO REDUCE THE *BENEFITS* TO GYNAECOLOGICAL OR NON-GYNAE PATHOLOGY, IN COMPARISON WITH THE OLDER HIGH-DOSE FORMULATIONS?

There has to be some real doubt about this and it will take years to resolve. The protection against functional cysts (see Q 4.59) is definitely reduced by such pills, though there is certainly no proof that it no longer exists. The modern more oestrogenic pills may well also be less protective against benign breast disease, fibroids and endometriosis which are benefited by relatively more progestogen. My own (theoretical) concern is particularly about the triphasics (see Q 4.174), which imitate (albeit imperfectly) the normal cycle. This may not be such a good idea, since eliminating the normal cycle seems, as we have just seen, to be relevant to the mechanism of the gynaecological benefits.

There is usually a downside: 'no such thing as a free lunch!' But we can be sure of one good thing: *any* oral contraceptive which regularly blocks ovulation ought to retain the protective effect against ovarian cancer.

4.58 BY HOW MUCH DOES THE COC PROTECT AGAINST PID AND WHAT IS THE MECHANISM?

The protective effect against symptomatic PID is large, a 50% or more reduction in the risk of hospitalization for the disease. This is such a major cause of subfertility (see Q 6.48), that in many parts of the world this is a significant non-contraceptive benefit of the pill.

Although suggestions that the COC might facilitate transmission of HIV have been largely discounted (see Q 4.243), there is nothing to suggest *protection* against any of the sexually transmitted viruses. (Except: there are data that all sexually transmitted infections (STIs) are important in promoting the sexual transmission of HIV. Hence the COC might reduce the risk of HIV infection *indirectly* through the reduced risk of PID.)

Mechanism

It seems likely that progestagens reduce not only the sperm penetrability of cervical mucus (see Q 4.4), but also its 'germ penetrability'. Indeed the two may even be connected, in that spermatozoa can act as 'biovectors': there is some evidence that sexually transmitted organisms such as *Chlamydia* and the gonococcus may actually 'hitch a lift', using the sperm as their means of transport to the upper genital tract!

Note that silent or less severe infection which can still occlude the tubes is not uncommon in pill-takers; and *Chlamydia* carriage is actually more frequent in COC-takers than controls (not easy to interpret as controls may use more condoms). Infection and sexual transmission of organisms are probably not impeded at the level of the cervix/vagina: the effect of the progestagen is one of protection of the upper genital tract. The 'bottom line' has to be to encourage condom use *as well*!

4.59 BY HOW MUCH DOES THE COC PROTECT AGAINST FUNCTIONAL OVARIAN CYSTS, AND WHAT IS THE MECHANISM?

The reduction has been shown in practically all studies. In a Boston study, pill-users were one-fourteenth as likely to develop such cysts as non-users. Although benign, such cysts often lead to surgery.

Functional cysts are caused by abnormalities of ovulation. Most of the time the COC abolishes all kinds of ovulation (both normal and abnormal). On the other hand the POP increases the risk of cyst formation (see Q 5.35; and also Q 4.57 above regarding the lowest-dose combined pills).

REVERSIBILITY OF THE COC

4.60 ARE COCs FULLY REVERSIBLE AS JUST STATED (SEE Q 4.55)? DO THEY IMPAIR FUTURE FERTILITY?

The short answers to these questions are yes to the first and no to the second. In the Oxford/Family Planning Association (FPA) study, for example, among previously fertile women who gave up contraception, by about 30 months over 90% of the ex-pill-users had delivered: a proportion which was indistinguishable from that for ex-users of the diaphragm and IUD. There was a definite delay of 2–3 months in the mean time taken to conceive, probably due in part to the advice pill-takers are often given (see Q 4.224). But a later analysis for *nulliparous* Oxford/FPA women stopping the pill *aged 30–35* showed a more marked delay of a year or so – though only affecting about half the population – in achieving delivery, relative to ex-diaphragm users. Despite this, conception rates became almost identical after 72 months: hence no evidence of permanent infertility.

4.61 WHAT THEN IS 'POST-PILL AMENORRHOEA' (PPA)?

The term should be abolished (see Q 4.62). It is commonly used to mean secondary amenorrhoea of more than 6 months' duration following discontinuation of the COC. Most authorities now believe that the association is casual rather than causal. Of 1862 inhabitants of Uppsala County, Sweden, 3.3% reported a history of amenorrhoea of longer than 3 months. Amenorrhoea of more than 6 months' duration occurred in 1.8% of the population, most frequently in women under the age of 24. So this is quite a common condition. If a woman is predisposed but instead takes the COC for many years, any episodes that would otherwise have been recognized will be masked by the regular withdrawal bleeds induced by her contraceptive. In such a woman, the pill could easily be unfairly blamed for her 'after pill' secondary amenorrhoea when it could in fact only be revealed 'after pill'.

Moreover, studies show that the probability of PPA is not associated with formulation, nor in most studies with duration of use. Professor Jacobs of University College London has shown that the distribution of diagnoses was the same in cases of secondary amenorrhoea post-pill as in non-post-pill cases; and in the two groups the types of treatment needed, the frequency with which they were employed, and the excellent outcome in terms of cumulative conception rates were all the same. All this argues very strongly against a specific pill-induced syndrome causing secondary amenorrhoea.

4.62 WHAT ARE THE BAD EFFECTS OF CONTINUING TO USE THE TERM 'POST-PILL AMENORRHOEA' AT ALL?

1 It leads to a tendency on the part of many doctors to defer investigation of patients with amenorrhoea which develops after the pill, thereby delaying the diagnosis and treatment of potentially serious conditions. Instead, since there is no specific syndrome, after 6 months without a period *all cases of secondary amenorrhoea should be referred* for investigation and appropriate treatment – whether they are 'post-pill' or 'post-condom'!

2 A second unfortunate result of accepting PPA as a real condition is that it deters doctors from prescribing oral contraceptives to women for whom they otherwise might be suitable. A past history of secondary amenorrhoea is good example (see Q 4.66). In some conditions, as we shall see, the COC can be positively beneficial and it is still frequently being needlessly withheld.

3 Thirdly, amenorrhoeic women often develop feelings of guilt that treatment with the pill has caused their amenorrhoea and has wrecked their chances of ever having a baby. In the first place it is most unlikely that the pill had anything to do with their problem; and secondly, even if it did, modern therapy of amenorrhoea is so effective that cumulative pregnancy rates approaching 100% can be confidently expected.

4.63 HOW ARE SUCH CASES OF SECONDARY AMENORRHOEA INVESTIGATED?

The Royal College of Obstetricians and Gynaecologists (RCOG) has issued (1998) valuable evidence-based Guidelines on the management of the infertile couple, in Primary and in Secondary care.

It is important for all concerned to be clear whether or not the women currently desires a pregnancy. It is crazy but not unheard of for high technology to be used to induce ovulation in a woman who promptly requests a termination when the resulting ovum is fertilized! (see Q 8.16).

It is beyond the scope of this book to go into details of hospital investigations for secondary amenorrhoea; but three of the most helpful tests are simple and non-invasive, and may be appropriately arranged by an interested general practitioner.

1 Weight and height, from which can be calculated the Body Mass Index (BMI): namely, weight in kg/height in metres squared. This is easily derived on a pocket calculator in the surgery, or from charts, and should normally be in the range 19–26.
2 The progestagen challenge test. This is usually performed by giving medroxyprogesterone acetate (MPA) 5 mg daily for 5 days. If this is followed by a WTB it means that the woman's oestrogen status is either normal or high. Absence of the WTB means subnormal oestrogen (see below).
3 The third of this trio of valuable and uninvasive tests is an ultrasound scan of the ovaries.

Other important tests – but not to be done in cycling women – are: plasma prolactin, thyroid function, FSH and LH.

4.64 WHAT ARE THE RISKS OF PROLONGED AMENORHOEA? HOW SHOULD THE WOMEN BE SUBSEQUENTLY TREATED IF THEY DO NOT WANT A PREGNANCY?

The management depends very much on the diagnosis and particularly on oestrogen status, as well as whether the woman is actually ready yet for fertility enhancement.

Prolonged *amenorrhoea and oligomenorrhoea* (say less than four periods a year) are *not by any means always innocuous conditions*, according to

Professor Jacobs. They should always be investigated, and management then depends on the diagnosis.

1 *Polycystic ovary syndrome (PCOS).* First of all this is *not* the same as just the finding of polycystic ovaries on ultrasound scan, which is a very common finding in more than 20% of normal women, studied both on the pill and off it. So far as we know it is only clinically of importance if the ultrasound finding is linked with symptoms: irregular or absent menses with, usually, evidence of excessive androgen (acne or hirsutes). These symptoms with the scan findings do then add up to the 'syndrome'. These women, even if amenorrhoeic, have *high* levels of both oestrogen and androgens, and with the latter goes a low level of sex hormone binding globulin (SHBG). Oddly enough their problem seems to be mediated through insulin-like growth factors, linked with carbohydrate and lipid metabolism (Syndrome X), and putting on weight sets up a number of vicious metabolic circles.

   The most important therapeutic point therefore is to help a non-overweight PCOS woman to stay slim, and if her BMI is above 30 she should benefit greatly by losing weight, with more unrefined carbohydrate intake and regular exercise. If hirsutes is a problem she may require a consultant-led high-dose cyproterone acetate and oestrogen regimen, followed by Dianette (Q 4.237) for maintenance.

   If acne alone is the problem, perhaps with some irregular menstrual cycling, there is no need to refer. Dianette may be prescribed, usually followed once the symptoms are controlled by the pill – this is an indication in my view for one of the modern 20–35 µg oestrogen varieties with desogestrel or gestodene. The intention of the combined treatment is to increase SHBG, so binding androgens, and to protect the endometrium from overstimulation.

   Be very cautious however if the BMI is above 30; and all ethinyloestradiol-containing products should normally be avoided above a BMI of 39.

2 *Secondary amenorrhoea in normal or underweight women.* This is often weight-related amenorrhoea and common in track athletes. The concern here is that they have no follicular oestrogen, little extraglandular oestrogen from peripheral conversion of androgen in fat depots, and moreover they have enhanced metabolism along the pathway which

degrades oestrogens to antioestrogens. All these mechanisms lead to low oestrogen levels and a serious risk of osteoporosis. If the amenorrhoea has continued for more than 6 months, a progestagen challenge test (see Q 4.57) and an oestradiol measurement should be arranged, with ideally also a bone scan if it is low (less than 100 pmol/l).

These women are theoretically also at risk of heart disease, like women with a premature menopause, if the hypoestrogenic state were to continue for a very long time. They should certainly stop smoking which also lowers plasma oestrogen, and be encouraged to put on weight. They are usually very opposed to taking hormones. But they might be better off healthwise on an oestrogen dominant and 'lipid friendly pill' (or opposed natural HRT oestrogens if preferred) than using barrier contraception alone.

3 *Hyperprolactinaemia.* This requires specialist treatment, e.g. with bromocriptine. Hypo-oestrogenism is not a problem in treated cases, if they are cycling and have normal libido. The COC is usable though relatively contraindicated, and the advice of the specialist in charge should be sought.

4 *Amenorrhoea but with normal oestrogenization* (positive progestagen challenge, ovaries show no ovulation but evidence of follicular activity). Here there is the contraceptive problem that at any time the woman might ovulate. There are no special grounds for using the COC, but neither is it contraindicated. The condom or cap or even just Delfen foam (Q 3.64) would be fine, if acceptable, until the first spontaneous period occurs. Since this suggests the return of ovulation, the woman would then be advised to consider transfering to a more effective method – not excluding the COC as an option.

4.65 IN SUMMARY, WHAT IS THE PLACE OF THE COC FOR WOMEN WITH AMENORRHOEA?

It is positively beneficial to use the COC in a number of these cases. Its oestrogen content helps where the oestrogen status is low, especially to prevent long-term problems such as heart disease and osteoporosis. And the progestagen content of the COC can also be of value in PCOS women with oestrogen excess and no endogenous progesterone, to protect their uterus from carcinoma of the endometrium.

4.66 WHAT ADVICE SHOULD BE GIVEN TO A HEALTHY WOMAN WHO GIVES A PAST HISTORY OF SECONDARY AMENORRHOEA BUT IS CURRENTLY SEEING NORMAL PERIODS?

All the evidence suggests that there is no reason to refuse the COC to such women, although they must understand that with or without the pill they might at some future time have difficulty in conceiving. Future fertility can never be proved in advance of becoming pregnant. Another important point is to *investigate* such a woman first if her current menses are in fact still erratic, for example, if she is experiencing *less than four periods per year*. She might well have the polycystic ovary syndrome (see above).

4.67 IN ORDER TO PRESERVE FUTURE FERTILITY, SHOULD PILL-USERS TAKE REGULAR BREAKS OF SAY 6 MONTHS, EVERY 2 OR EVERY 5 YEARS?

The answer here is an unusually confident no. This follows from Q 4.60: the pill is a reversible means of birth control, whose reversibility is not dependent on duration of use. Too often breaks demonstrate very well to the woman that her fertility is unimpaired – by an unplanned pregnancy! See also Qs 4.29, 4.30 and 4.247 which add a health (rather than fertility-related) perspective to this same issue, of duration of use/taking breaks.

4.68 CONTRARY TO THE COMMON MYTH ABOUT ITS REVERSIBILITY, DOESN'T THE COC IN FACT MUCH REDUCE THE LIKELIHOOD OF INFERTILITY?

Yes. See Q 4.55. Many of the benefits of the pill relate to conditions which can readily impair fertility and childbearing, specifically:

1 less *pelvic infection*;
2 fewer *ectopics*;
3 less *endometriosis*;
4 less growth of *fibroids*, a cause of miscarriage;
5 less functional *ovarian cysts*, a cause of unnecessary surgery;
6 less surgery altogether, for all the conditions listed here, a frequent cause of *pelvic adhesions* and consequent infertility;

7 less unwanted *pregnancies*: which can lead in various ways to secondary infertility (e.g. by infected abortions of all kinds, or by puerperal infection).

For the same reasons there is no logic in pill-takers being specially earmarked for a regular annual bimanual examination (see Q 4.182).

MAIN DISADVANTAGES AND PROBLEMS

4.69 WHAT ARE THE MAJOR ESTABLISHED UNWANTED EFFECTS OF COCS?

These are summarized here before more detailed consideration. They are under four main headings:

CIRCULATORY DISEASES (See QS 4.92–4.113)

LIVER DISEASE
1 liver adenoma (see Q 4.91), or carcinoma (see Q 4.90);
2 cholestatic jaundice (see Q 4.211);
3 gallstones (see Q 4.213).

ADVERSE EFFECTS ON SOME CANCERS (See Qs 4.70–4.90)

UNWANTED SOCIAL EFFECTS
These are hotly debated. Discussion ranges over whether removal of the fear of pregnancy has in some societies tended to promote intercourse with multiple partners with its consequences on marital and emotional stability, STIs etc., etc. – or whether other simultaneous changes such as the decline in religious belief have been more important factors.

> **NOTE:** There are many other possible adverse effects which are important and relevant but either less well established or less serious. They are considered below, either under 'Indications and Contraindications' or in the sections on 'Dealing with other side-effects and events'. See also Qs 4.155 and 4.156.

THE COC AND NEOPLASIA
(BENIGN AND MALIGNANT)

4.70 DOES THE COC INFLUENCE THE RATES OF BENIGN AND MALIGNANT NEOPLASMS?

It should not be surprising that artificial hormones can influence neoplasia; but recent research has confirmed the expectation that the effect of hormones would not be all in one direction. Some benign neoplastic conditions are benefited by OC use (e.g. benign breast disease), some are promoted (e.g. liver adenomas). Similarly two cancers are now clearly shown to be less frequent in pill-users (carcinoma of the ovary and endometrium); whereas the COC may possibly act as a co-carcinogen in the case of two other common cancers (cervix and breast). The literature is complex and this story is still a long way from being fully told.

4.71 WHY HAS IT TAKEN SO LONG TO BEGIN TO SHOW ASSOCIATIONS BETWEEN THE PILL AND NEOPLASIA?

1 The main reason is summarized in the word *latency*. There can be up to 30 years between first exposure to an agent and its manifestation in the incidence of tumours. Even the largest prospective studies tend to have too few numbers and take too long to give an answer. Hence data have been obtained mainly from case-control studies, which are notoriously subject to bias. Other problems relate to the following:

2 The specificity of any co-carcinogen to the species, to the tissue and to tumour histology.

3 Time of life is relevant – in animal models chemicals can have contrary actions, promoting or inhibiting tumours according to when in the life of the individual exposure takes place.

4 Formulation: not only differing ratios of progestagen to oestrogen, but also different progestagenic chemicals, are used around the world. It is particularly unfortunate that most studies cannot disentangle the effects of specific formulations (apart from generally showing that low oestrogen pills usually have a lesser effect).

4.72 WHAT IS THE BENEFIT/RISK BALANCE SHEET FOR NEOPLASIA AND THE PILL, SO FAR AS IS CURRENTLY KNOWN?

See Figure 4.6. The situation can best be explained to a patient in terms of 'swings and roundabouts'. Some cancers are definitely less frequent in

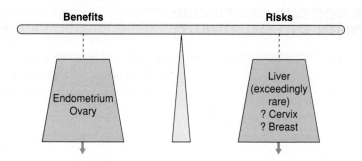

Figure 4.6 Cancer and the pill. Q 4.72 *Note*: there is much more uncertainty about the adverse than the beneficial effects.

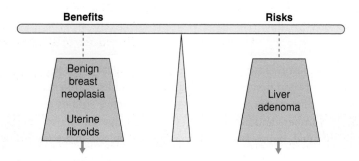

Figure 4.7 Benign neoplasia and the pill. Q 4.91

pill-users (endometrium and ovary). Others may be more frequent (but in none of those shown is a causative link proven beyond doubt). For all remaining common malignancies (e.g. of the respiratory, gastrointestinal or renal tracts), there seems no association, or certainly no adverse association, at all. A similar balance sheet can be struck for benign neoplasia (see Fig. 4.7).

The 'bottom line' in counselling is:

Populations using the pill may develop different benign or malignant neoplasms from non-users, but computer models using the best currently accepted data and assumptions do not so far indicate that the overall risk of tumours is increased. (There is no proof of an overall reduction of risk either.) Now let us consider some of the details.

4.73 WHAT IS THE INFLUENCE OF COCs ON CARCINOMA OF THE OVARY?

Good news! Many studies have yielded results pointing in the same direction, namely that epithelial ovarian tumours are less frequent in COC-users. Overall the risk is reduced by about half. There is increasing protection with increased duration of use amounting to a two-thirds reduction after more than 5 years, and the largest study shows that the protective effect lasts for at least 15 years after pill-taking ceases. This is good news indeed as ovarian cancer carries a high mortality.

4.74 WHAT IS THE INFLUENCE OF COC USE ON CARCINOMA OF THE ENDOMETRIUM?

More good news, the risk of this cancer in ever-users is again reduced by about 50%. Four studies show increasing protection with increasing duration of use and three studies show some degree of persistence of the effect after stopping the method, lasting according to one of them for at least 15 years.

The similarity of the beneficial effects of the COC on these two cancers is striking, but not surprising (see Q 4.56).

4.75 WHAT IS THE INFLUENCE OF THE COC ON TROPHOBLASTIC DISEASE (HYDATIDIFORM MOLE)?

There is no evidence that the incidence of any form of this tumour of pregnancy is increased by past pill-use.

However, workers at Charing Cross Hospital in London have shown that usage of the combined pill after this diagnosis and before human chorionic gonadotrophin (hCG) has reached undetectable blood levels, doubles the likelihood that the patient will require chemotherapy for incipient choricarcinoma. Other researchers, notably from America, have failed to show this association: but their chemotherapy policy is far more aggressive.

The London team remains convinced of a causative link. Since it is not clear if the effect is due more to the progestagen than the oestrogen, they therefore continue to recommend that *all* hormonal methods are avoided (WHO 3, see Q 4.130) until the hCG levels are undetectable, in urine at first, then confirmed in the blood (then WHO (1)). IUDs are WHO 3 while hCG levels are high (a scan should first exclude invasive cancer involving the uterine wall). Fortunately, in the vast majority of cases the hCG levels do become undetectable within 2 months of evacuation of the mole. The prohibition against hormonal methods, which is only precautionary (and in the USA only a relative contraindication), is therefore usually short-lived and *not* as long as until the next conception – which may be planned for 6 months after no hCG is detectable. Re emergency contraception, see Q 7.29.

4.76 WHAT IS THE INFLUENCE OF THE COC ON CARCINOMA OF THE CERVIX?

Evidence exists of a modest increased risk of both squamous cell and the much rarer adenocarcinoma of the cervix. Studies on cervical cancer are complicated by confounding with the sexual variables: i.e. by the problem of getting accurate information about different patterns of sexual activity, both for women and their partners. The prime carcinogen is clearly sexually transmitted, probably a virus or combination of viruses (specific strains of the human papillomavirus being likely candidates). Co-factor(s) are important: for that role, cigarette smoking currently stands most accused.

Most studies, in different populations, do show an association between incidence of and (in the RCGP study) mortality from this cancer, plus its premalignant forms, and use of the COC. But is the association causative or casual? The Oxford/FPA cohort study seems at first to support the former view by demonstrating an effect of duration of pill-use among nearly 7000 parous women. No effect of duration of IUD-use was found among over 3000 users of that method with whom they were compared. The incidence of all forms of cervical neoplasia combined rose from 0.9/1000 woman-years in those with up to 2 years' pill-use to 2.2/1000 woman-years after 8 years. In the first report of this study all 13 cases of invasive cancer occurred in women in the oral contraceptive group. The frequency of taking cervical smears for cytology was similar but it was not possible to control for exposure to the sexually transmitted carcinogen – there was no information about the number of sexual partners of the woman, leave alone those of her man. ...

4.77 WHAT IS YOUR OVERALL ASSESSMENT OF THE ASSOCIATION WITH NEOPLASIA OF THE CERVIX?

It remains possible that the link with the COC is entirely caused by confounding, with sexual activity. But it may well also be a weak co-factor, certainly weaker than cigarette smoking: possibly, according to more than one study, speeding transition through the preinvasive stages.

The COC is not the true carcinogen for this cancer. Its influence is clearly many times less than the influence of sexual lifestyle. Users should have regular cervical smears. Three-yearly is still considered adequate to enable preventive action before invasive cancer develops (see also Q 4.78), unless there are other risk factors. (If resources were to permit, the first wider category to be offered more frequent smears should be all smokers, ahead of pill-takers except those who also smoke.)

4.78 SHOULD WOMEN DISCONTINUE COC USE ONCE AN ABNORMAL CERVICAL SMEAR HAS BEEN DETECTED?

It is currently entirely acceptable to continue COC use during the monitoring of a mildly abnormal cervical smear, during definitive treatment of cervical intraepithelial neoplasia (CIN), and subsequently. These are very weak, relative contraindications (WHO 1–2, see Q 4.130): though the recurrence risk for the problem would of course be minimized if the couple were prepared to use a barrier method instead or as well (see Qs 2.26 and 3.17).

4.79 WHAT IS THE ASSOCIATION BETWEEN BREAST CANCER AND COC USE?

The incidence of this disease is high and therefore it must inevitably be expected to develop in women whether they take COCs or not. Since the recognized risk factors include early menarche and late age of first birth, use by young women was rightly bound to receive scientific scrutiny. However if there is a real causative link with pill-use, use by older women will obviously lead to more attributable cases since the incidence rises steeply with age above 35 years, as shown in Figure 4.8.

The literature to date is copious, complex, confusing and contradictory! Research is complicated by the problems related to: *latency, changes in formulation, time of exposure, and high-risk groups.*

4.80 WHAT LIGHT IS SHED BY THE 1996 PAPER BY THE COLLABORATIVE GROUP ON HORMONAL FACTORS IN BREAST CANCER? (CGHFBC)

They have shed much light, indeed the new model they propose is the one now most widely accepted. They succeeded in re-analysing original data which relates to over 53 000 women with breast cancer and over 100 000

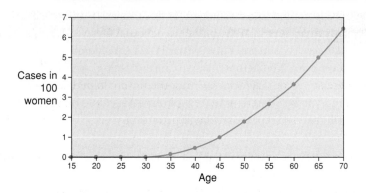

Figure 4.8 Background risk: cumulative number of breast cancers per 100 women, by age.

controls from 54 studies in 25 countries. This is 90% of the world epidemiological data. It has changed the 'model' described in earlier editions of this book, in which the pill-associated increased risk was for breast cancer occurring at a young age, and that it might or might not diminish or disappear at older ages.

This new model does show disappearance of the risk in ex-users, but now recency of use of the COC is the most important factor: with the odds ratio unaffected by age of initiation or discontinuation, use before or after first *full term* pregnancy, or duration of use. The main findings are summarised in Table 4.5 and below.

TABLE 4.5   THE INCREASED RISK OF DEVELOPING BREAST CANCER WHILE TAKING THE PILL AND IN THE 10 YEARS AFTER STOPPING

User status	Increased risk
Current user	24%
1–4 years after stopping	16 %
5–9 years after stopping	7 %
10 plus years an ex-user	No significant excess

(Collaborative Group on Hormonal factors in Breast Cancer, 1996)

4.81 SO WHAT IS THE GOOD NEWS IN THE NEW MODEL OF BREAST CANCER AND THE COC?

Combined oral contraceptive (COC) pill users can be reassured that:

- while the small increase in breast cancer risk for women on the pill noted in previous studies is confirmed, the odds ratio of 1.24 signifies an increase of 24% only while women are taking the COC and for a few years thereafter, diminishing to zero after 10 years;
- beyond 10 years after stopping there is no detectable increase in breast cancer risk for former pill users;
- the cancers diagnosed in women *who use or have ever used* COCs are *clinically less advanced* than those who have never used the pill; and are less likely to have spread beyond the breast;
- this re-analysis shows that these risks are not associated with duration of use, the dose or type of hormone in the COC, and there is no synergism with other risk factors for breast cancer (e.g. family history – see below);
- the risks for progestagen only contraceptives (POP and injectables) failed to reach statistical significance. (However this does not exclude a real effect, which in that case would be very similar for those methods to the model for the COC.)

4.82 WHAT IS THE NOT-SO-GOOD NEWS?

Mainly, this affects use by those with pre-existing risk factors and older women, who are now permitted to use the COC to age 50 if they choose to do so, provided they are fully healthy non-smokers (Q 4.250). If the background risk for the individual is larger, whether because of increased age or a family history, the applicable percentage increase in Table 4.5 necessarily means more attributable cases (than in younger women without any breast cancer risk factor).

As Figure 4.8 shows, irrespective of the use of hormonal contraception the cumulative risk of breast cancer in young women is very small, being 1 in 500 in women up to age 35. But the cumulative risk increases with age thereafter, to 1 in 100 at age 45 and 1 in 12 by age 75. The increase in attributable cases as age of last use increases has been calculated, and is shown in Table 4.6. Most importantly, for a given age at last use the excess risk is little affected by a women's prior duration of oral contraceptive use. Everything seems to depend on **recency** of use (i.e. current or within 10 years) at the given age.

TABLE 4.6 CUMULATIVE RISK OF BREAST CANCER BY RECENCY OF USE.
Showing usage in different age groups, the cumulative numbers of breast cancer cases per 10 000 women in never-users of oral contraception and the cumulative number per 10 000 women who had use oral contraception for 5 years and who were followed up for 10 years after stopping

Pill use for 5 years or any duration*	To age 20	To age 25	To age 30	To age 35	To age 40	To age 45
Breast Cancers diagnosed by:	Age 30	Age 35	Age 40	Age 45	Age 50	Age 55
Never-users:	4	16	44	100	160	230
Users who stopped 10 years earlier	4.5	17.5	49	110	180	260
Excess number of cases of breast cancer per 10 000 women	0.5	1.5	5	10	20	30

*Since the researchers state that for a given age at last use the excess risk is little affected by a women's prior duration of oral contraceptive use.

4.83 MIGHT THESE FINDINGS BE EXPLAINED BY SURVEILLANCE BIAS?

The collaborative group do concede that their findings, of less advanced cases being identified in ever-takers of the pill but more of them being found at each given age, could actually be explained wholly or in part by surveillance bias (through pill-takers both during *and after* the years of use of the method perhaps being more 'breast aware' than non-takers).

However the consensus interpretation which I personally accept for the present is that the pill is a weak co-factor acting after some other initiating factor(s) for this cancer; but that for some reason (as has also been found with HRT) the resulting tumours are less aggressive.

4.84 SO WHAT ARE THE CLINICAL IMPLICATIONS FOR ROUTINE PILL-COUNSELLING

The Faculty of Family Planning in the UK has concluded that pill-users should be informed of/counselled about the new data summarized in

Tables 4.5 and 4.6 but reiterates the advice given by the UK Committee on Safety of Medicines that there need be no fundamental change in prescribing practice.

- The breast cancer issue should now normally be addressed, in a sensitive way, as part of routine pill counselling for all women. This discussion should be initiated opportunely, and not necessarily at the first visit if not raised by the woman; along with encouragement to report promptly any unusual changes in their breasts at any time in the future ('breast awareness'). (There is no evidence that either professionally taught self-examination or periodic clinical examination reduce mortality from breast cancer).
- The balancing protective effects against at least two malignancies (ovary and endometrium), see above should also be mentioned.
- *The known contraceptive and non-contraceptive benefits of COCs may seem so great to many (but not to all), as to compensate for almost any likely lifetime excess risk of breast cancer.*

4.85 HOW DO YOU EXPLAIN THE COMPLEXITIES OF TABLE 4.6 TO A PILL-TAKER?

- I use the fourth column of Table 4.6, dividing the numbers by 10, and ask her to visualize two concert halls each holding 1000 women. Imagine that the first is filled with 1000 pill-takers, all now aged 45, but all having used the COC for varying durations of time then stopping when they reached age 35 (a common situation). The (cumulative) number of cases of breast cancer would be 11 in Concert Hall 1. However, in Hall 2 which is filled with never-takers of the pill also all currently aged 45 there would be 10 cases; i.e. there is only one extra pill-attributable case/1000 in Hall 1. See Figure 4.9.
- Moreover if the pill is acting only as a co-factor (see above) it is very possible that she was a woman who would have developed the disease without the pill at a later age anyway.
- And the remaining 989 women in Hall 1 will from this time on have only the same risk of breast cancer as the women of Hall 2, i.e. *no ongoing added risk because it is over 10 years since their last pill.* This is a very important point to explain, with the overall risk rising so much with age.
- Finally, the cancers diagnosed among the pill-takers in Hall 1, already and in future, will tend to be less advanced than those in Hall 2.

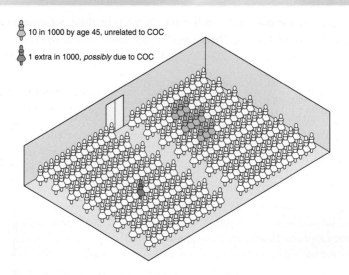

10 in 1000 by age 45, unrelated to COC

1 extra in 1000, *possibly* due to COC

Figure 4.9 Cumulative incidence of breast cancer during, plus after, use of COC until age 35. From: Guillebaud J (1998) *Contraception Today* (3rd ed) p. 10, London: Martin Dunitz. With permission.

4.86 WHAT ABOUT PILL-USE BY AN OLDER WOMAN?

As Table 4.6 shows, without a change in relative risk there is an increased attributable risk with age. For example, there are 30 extra cases per 10 000 for ex-users now aged 55 who stopped the COC 10 years before, rather than the 10 extra cases of column 4 (which was the basis for Figure 4.9). This must be explained and may be acceptable to many with the balancing from the established protection against cancer of the ovary and endometrium. But to my mind these new data will increasingly lead to more older women choosing from other options which are now available (especially IUDs and the IUS).

4.87 WHAT ABOUT COC USE IN HIGH-RISK GROUPS FOR BREAST CANCER, SPECIFICALLY (A) THOSE WITH A *FAMILY HISTORY* OF A YOUNG (UNDER 40) FIRST-DEGREE RELATIVE WITH BREAST CANCER? AND (B) WOMEN WITH BENIGN BREAST DISEASE (BBD)?

Here we see the effect of having a larger background risk than the generality of women: rather as just discussed for older women. The 24% increment is not greater, but when applied to a bigger background risk will obviously mean more attributable cases. Therefore both these are *relative contraindications* (Q 4.133). However, if a past breast biopsy showed epithelial atypia this in my view is WHO 4 (Q 4.130) or maybe WHO 3, after discussion with an oncologist.

Different women will react differently to the same information, given as it should always be in a balanced way. Some will ask for a method where no possible increase in breast cancer risk has been suggested, above that she has to live with. If however the woman chooses the COC as she is entitled to do, given its benefits, it should be a low oestrogen formulation for a limited duration, with specific counselling and reassessed every 5 years or so.

4.88 WHAT IS THE PROGNOSIS IF A WOMAN DEVELOPS BREAST CANCER WHILE ON THE COC? SHOULD WOMEN WITH THIS HISTORY EVER USE HORMONAL METHODS IN FUTURE?

The prognosis is better than for a condom-user (see above). Nevertheless most authorities advise that the pill should be discontinued, and women with a history of this cancer should normally avoid *combined* OCs thereafter. Progestagen-only methods are acceptable during remission, following discussion with the oncologist and with continued surveillance.

4.89 HAS THE LAST WORD BEEN SPOKEN ON THIS ISSUE?

No way! Research continues. There remain doubts, especially about the cohort of women who started the COC as teenagers (before first full-term pregnancy) and have not yet reached the age of maximum incidence of breast cancer in large numbers. But the available data on this long latency, a concern often highlighted by Professor McPherson of London, is reassuring: thus far. ...

4.90 WHAT IS THE INFLUENCE OF THE COC ON OTHER CANCERS?

1 *Primary hepatocellular carcinoma.* Case reports and three case-control studies have suggested that COC-use may promote this rare cancer. The annual attributable risk is estimated as less than 4 per million users. The pill association is not established in hepatitis B-infected livers, fortunately, since that is the main risk factor. Once again smoking 'rears its ugly head': increasing the relative risk of this cancer by a factor of 4 even without the COC. A past history of liver tumours (benign as well as malignant) absolutely contraindicates the COC thereafter.

151

2 *Malignant melanoma of the skin.* An increased risk, particularly of the superficial spreading type of this cancer, was suggested among COC-users. Most other studies show no link. It is becoming increasingly probable that the association is not causal, related to the pill itself, but to the confounding variable of exposure to ultraviolet light.

Women in long-term remission after melanoma, and also after apparent cure following conservative treatment for cancer of the ovary and cervix may use COCs – provided their oncologist agrees.

3 No association has been shown with malignancy involving any other organ or tissue.

4.91 WHAT IS THE INFLUENCE OF THE COC ON BENIGN NEOPLASMS?

See Figure 4.7, page 142.

1 *Benign breast disease (BBD).* A definite protective effect has been shown which increases with duration of use and is probably attributable to the progestagen component of the pill. The protection in some studies seems to be restricted to the commonest but less serious forms of the disease without epithelial atypia, the latter being considered the premalignant variety (see Q 4.87). This may explain the paradox that COCs protect against BBD developing in the first place but have no demonstrable protective effect against breast cancer.

2 *Hepatocellular adenoma.* This tumour occurs about 10 times more frequently in users of modern <50 µg COCs than in other women, but the background prevalence is so low that the incidence among COC-users is still tiny (around 1/100 000 users per year). The risk is greatest in older women using relatively high-dose pills for a long period of time (see Q 4.215).

Focal nodular hyperplasia (FNH) of the liver has also been linked, and may regress with COC – withdrawal. See Q 4.131 for prescribing implications.

3 *Other benign tumours showing no association.* These include benign trophoblastic disease (but see Q 4.75) and prolactinoma of the pituitary gland. For some years it was widely held that COC-use increased the risk of the latter, but two good case-control studies have provided strong evidence against the association.

4 *Fibroids.* While older high oestrogen OCs were believed to cause fibroids to increase in size, current more progestagen-dominant brands have been shown to reduce the risk of hospital referral for fibroids.

THE COC AND CIRCULATORY DISEASES

4.92 WHICH CIRCULATORY DISEASES HAVE BEEN SHOWN TO BE COMMONER IN COC-USERS?

To expand from Q 4.69:

1 *Systemic hypertension* – this is not really a disease in its own right: it predisposes to and does its damage through the arterial circulatory diseases below.
2 *Venous disease*:
   (a) deep venous thrombosis;
   (b) pulmonary embolism;
   (c) rarely thrombosis in important single veins, e.g. mesenteric, hepatic or retinal.
3 *Arterial diseases.* These include:
   (a) myocardial infarction;
   (b) thrombotic strokes;
   (c) haemorrhagic strokes;
   (d) other arterial events affecting solitary but vital vessels, such as mesenteric or retinal arteries.

4.93 CAN ANY OF THESE RISKS BE EXPLAINED BY KNOWN METABOLIC CHANGES INDUCED BY THE ARTIFICIAL HORMONES OF THE COC? IN PARTICULAR, WHAT IS THE INFLUENCE OF THE OESTROGEN CONTENT?

Over the years, biochemistry has been of only very limited help. Very many studies have been done but the true meaning of many of the findings has been difficult to interpret – particularly those thought to relate to arterial disease (Q 4.94). See Table 4.7.

1 Oestrogen induces alterations in clotting factor levels which may be thrombogenic. More important changes include reduced levels of antithrombin III, but increased levels of fibrinogen and several of the vitamin K-dependant coagulation factors. These changes help to explain the increased risk of *venous* thrombosis, particularly if the woman already has a congenital or acquired predisposition such as Factor V Leiden (see Q 4.108).

   However, it is likely that if there is already significant arterial wall disease, oestrogen may also promote superimposed arterial thrombosis.

There is evidence of a compensatory increased fibrinolytic activity, also an oestrogen effect.

> **NOTE:** This protective fibrinolysis is impaired by heavy smoking.

This may in part explain the rarity of overt disease, especially arterial disease, in non-smoking pill-users.

2 Hepatic secretion of many different proteins is stimulated by oestrogens. These proteins are involved in: the transport of hormones, vitamins and minerals, the control of blood pressure and immunological processes. When oestrogen is given the stimulatory effect can sometimes be suppressed by concomitant administration of a progestagen. But the interactions are complex: there may also be synergism or independence of the effects, and differences between progestagens. See Table 4.7.

3 Finally, synthetic oestrogens have been shown to raise arterial blood pressure both in short-term challenge experiments and in longer-term studies.

4.94 WHAT IS THE INFLUENCE OF THE PROGESTAGEN CONTENT ON METABOLISM AND RISK?

1 The risk of venous thromboembolism may be modified in some way as yet unexplained (see Qs 4.102–4.107), though the epidemiology suggesting this remains contentious!

2 Provided oestrogen is also given, increasing the dose of progestagen leads to an increased rate of diagnosis of clinical hypertension. (On the other hand when given without oestrogen, as in the POP or DMPA, progestagens have no important adverse effect on blood pressure.)

3 When oestrogen was kept constant, the incidence of arterial diseases, both as a group and individually, was correlated with the progestagen dose in some early epidemiological studies. This has only been shown for norethisterone-levonorgestrel group progestagens, often unhelpfully referred to as the 'second generation'.

4 Many studies including an RCT at my Centre have shown that if a constant dose of oestrogen is given the potential oestrogen-induced HDL-cholesterol increase is reversed by LNG- and NET-containing pills, whereas it is permitted by DSG or GSD if present (see Q 4.106). Prior to

TABLE 4.7 SOME METABOLIC EFFECTS OF COMBINED ORAL CONTRACEPTIVES

	Blood level	Remarks
Liver		
Liver functioning	Altered	These many changes cause no
(a) generally	in all users	apparent long-term damage to the
(b) specifically		liver itself. The liver is involved,
Albumen	↓	however, in the production of most
Transaminases	↑	of the changes in blood levels of
Amino acids	Altered	substances shown elsewhere in
Homocysteine	↑	this table, including the important
		changes in carbohydrate and lipid
		metabolism, and coagulation factors
Blood glucose after		These changes, barely detectable
carbohydrate ingestion	↑	with the latest pills, may partly
Blood lipids	Altered, mostly↑	explain the increased risk of
HDL-cholesterol – in low		arterial disease with earlier
oestrogen/progestogen-		preparations
dominant COCs	↓	
Clotting factors		
(a) generally	Mostly ↑	Both the pill and smoking affect
(b) specifically		these interrelated systems.
Antithrombin III		Fibrinolysis is enhanced by COC
(anti-clotting factor)	↓	in the blood, but reduced in the
Fibrinolysis	↑	vessel walls
Tendency for platelet	↑	
aggregation		
Hormones		
Insulin	↑	These hormone changes are
Growth hormone	↑	related to those affecting blood
Adrenal steroids	↑	sugar and blood lipids (above)
Thyroid hormones	↑	
Prolactin	↑	
LH	↓	These effects are integral to
FSH	↓	contraceptive actions. However, the
Endogenous oestrogen	↓	first three tend to rise in some
Endogenous progesterone	↓	women during the pill-free week.
		Hence any effective lengthening of
		the pill-free time may lead to an
		LH surge and ovulation

Table 4.7 continued

TABLE 4.7 *(cont'd)*

	Blood level	Remarks
Minerals and vitamins		
Iron	↑	This is a good effect for women prone to iron deficiency
Copper	↑	
Zinc	↓	Effects unknown, but not believed
Vitamins A, K	↑	to cause any health risk for most
Riboflavin, folic acid	↓	pill-users. Pyridoxine is discussed
Vitamin B_6 (pyridoxine)	↓	at Q 4.199
Vitamin B_{12} (cyanocobalamin)	↓	
Vitamin C (ascorbic acid)	↓	
Binding globulins (including SHBG)	↑	These globulins carry hormones and minerals in the blood. Because their levels increase in parallel with the latter, the effective blood levels of the hormones or minerals are usually not much altered
Blood viscosity	↑	
Body water	↑	This retention of fluid explains some of the weight gain blamed on the pill
Factors affecting blood pressure	Altered	
Renin substrate		Charges do not correlate as well
Renin activity		as expected with the incidence of
Angiotensin II	↑	frank hypertension
Cardiac output		
Immunity/allergy		
Number of leucocytes	↑	See Qs 4.242–4.244
Immunogobulins	Altered	
Function of lymphocytes	Altered	

Notes:

1 In the table ↑ means the level usually goes up, ↓ down.

2 'Altered' means that the changes are known to be more complex, with both increases and decreases occurring within the system.

3 The changes are generally (a) within the normal range, (b) similar to those of normal pregnancy.

4 These effects are obviously highly relevant to the interpretation of many laboratory tests. See Q 4.254.

the CSM's letter of October 1995 and the subsequent 'pill-scare', it was widely thought and promoted by the relevant manufacturers that lack of reduction of HDL-cholesterol would be beneficial (to the arterial walls). This view is now less confidently held – for women without risk factors, anyway – since there is increasing evidence that no formulation of COC is atherogenic (or in particular promotes heart attacks) unless there is an arterial risk factor such as smoking.

5 *When arterial risk factors are present*, however, it remains a tenable hypothesis that these apparently 'lipid-friendly' products *may* reduce arterial disease risk, relative to other products. See below Q 4.111.

4.95 GIVEN THE IMPORTANCE OF BLOOD PRESSURE IN ARTERIAL DISEASE, WHAT EFFECTS DOES THE COC HAVE?

In the majority of combined pill-users there is a slight, measurable increase in both systolic and diastolic blood pressure, within the normotensive range. Early large studies showed a 1.5–3 times higher relative risk of clinical hypertension. Modern varieties with reduced biological impact of the oestrogen and progestagen (both are relevant since there is synergism once oestrogen is being taken) have reduced but not eliminated this risk.

Predisposing factors include strong family history, and a tendency to water retention and obesity. Past pregnancy-associated hypertension (toxaemia) does not predispose to hypertension during OC use, in controlled studies. But the RCGP study showed that *past toxaemia history* (which may be a 'marker' for essential hypertension, not diagnosed before the pregnancy) does strongly predispose to myocardial infarction, especially in smokers (see Q 4.133).

Hypertension is an important risk factor for the arterial diseases to be considered in detail below, especially heart disease and both types of stroke.

4.96 AS OF 1999, WHAT DO WE REALLY KNOW ABOUT HOW THE COC MAY AFFECT THE VARIOUS CARDIOVASCULAR DISEASES?

A most useful summary of the worldwide epidemiological findings was published by the WHO in 1998 in their periodical *PROGRESS in Human Reproduction Research* (which also contains all the most important references). In view of the amount of heat that has been generated on this subject since October 1995, I feel the best way to answer the above question is to reproduce much of this (with permission, slightly rearranged/shortened and with a few comments of my own). In comparison with the others in this book this will be a very long answer!

CARDIOVASCULAR DISEASE AND
STEROID HORMONE CONTRACEPTIVES

Steroid hormone contraceptives have been available since the 1960s and are now used by more than 100 million women worldwide. Reports linking combined oral contraceptives with cardiovascular side-effects (venous and arterial thrombotic events) appeared soon after these products were first marketed. Since then a large number of epidemiological studies have investigated whether users of combined oral contraceptives are at increased risk of cardiovascular disease. Information is now available about the effects of more recently introduced combined oral contraceptives from several large, recently completed studies, including the WHO Collaborative Study of Cardiovascular Disease and Steroid Hormone Contraception (which was conducted in 21 centres in different countries in Africa, Asia, Europe and Latin America).

On 3–7 November 1997, the Programme convened in Geneva a Scientific Group Meeting on Cardiovascular Disease and Steroid Hormone Contraception.

In its discussions the Scientific Group relied mainly on published data, although it also considered unpublished information from several new studies. Acknowledging the major changes that have taken place in the hormonal content of combined oral contraceptives and prescribing patterns, the Scientific Group paid particular attention to studies which included data collected after 1980.

The Scientific Group concluded that the incidence and mortality rates of all cardiovascular diseases (stroke, myocardial infarction, and venous thromboembolism) in women of reproductive age are very low. Any additional cardiovascular disease incidence or mortality attributable to oral contraceptives is very small if the users do not smoke and do not have other cardiovascular risk factors.

Although the focus of the Scientific Group deliberations was on the cardiovascular effects of steroid contraceptives, other considerations also influence women and couples when they make their choice of contraceptive method. These factors include real and perceived risks and benefits associated with each method of contraception. Social, economic, psychological and cultural factors are also important. The conclusions and recommendations of the Scientific Group should not, therefore, be taken in isolation. Instead, they should form part of the detailed information needed when making informed choices in this important area of preventive health care. The background papers prepared for the meeting have been published in the journal *Contraception* (volume 57, March 1998). The final report of the Scientific Group Meeting has been published in 1998 by WHO (Technical Report Series, No 877).

Venous thromboembolism (VTE)

The first epidemiological evidence implicating use of combined oral contraceptives with an increased risk of venous thromboembolism (blood clots in veins) appeared in 1967. All of the studies conducted since then have found that current users of combined oral contraceptives have a higher risk of venous thromboembolic disease than women not using oral contraceptives. In most studies the relative risks were statistically significant.

The consistency of the findings, the size of the relative risks, and the lack of plausible explanation in terms of bias, confounding or chance, strongly suggest a causal relationship between current use of combined oral contraceptives and venous thromboembolic disease. The absolute risk, however, remains very low.

Earlier studies of use of oral contraception and venous thromboembolism found little change in risk with increasing duration of use. The WHO study showed little evidence overall of an appreciable change in risk with duration of use, although the size of the relative risk diminished slightly during the first few years. A comparison between women who had used combined oral contraceptives for the first time and those who had never used them in the Transnational Study indicated a 10-fold increased risk during the first year of use which fell to a twofold increase in subsequent years. [JG's comment: this is an expected effect since some women, with a congenital predisposition to VTE, will suffer the event relatively soon after first exposure to the added prothrombotic factor of the COC.] Past users of combined oral contraceptives are not at greater risk of venous thromboembolic disease than women who have never used them. The risk among current users falls to that among non-users within 3 months of stopping oral contraceptives. [JG: probably within 2–4 weeks, in fact.]

The *relative risk* of venous thromboembolism associated with current use of oral contraceptives does not appear to vary with age. The *incidence* of venous thromboembolic disease, however, rises with age. This means that the *absolute risk* [see Q 4.97] of venous thromboembolic disease attributable to oral contraception is higher in older than in younger women. In the WHO study, oral contraceptive users who were obese had a higher relative risk than did users who were not obese, in both developing and developed countries.

Recent studies have shown that women with hereditary clotting defects are at a much higher risk of venous thromboembolism if they use oral contraceptives. Current users of oral contraceptives with factor V Leiden mutation had a relative risk of deep vein thrombosis of 35 compared with non-users without this mutation. Even with such a high relative risk, however, the absolute risk was still low: around three additional cases of venous thromboembolism per year per 1000 users with factor V Leiden mutation compared with users without this defect [see Q 4.108–4.109].

Early studies suggested that reduction in the oestrogen content of combined oral contraceptives might lower the risk of deep vein thrombosis and pulmonary

4.96 continued

embolism; however, the evidence was not entirely consistent. There is no convincing evidence that the risks have declined substantially over time, or with reductions in oestrogen content. [**i.e. further reductions below 50 µg.**] The influence of the progestogen component of combined oral contraceptives on the risk of venous thromboembolism has, until recently, received comparatively little attention.

Since the end of 1995, four studies have reported that users of low-dose (< 50 µg of oestrogen) combined oral contraceptives containing desogestrel or gestodene have a higher risk of venous thromboembolic disease than users of low-dose contraceptives containing levonorgestrel. Comparison between results has been complicated by the use of different reference groups.

The Scientific Group concluded that:

- Current users of combined oral contraceptives have a low absolute risk of venous thromboembolism, which is none the less 3–6 times that in non-users. The risk is probably highest in the first year of use and declines thereafter, but persists until discontinuation.
- After use of combined oral contraceptives is discontinued, the risk of venous thromboembolism drops rapidly to that in non-users.
- Among users of combined oral contraceptive preparations containing less than 50 µg of ethinyloestradiol, the risk of venous thromboembolism is not related to the dose of oestrogen. [**JG: rather, this expected link has not been shown.**]
- Combined oral contraceptives containing desogestrel or gestodene probably carry a small risk of venous thromboembolism beyond that attributable to combined oral contraceptives containing levonorgestrel. [**JG: This is still debated, since bias and 'attrition of susceptibles' (see Q 4.103) explain some, maybe most, of the difference, and more recent studies – notably by Farmer *et al.* – are not confirmatory.**] There are insufficient data to draw conclusions with regard to combined oral contraceptives containing norgestimate.
- The absolute risks of venous thromboembolism attributable to use of oral contraceptives rise with increasing age, obesity, recent surgery, and some forms of thrombophilia.
- Cigarette smoking and raised blood pressure, which are important risk factors for arterial disease, do not appear to elevate the risk of venous thromboembolic disease. [**JG: Farmer's data (1999) from a large general practice database suggest otherwise: that smoking about doubles the risk in pill-takers.**]
- There are insufficient data to conclude whether there is a relation between venous thromboembolism and the use of progestogen-only contraceptives.
- The relative risks of venous thromboembolic disease observed in users of combined oral contraceptives in developed countries appear to be applicable to developing countries.

Acute myocardial infarction (AMI)

Myocardial infarction is uncommon in women of reproductive age. Because of this, studies of large populations are needed to determine factors that cause this condition in this population group. Data are available which show that age, cigarette smoking, diabetes, hypertension and raised total blood cholesterol are important risk factors for myocardial infarction in young women.

Most contraceptive users are healthy with a low incidence of major disease. Thus, even though serious adverse events occur infrequently in contraceptive users, they tend to have greater implications than adverse events arising during the treatment of sick patients. In addition, the very large number of women using steroid hormone contraceptives throughout the world means that even a modest rise in risk has the potential to affect a large number of women.

The first report of coronary thrombosis in an oral contraceptive user was published in 1963. The results of the first epidemiological studies of vascular disease in oral contraceptive users were published in the late 1960s but only two presented data on myocardial infarction and neither found an elevated risk in current users of oral contraceptives. Subsequent studies, however, suggested such risk may be present.

The WHO Collaborative Study of Cardiovascular Disease and Steroid Hormone Contraception reported a relative risk of myocardial infarction in current users of combined oral contraceptives of 5.0 in Europe and 4.8 in developing countries. A Transnational Study conducted in 16 centres in six European countries reported a relative risk of myocardial infarction in current users of combined oral contraceptives of 2.4. The Scientific Group concluded that this variation in relative risks reported by the different studies may be due to differences in the prevalence of smoking, especially heavy smoking, and the checking of blood pressure, and to the use of hospital-based rather than community-based controls. The Group found no substantive evidence of increased relative risk of myocardial infarction among previous users of combined oral contraceptives compared with women who have never used them.

A number of studies have tried to determine whether women with established risk factors for myocardial infarction are at especially increased risk if they use combined oral contraceptives. Studies comparing the risk in younger and older users of oral contraceptives found that, while the incidence of myocardial infarction increases with age, there is no convincing evidence that the relative risk of myocardial infarction among current users of oral contraceptives differs with age. Research shows that cigarette smoking increases the relative risk of myocardial infarction, irrespective of a woman's use of oral contraception. Studies of current users of combined oral contraceptives who were smokers found substantially higher relative risks among those who were heavy smokers than among those who were light smokers or non-smokers.

4.96 continued

In the Transnational Study, there was no difference in risk between users of oral contraceptives who did not smoke and non-users who did not smoke. In the WHO study, current users at low risk of cardiovascular disease who did not smoke and who reported having their blood pressure checked before the current episode of use had the same risk of myocardial infarction as non-users who did not smoke. Similar results were found in both developing and European countries.

Two recent studies confirmed that current users of oral contraceptives with a history of high blood pressure have higher relative risks of myocardial infarction than users without such a history. In both the WHO and the Transnational Studies, current users of oral contraceptives who reported not having had their blood pressure checked prior to the current episode of use had higher relative risks of myocardial infarction than current users whose blood pressure had been checked.

The amount of increase in blood pressure that increases the risk of myocardial infarction could not be determined in the above case-control studies. Owing to the high background risk of myocardial infarction in women with hypertension, and to the possible enhanced risk of myocardial infarction in such women from the use of combined oral contraceptives, women with known hypertension should be prescribed oral contraception only after careful clinical assessment.

Studies of the influence of the hormonal content of combined oral contraceptives are complicated by the interrelationship between the dose of oestrogen and the type and dose of the accompanying progestogen. Early studies suggested a direct relationship between the dose of oestrogen and risk of cardiovascular disease. In other studies, conflicting results were found.

The Scientific Group concluded that:

- The incidence of fatal and non-fatal myocardial infarction is very low in women of reproductive age in both developed and developing countries. Women who do not smoke, who have their blood pressure checked, and who do not have hypertension or diabetes, are at no increased risk of myocardial infarction if they use combined oral contraceptives, regardless of their age. [JG: **Indeed in every study, including the four main cohort studies and the 1999 MICA case-control study, this disease has effectively not been reported in a pill-taker unless she also smoked or had another arterial risk factor, and regardless of pill-formulation.**]
- There is no increase in the risk of myocardial infarction with increasing duration of use of combined oral contraceptives. There is no increase in the relative risk of myocardial infarction in past users of combined oral contraceptives. [JG: **This is not the pattern to be expected if the COC, alone, in the absence of arterial risk factors, were atherogenic – and most of these data relate to pills with 'second generation' progestagens.**] These conclusions appear to apply equally to women in developed and developing countries.

- Women with hypertension have an increased absolute risk of myocardial infarction. The relative risk of myocardial infarction in current users of combined oral contraceptives with hypertension is at least three times that in current users without hypertension. This conclusion appears to apply equally to women in developed and developing countries.

- The increased absolute risk of myocardial infarction in women who smoke is greatly elevated by use of combined oral contraceptives, especially in heavy smokers. This conclusion appears to apply equally to women in developed and developing countries. The relative risk of myocardial infarction in heavy smokers who use combined oral contraceptives may be as high as 10 times that in non-smokers who do not use combined oral contraceptives. [JG: See Table 4.8.]

- Although the *incidence* of myocardial infarction increases exponentially with age, the *relative risk* of myocardial infarction in current users of combined oral contraceptives does not change with increasing age.

- The available data do not allow the effect of the dose of oestrogen on the relative risk of myocardial infarction to be evaluated independently of the type and dose of progestogen.

- There are insufficient data to assess whether the risk of myocardial infarction in users of low-dose combined oral contraceptives is modified by the type of progestogen. The suggestion that users of low-dose combined oral contraceptives containing gestodene or desogestrel may have a lower risk of myocardial infarction than users of low-dose formulations containing levonorgestrel remains to be substantiated. [JG: The Transnational Study did show this, a statistically significant effect, the relative benefit probably focused – if the effect is real – in the smokers (Q 4.111). But the MICA study (1999) was not confirmatory.]

Ischaemic stroke

The relationship between use of combined oral contraceptives and ischaemic stroke has been demonstrated in a number of epidemiological studies. Most found current use of combined oral contraceptives to be associated with an overall increased risk of ischaemic stroke which was roughly three times that of non-users.

Studies that have looked for a relationship between increased risk and duration of use have found little evidence of one. Some studies reported no significantly elevated risk of ischaemic stroke among past users of combined oral contraceptives compared with women who had never used them.

Various studies have observed that age, smoking, hypertension and migraine are independently associated with the risk of ischaemic stroke in women. It is likely that the risk of ischaemic stroke varies among users of combined oral contraceptives, depending on their characteristics. [JG: and it is unfortunate that in the important factor of migraine the influence of different symptomatology features so little in the epidemiological studies – see Qs 4.147–4.154.]

4.96 continued

The WHO study reported higher relative risks among users of combined oral contraceptives who were aged 35 years or more than among those who were under 35, but this difference was attenuated among women who had their blood pressure checked. Substantially higher relative risks among older users were also reported in a case control study in Italy. The age-related effects may have been due to changes in the prevalence of hypertension among older women.

In the WHO study and the Collaborative Group study in the USA in the 1970s, users of oral contraceptives with a history of hypertension had a substantially greater relative risk of ischaemic stroke than users without hypertension. Compared with women without a history of hypertension who were not using combined oral contraceptives, the relative risk among women in the WHO study who were current users and who had a history of hypertension was 14.5 in developing countries and 10.7 in Europe; the relative risk associated with current use of oral contraception by women without hypertension was 2.7 in developing countries and 2.7 in Europe. The WHO and Transnational Studies both found smaller relative risks among women who reported having had their blood pressure checked prior to their current episode of oral contraceptive use. Taken together, these findings suggest that blood pressure may have an important role in the risk of ischaemic stroke associated with use of oral contraceptives.

In the WHO and Transnational studies use of oral contraceptives containing less than 50 µg of oestrogen was associated with a smaller relative risk than was use of higher-dose preparations in European countries.

Neither the dose nor the type of progestogen in combined oral contraceptives was found to have a consistent effect on relative risk in women recruited to the WHO study. However, the number of women using the more recently introduced preparations containing desogestrel, gestodene or norgestimate was very small.

The Scientific Group concluded that:

- The incidence of fatal and non-fatal ischaemic stroke is very low in women of reproductive age in both developed and developing countries.
- The reported estimates of relative risk of ischaemic stroke associated with use of combined oral contraceptives have decreased since the earliest epidemiological studies linking use of oral contraceptives with stroke.
- In women who do not smoke, who have their blood pressure checked, and who do not have hypertension, the risk of ischaemic stroke is increased about 1.5-fold in current users of low-dose combined oral contraceptives compared with non-users. There is no further increase in the risk of ischaemic stroke with increasing duration of use of combined oral contraceptives. Women who have stopped taking combined oral contraceptives are at no greater risk of ischaemic stroke than women who have never used oral contraceptives. These conclusions appear to apply equally in developed and developing countries.

- Women with hypertension have an increased absolute risk of ischaemic stroke. The relative risk of ischaemic stroke in current users of combined oral contraceptives with hypertension appears to be at least three times that in current users without hypertension. This conclusion appears to apply equally in developed and developing countries.
- The absolute risk of ischaemic stroke in women who smoke is about 1.5–2 times that in non-smokers; this risk is multiplied by a factor of 2–3 if such women are current users of combined oral contraceptives. This conclusion appears to apply equally in developed and developing countries.
- The risk of ischaemic stroke in users of combined oral contraceptives containing high doses of oestrogen is higher than that in users of combined oral contraceptives containing low doses of oestrogen.
- There are insufficient data to allow any conclusion to be drawn about whether the risk of ischaemic stroke is related to the type or dose of progestagen contained in low-dose combined oral contraceptives.

   [JG: careful prescribing in relation to headaches and focal neurological aura symptoms (Qs 4.147–4.154) should further reduce the risk of this catastrophic complication, but we need more data.]

Haemorrhagic stroke

Most recent studies have found smoking and hypertension to be important independent risk factors for haemorrhagic stroke. Only the WHO study, however, had sufficient statistical power to examine the risk of haemorrhagic stroke in women with different characteristics. In both developing and European countries, current users of combined oral contraceptives aged 35 years or more had a significantly increased relative risk of haemorrhagic stroke compared with non-users, but younger users did not. The relative risk of haemorrhagic stroke in current users of combined oral contraceptives who smoked was 3–4 times that of non-users who did not smoke. Compared with non-users without a history of hypertension, current users with such a history had a substantially higher relative risk of haemorrhagic stroke.

The Scientific Group found no evidence to date that either the oestrogen or the progestagen constituents of the combined oral contraceptives affect the risk of haemorrhagic stroke. Sufficient data were also not available on the risk of haemorrhagic stroke associated with use of the various types of progestagen-only contraceptives.

The Scientific Group concluded that:

- The incidence of fatal and non-fatal haemorrhagic stroke is very low in women of reproductive age in both developed and developing countries. In women aged less than 35 years, who do not smoke, and who do not have hypertension, the

4.96 continued

relative risk of haemorrhagic stroke associated with use of combined oral contraceptives is not increased. There is no increase in the risk of haemorrhagic stroke with increasing duration of use of oral contraceptives. Women who have previously used oral contraceptives are at no greater risk of haemorrhagic stroke than women who have never used them. These conclusions appear to apply equally in developed and developing countries.

- Women with hypertension have an increased absolute risk of haemorrhagic stroke. The relative risk of haemorrhagic stroke in current users of combined oral contraceptives with hypertension may be 10 times that in current users without hypertension. This conclusion appears to apply equally in developed and developing countries.
- The risk of haemorrhagic stroke in women who smoke is up to twice that in non-smokers; in women who are current users of combined oral contraceptives and who smoke, the relative risk is about 3. This conclusion appears to apply equally in developed and developing countries.
- The incidence of haemorrhagic stroke increases with age, and current use of combined oral contraceptives appears to magnify this effect of ageing.
- There is no evidence that either the oestrogen or the progestagen constituent of combined oral contraceptives is related to the risk of haemorrhagic stroke.

See Table 4.8, page 170.

POSSIBLE BIOLOGICAL MECHANISMS FOR CARDIOVASCULAR EFFECTS

The complexity of the mechanisms underlying cardiovascular disease has been increasingly recognized over recent years. Combined oral contraceptives affect lipoprotein and carbohydrate metabolism, haemostasis, and mechanisms regulating blood pressure. An influence on the functioning of the endothelium of blood vessels and arterial tone also seems likely. The Scientific Group suggested that the potential significance of these changes should be investigated and interpreted using new models of vascular pathophysiology.

The Scientific Group concluded that:

- Epidemiological observations are more likely to be accepted if they are biologically plausible, although the absence of such an explanation does not exclude a causal relationship.
- The biological mechanisms underlying cardiovascular disease involve a complex interplay between lipoprotein metabolism, humoral regulators such as insulin, coagulation and fibrinolysis, the renin–angiotensin–aldosterone system, and the functioning of the endothelium of blood vessels.
- Combined oral contraceptives do not increase the risk of developing diabetes mellitus. They have little effect on fasting plasma concentrations of glucose and

insulin, but cause modest elevations in the plasma levels of glucose and insulin after an oral glucose challenge and may increase insulin resistance. The clinical significance of such changes in otherwise healthy young women is unknown, especially in relation to arterial disease.

The changes in metabolism of lipoproteins in plasma induced by use of combined oral contraceptives have been extensively studied. Low-dose combined oral contraceptives increase fasting plasma levels of triglycerides but have only minor effects on low-density lipoproteins, lipoprotein or total cholesterol. The effect on high-density lipoproteins depends on the balance of oestrogen and progestagen. The clinical significance of such changes is uncertain in the context of current low-dose formulations. Combined oral contraceptives alter the plasma concentrations of many components (including their activation markers) of both the coagulation and fibrinolytic systems. These changes are less marked with combined oral contraceptives containing low doses of ethinyloestradiol and even less so with progestagen-only contraceptives. Hereditary conditions such as antithrombin III defect and factor V Leiden mutation predispose women to venous thromboembolism. These disorders may underlie a large proportion of idiopathic venous thromboembolic events, perhaps one-third of those seen in Caucasian women. This effect is increased in women using combined oral contraceptives.

The prevalence of hereditary conditions such as antithrombin III defect and factor V Leiden mutation is about 5% in caucasian women but is lower in other populations. The positive predictive value of screening for these disorders is very low. [JG: see Q 4.108–4.109]

Even low-dose combined oral contraceptives cause modest elevations in blood pressure which may increase the risk of arterial disease. In healthy young women with a low background risk of arterial disease, small increases in blood pressure attributable to use of combined oral contraception are likely to have minimal effects on the absolute risk of arterial disease.

Comparative studies of users of low-dose combined oral contraceptives suggest that the dose and type of the progestagen component influence the effect of these preparations on lipid and lipoprotein metabolism and haemostasis. The clinical significance of these differences is uncertain.

RECOMMENDATIONS FOR FURTHER RESEARCH

The Scientific Group made a number of recommendations regarding areas of future research related to the risk of cardiovascular disease and the use of steroid contraception:

Further research is needed on the prevalence of risk factors predisposing women of reproductive age to cardiovascular disease in developing and developed countries.

- More research is needed on the pathogenesis of arterial disease in women of reproductive age.
- The effect of the use of steroid contraceptives by women with diabetes on their risk of cardiovascular disease needs to be studied, perhaps using surrogate end-points.
- More epidemiological research about the risks of cardiovascular disease among users of combined oral contraceptives in developing countries is required because current conclusions about the effects of the various formulations are based on only one study which finished data collection in 1993. Many developing countries, moreover, are experiencing rapid changes in the prevalence of risk factors that affect the incidence of cardiovascular disease.
- The effects of different oral contraceptives on endothelial function requires study. This might involve measuring plasma levels of biological markers of endothelial function as well as using non-invasive techniques in human subjects.
- Further studies are required on the influence of steroid hormones on systems regulating blood pressure and on the mechanisms by which these hormones affect the interplay between plasma lipoproteins and haemostatic factors.
- The role of the structure of the progestagen molecule in determining haemostatic effects needs to be elucidated.
- More data are needed on the risk of cardiovascular disease among users of progestagen-only preparations, especially injectables and implants, in developed as well as developing countries.
- Further research is needed in different health settings to determine the levels of blood pressure at which steroid hormones can be used safely, and to evaluate the optimal frequency of monitoring of blood pressure during use of steroid contraceptives.

MAKING INFORMED CHOICES ABOUT COMBINED ORAL CONTRACEPTIVES

Any assessment of the risk of cardiovascular disease associated with combined oral contraceptives is complex. Nevertheless, it is clear that mortality rates from cardiovascular disease are extremely low among women of reproductive age, and that the added risk of using steroid contraceptives is also very low. Within the context of the everyday risks of modern life, steroid contraceptives are safe. Factors which need to be taken into account when determining a woman's risk of cardiovascular disease while using combined oral contraceptives include:

- the age-specific incidence of each cardiovascular condition;
- the strength of the association between use of combined oral contraceptives and each cardiovascular outcome;

the woman's age and presence of other risk factors for cardiovascular disease such as smoking and a history of hypertension;
- whether there are important differences in risk between particular formulations of combined oral contraceptive and, if so, the choice of formulation.

At the population level, the impact of combined oral contraceptives on cardiovascular disease within any country depends on:

the age-specific prevalence of use of combined oral contraceptives;
- the characteristics of the users;
- if there are important differences between formulations, and the proportion of women using each formulation at different ages.

The number of cardiovascular events attributable to the use of combined oral contraceptives is very small, especially among users of all ages who do not smoke and among younger users who smoke. [JG: this is shown very clearly in Table 4.8 here, which comes from the same WHO publication, especially as the numbers shown are per *million* women per year.] The number of associated deaths is even smaller and, again, is highly dependent on whether the user is a smoker. Any small increase in risk of cardiovascular disease must be considered against the very high contraceptive efficacy of combined oral contraceptives and the rapid reversibility of this effect after they are stopped. The use of less reliable alternative methods of contraception (or the avoidance of any contraception) exposes women to an increased risk of pregnancy, a condition which is associated with a higher incidence of venous thromboembolic disease than that associated with the use of any of the currently available low-dose combined oral contraceptives. In addition, combined oral contraceptives are associated with many non-contraceptive benefits, including a reduced risk of endometrial and ovarian cancer. By any standards, all of the currently available low-dose combined oral contraceptives can be regarded as safe.

The Study Group concluded that:

- The incidence and mortality rates of all cardiovascular diseases (stroke, acute myocardial infarction and venous thromboembolic disease) in women of reproductive age are very low (**Table 4.8**).
- Any increase in incidence of, or mortality from, cardiovascular disease attributable to use of combined oral contraception is very small if users do not smoke and do not have other risk factors for cardiovascular disease. For example, among users of combined oral contraceptives who do not have risk factors for cardiovascular disease, the annual risk of death attributable to use of oral contraceptives is approximately 2 deaths per million users at 20–24 years of age, 2–5 per million users at 30–34 years of age and approximately 20–25 per million users at 40–44 years of age. [JG: in Figure 4.11 below I use a summary risk of 10 per million (=1:100 000) for the total all-age and all-cause mortality risk of the COC.]

TABLE 4.8 ESTIMATED NUMBER OF CARDIOVASCULAR EVENTS AT DIFFERENT AGES AMONG NON-USERS AND USERS OF COMBINED ORAL CONTRACEPTIVES IN DEVELOPED COUNTRIES, BY SMOKING HABITS

Non-smokers – Non-users

Number of events (per million woman-years)	Age (years) 20–24	30–34	40–44
Acute myocardial infarction	0.13	1.69	21.28
Ischaemic stroke	6.03	9.84	16.05
Haemorrhagic stroke	12.73	24.28	46.30
Venous thromboembolism	32.23	45.75	59.28
Total	51.12	81.56	142.9

Non-smokers – Users*

Number of events (per million woman-years)	Age (years) 20–24	30–34	40–44
Acute myocardial infarction	0.20	2.55	31.92
Ischaemic stroke	9.04	14.75	24.07
Haemorrhagic stroke	12.73	24.28	92.60
Venous thromboembolism	96.68	137.30	177.80
Total	118.70	178.90	326.40

Smokers – Non-users

Number of events (per million woman-years)	Age (years) 20–24	30–34	40–44
Acute myocardial infarction	1.08	13.58	170.20
Ischaemic stroke	12.06	19.67	32.09
Haemorrhagic stroke	25.46	48.55	138.90
Venous thromboembolism	32.23	45.75	59.28
Total	70.83	127.60	400.50

Smokers – Users*

Number of events (per million woman-years)	Age (years) 20–24	30–34	40–44
Acute myocardial infarction	1.62	20.36	255.30
Ischaemic stroke	18.09	29.51	48.14
Haemorrhagic stroke	38.19	72.83	231.50
Venous thromboembolism	96.68	137.30	177.80
Total	154.60	260.00	712.70

*Blood pressure was checked in users.

Source: Farley TMM, Collins J, Schlesselman JJ. Hormonal contraception and risk of cardiovascular disease: an international perspective. *Contraception*, 1998, 57:211–230.

- The risk of mortality from cardiovascular disease attributable to use of oral contraception is much greater (up to 10-fold) among women aged 40–44 years than among women aged 20–24 years.
- At any given age a woman who smokes but who does not use oral contraceptives is at greater risk of death from arterial disease than a user of oral contraceptives who does not smoke. [JG: worth saying this to some women – and men!] The benefits of blood-pressure measurement in reducing the risk of cardiovascular disease attributable to use of oral contraception increase with the age of the user. [JG: and WHO found that not having BP taken at all is a good surrogate for poor healthcare of pill-takers!]
- Venous thromboembolic disease is the most common cardiovascular event among users of oral contraceptives. However, it contributes very little to any increase in the number of deaths since the associated mortality is relatively low compared with that associated with arterial diseases. Long-term disability from non-fatal venous thromboembolic disease is also low.

4.97 WHAT IS THE DIFFERENCE BETWEEN RELATIVE RISK AND ABSOLUTE OR ATTRIBUTABLE RISK?

This is a most important distinction, which is not often understood by either patients or journalists, notably in relation to venous thromboembolism (VTE). Twice almost nothing out of a million is still almost nothing! Absolute risk came up several times above, in the long *WHO 'PROGRESS'* quotation, and will be very relevant in what follows:

> A small relative risk may easily cause more attributable cases than a large one, if the background prevalence is high – and vice versa.

In Table 4.9 the first set of figures (A) actually apply to the frequency of hepatocellular adenoma in controls as compared with COC-users using older 50-μg-plus pills. The second set (B) come from Table 4.8 (Q 4.96) which itself is from the 1998 report of the WHO's special Scientific Group. They apply to *smokers* aged 40–44, who would have an increase in relative risk of acute myocardial infarction (AMI) of only 1.5 if they additionally took

TABLE 4.9 ATTRIBUTABLE RISK

Background prevalence	Relative risk	No. of cases	No. of cases attributable
(A) 1 in 10^6	$\times 20$	20	19
(B) 170 in 10^6	$\times 1.5$	255	85

Note: Even as much as ten times an infinitesimal risk can still be infinitesimal. See Q 4.97.

the modern low-dose pills at that age; but the attributable number of extra cases (absolute risk) is 85 per million. Contrast only 19 extra cases of hepatoma in the first set of figures (A), despite a 20-fold greater relative risk

Neither statistic is good news (both are dangerous conditions). But the difference in the excess number of cases caused by the method explains why it was reasonable to accept, for 50-μg-plus pills, a 20-fold increase in the risk of benign liver tumours. However a mere 50% increase in AMI through more modern pills is widely considered unacceptable for smokers above age 40.

> **4.98 PATIENTS ARE NATURALLY ANXIOUS ABOUT THE KNOWN ADVERSE EFFECTS OF THE COMBINED PILL ON CANCER AND CIRCULATORY DISEASE. ASSUMING THEY OTHERWISE WISH TO USE THE METHOD, HOW MAY THIS ANXIETY BE REDUCED?**

See Q 4.96, the section on 'making informed choices', and Figures 4.10 and 4.11 here. The media do the general public a disservice by tending to exaggerate the bad systemic effects, and by not pointing out the counterbalancing non-contraceptive benefits, aside from the advantages of efficacy, reversibility and convenience. Another form of counterbalancing is shown on the right-hand side of Figure 4.10, namely the comparison with the risks of pregnancy (so effectively avoided by the COC) and the avoidance of the risk and inconvenience of the alternative methods.

Potential users can be reminded that there are many other risks in life. However intelligent and educated, most of us are amazingly 'risk-illiterate'.

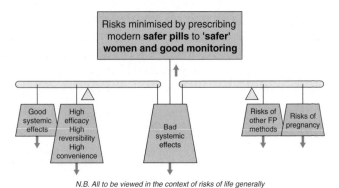

N.B. All to be viewed in the context of risks of life generally

Figure 4.10 The risks versus the benefits of hormonal contraception. Q 4.98. (See Fig. 4.11 for 'the risks of life generally')

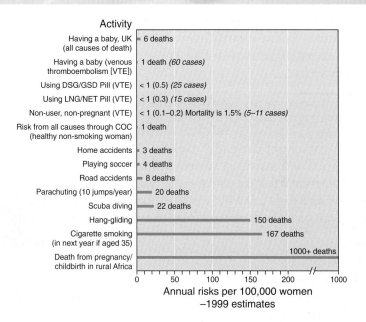

Figure 4.11   The risks of various activities (annual number of deaths per 100 000 exposed) See Q 4.98. With regard to cancer, in this Figure excess cancer mortality is assumed to be zero – See Q 4.72 and Figure 4.6. Sources: Dinman BD (1980) *JAMA* 244: 1226–8; Mills A et al (1996) *BMJ* 312: 121; Anon (1991) *BMJ* 302: 743. Strom B (1994) *Pharmacoepidemiology* (2nd ed) pp. 57–65, Chichester: Wiley. Guillebaud JG (1998) *Contraception Today* (3rd ed) p. 20, London: Martin Dunitz

Many risks are far greater than pill-taking, yet cause minimal concern: for example having babies or travelling by car (Fig. 4.11) – let alone smoking!

For the many who are not very numerate risks are best expressed in relative terms. The risk of dying through pill-taking is 'less than one hundredth of the risk of death through smoking 20 cigarettes a day', for example.

Life is pretty risky: believe it or not, each year one has a 1:1000 chance of having to visit a Casualty Department through being injured by a bottle or a can. At least three deaths have been reported from the Brompton hospital through allergy to hamsters. ...

Among one million men, the risk of dying (from all natural causes) is one in a million:

- in the next 7.5 hours if aged 40;
- in the next 5 minutes if aged over 65!

Finally, prospective pill-takers can be reminded that the tiny risks of the COC can be further reduced: by careful prescribing of lower-dose preparations, with good subsequent monitoring (see Qs 4.114–4.131, 4.133 and 4.180).

4.99 WHAT EFFECT DOES SMOKING HAVE ON THE MORTALITY OF ARTERIAL DISEASE IN PILL-USERS?

Given the relevance of smoking as a serious risk people take for granted: it is salutary to note that the 1983 report of the RCGP showed (and later data are congruent) that the pill-user who also smoked was not only more likely to suffer a heart attack but was also much more likely to die as a consequence – a higher case-fatality rate was noted in smokers.

4.100 HOW CAN A BUSY DOCTOR EVER CONVEY ENOUGH INFORMATION ABOUT COCs TO ENABLE WORRIED WOMEN TO MAKE A FULLY INFORMED DECISION?

So much is now known about the method that this is becoming ever more difficult to do. The advice of the Medical Defence Societies is:

A doctor has the duty to give such warnings and carry out such checks as are considered by his/her peers to be necessary having regard to the relevant circumstances of the case. There is no obligation to explain every risk but there is the need to be forthright in explaining risks.

In other words, you should be frank about what is known and honest about what is not yet known; communicate the main pros and cons of the method as in Qs 4.55, 4.69–4.98; explain the practicalities, rules for missed pills, minor side-effects – most especially breakthrough bleeding; and allow time for questions to be asked and answered. Full records should be kept. A pretty tall order!

For most busy practitioners who wish to maintain high standards 'allow time' means more accurately *'make time', plus delegate.* In the real world, how do they present? In the middle of a busy surgery, as like as not needing postcoital contraception (see Ch. 7, a whole chapter to take account of there!) first, and then to start the COC before their follow-up visit. ... Can all this ever be well done without the availability of counselling by a (family planning-trained) nurse, supplemented by you perhaps at the end of your surgery or during the next dedicated family planning session? See Q 8.16.

4.101 WHAT ELSE IS IMPORTANT AS AN ADJUNCT TO GOOD COUNSELLING?

The written word! In my view *counselling should always be supplemented by a leaflet*, and I think the best is still 'Choosing and using the combined pill', published by the UK FPA. Among other things this has advice for missed pills and a medicolegally important list of those side-effects which should lead the woman to seek urgent medical advice (see Q 4.191).

Finally, much medical time may be saved if those women who desire the impossible, a 2-hour consultation about oral contraception, are referred to my comprehensive paperback entitled *The Pill* (see Further Reading)!

A MORE DETAILED APPRAISAL OF THE CONTROVERSY ABOUT VENOUS THROMBOEMBOLISM (VTE) AND ITS IMPLICATIONS FOR PRESCRIBERS

4.102 NOW THAT THE DUST HAS SETTLED, WHAT IS YOUR ASSESSMENT OF THAT LETTER FROM THE UK COMMITTEE ON THE SAFETY OF MEDICINES (CSM) ON 18 OCTOBER 1995 REGARDING VTE?

There is a range of expert views about the four publications on combined oral contraceptives and venous thromboembolism (VTE) actually published in December 1995 and January 1996, mentioned above in the long WHO extract. They were carefully performed and reasonably congruent with each other. They reported a doubling of the odds ratio for users of desogestrel/gestodene-containing products (DSG/GSD-containing or so-called '3rd generation' progestagens) in comparison with the '2nd generation' levonorgestrel or norethisterone-containing ones (here termed LNG/NET pills).

The 'generation' terminology is ambiguous and best avoided.

4.103 YET HAS NOT THE ACCURACY OF THIS FINDING BEEN QUERIED?

Indeed: by many authorities in the USA and especially in continental Europe – including those involved in the Transnational study, one of the pivotal studies just mentioned. On more thorough reanalyses of their original data (especially looking at first-time pill users) they do not believe their own study shows any real excess risk of VTE with DSG/GSD products. They believe that the whole of the apparent association might be explained not by cause-and effect but by:

- prescriber bias (prescribers being selectively more likely, prior to October 1995, to use DSG/GSD products for first-timers and women thought to be at risk of VTE);
- the 'attrition of susceptibles' or 'healthy user effect' (LNG/NET pills being more commonly used by longer term users and parous women who would be less likely as a population to suffer a VTE, since those who had had this disease would no longer be using the method);
- diagnostic bias resulting from prescriber bias, in that women on DSG/GSD pills because of a perceived higher risk might then be also more likely to be referred for accurate investigations leading to this easily-overlooked diagnosis being made more often than among LNG/NET pill-users.

Evidence for these alternative explanations for the finding comes from:

1 Lewis and co-workers from the Transnational Study showed in 1996 a significant trend of increasing risk of VTE for the progestagens in COCs, related solely to the recency of their introduction to the market.
2 There is also the very odd WHO finding that Mercilon with 20 μg of EE, the artificial oestrogen well-recognized as creating prothrombotic coagulation changes, was significantly associated with more cases of VTE than Marvelon with 30 μg!

Neither of the above are biologically plausible, yet they may be readily linked to prescriber bias and the healthy user effect.

But for honest seekers after the truth (you the reader and I!) the question remains whether there could be *some* real difference between DSG and GSD versus LNG or NET combined products in allowing EE to cause VTE events *despite* the non-causative explanations – though clearly these must apply in part (see below).

4.104 WHAT ABOUT MORE RECENT STUDIES, SINCE EARLY 1996?

During 1996–99, a countrywide study from Denmark (Lidegaard) and especially several large general practice database studies led by Professor Farmer of London, have failed (in Farmer's case with improved matching of cases to controls by exact year of birth) to show a statistically significant difference between the 'generations' of COCs, however defined. Farmer's group also and probably more importantly, failed with reasonable statistical power to show a difference between different individual DSG and GSD combined formulations and the reference LNG product Microgynon 30.

4.105 SO, IN YOUR OPINION, WHERE DOES THAT LEAVE US AS PRESCRIBERS?

At the time of writing (July 1999), personally, I am sure the apparent doubling is a 'worst case scenario': because of the exaggerating effects of the above biases and confounders. But even allowing for them, I am prepared to accept some difference of VTE risk when comparing the DSG/GSD pills with the levonorgestrel (LNG) norethisterone (NET) ones: see Q 4.106.

4.106 IS IT BIOLOGICALLY PLAUSIBLE THAT THE SAME 30 μG DOSE OF ETHINYLOESTRADIOL WOULD HAVE DIFFERENT EFFECTS WHEN COMBINED WITH THE TWO DIFFERENT TYPES OF PROGESTAGENS?

There is a degree of biological plausibility, yes, since we have known for years that LNG in particular behaves in some respects as an anti-oestrogenic progestogen:

- A dose of 30 μg of ethinyloestradiol (EE) raises sex hormone binding globulin (SHBG), raises HDL-cholesterol and tends to improve acne.
- In a randomized controlled trial at the Margaret Pyke Centre we have found that if LNG 150 μg is combined with the same 30 μg dose of ethinyloestradiol (EE), as in Microgynon/Ovranette: SHBG goes up less than with EE alone, HDL-cholesterol is actually slightly lowered, and, clinically, acne may be worsened. Therefore levonorgestrel (and, in high enough dose, norethisterone) is clearly capable of opposing the oestrogenicity of ethinyloestradiol, in its biochemical effects (e.g. SHBG) and in some of its somatic effects (e.g. acne).
- However, combined with desogestrel 150 μg as in Marvelon, the same dose of EE raises SHBG more, raises HDL-cholesterol and tends to improve acne – all very like EE would on its own.

Thus on those three criteria (among others) DSG/GSD pills allow EE to have more of its oestrogenic effects than LNG ones do. Since prothrombotic coagulation changes are also primarily oestrogen-related, a similar difference in VTE potential has always been *possible*, though not necessarily actual!

4.107 BUT SURELY NO-ONE HAS BEEN ABLE TO SHOW A CONSISTENT DIFFERENCE IN THE EFFECTS OF THE TWO TYPES OF PILL ON COAGULATION?

True, which is why the manufacturers of DSG/GSD pills have been reluctant to accept that they have any greater VTE risk-increasing effect than the LNG/NET ones. But the lack of data is not fully reassuring: the haemostatic system is immensely complicated. At least half of idiopathic cases of VTE are not explainable by modern coagulation testing. Therefore it may be that the right measurements to show a real difference are not available. There could be important real differences especially in the earliest stages of the coagulation cascade: which is the point of action of the important natural anticoagulants which cause the known hereditary predispositions to VTE (see below). This possibility is now being actively researched.

4.108 WHAT ARE THE MAIN HEREDITARY PREDISPOSITIONS TO VTE? AND WHAT ACTION SHOULD BE TAKEN IF ONE IS SUSPECTED?

Women with possible hereditary thrombophilia in a first degree relative under age 45 (Table 4.10) should in my view not be prescribed any combined oral contraceptive until thrombophilia has been excluded. The main abnormalities are Factor V Leiden (the genetic cause of Activated Protein C Resistance) which is the most prevalent; and deficiencies of Protein C, Protein S and Antithrombin III. Any of these, once known about, absolutely contraindicate all EE-containing pills (although actually, given the background rarity of VTE, the attributable risk from having any of them is not great, see Qs 4.97 and 4.109).

Even if they are not found the woman cannot be totally reassured, since by no means all the predisposing abnormalities of the complex haemostatic system have yet been characterized. Therefore the COC remains relatively contraindicated for a woman with a positive family history but negative test results. She may indeed use the pill method, but should be specifically advised about the early symptoms of thromboembolism. Like all with a single relative contraindication for venous thromboembolism (VTE) she should receive a LNG/NET pill.

4.109 IF RESOURCES ARE AVAILABLE, WHY DO WE NOT JUST SCREEN EVERYONE WHO ASKS TO GO ON THE PILL FOR A PREDISPOSING FACTOR TO VTE?

Because it is neither cost-effective nor good practice to screen for the hereditary thrombophilias in cases without well-defined family history criteria (thrombophilia in family, or idiopathic thrombosis in parent or sibling under 45). Given that each year so many – 997 of 1000 with the main predisposition – never actually get a thrombosis (see page 159: they prove to be in reality 'false positives') and that other predispositions exist which are not yet measurable (leading to many 'false negatives'): more harm than good would result.

4.110 WHAT ARE THE ACQUIRED THROMBOPHILIAS, AND WHEN SHOULD THEY BE LOOKED FOR/SCREENED FOR?

Antiphospholipid antibodies (such as the unhelpfully-named lupus anticoagulant) may appear in various connective tissue disorders, especially systemic lupus erythematosus (SLE). They should be looked for whenever such a disorder is suspected, and are often routinely sought by laboratories. But once again screening for these in healthy women is not cost-effective because of the number of false positives (women with a detectable abnormality who never get a thrombosis, even during years of pill-taking) and false negatives (women who suffer an idiopathic thrombotic event with or without the COC yet have no congenital or acquired abnormality which modern technology can detect). The latter, in most series, account for up to 50% of hospitalized idiopathic thromboses. Here we have a major research challenge for the haematologists!

Antiphospholipid antibodies increase the risk of both VTE and arterial disease and therefore if present they absolutely contraindicate the COC – but not any of the progestagen-only methods.

4.111 WHICH PROGESTAGENS MIGHT BE BEST FOR THE LEAST ARTERIAL WALL DISEASE RISK? (CHIEFLY MYOCARDIAL INFARCTION AND STROKES)

There remains the possibility of a relative benefit to the arterial walls and hence arterial disease from what appear to be the 'good' effects of DSG/GSD brands on lipids: they do not lower HDL-cholesterol as some of the higher dose LNG and NET brands do. Being more oestrogen-dominant they allow EE to exert more of its effects, and on the model of oestrogen used as HRT after the menopause it would be expected that this would be relatively beneficial to arterial wall disease.

Some epidemiological data on *acute myocardial infarction* (AMI) are now available, but not enough to be conclusive. Lewis *et al.* (from the Transnational OC study) reported in 1996 no significant increase in this risk in users of DSG/GSD pills compared with women not using the pill. Smokers using LNG/NET brands had 11.1 times the risk of non-smoking women not using the pill (a significant difference). And, in 1997, the same group reported a three-fold reduction in the relative risk of AMI for women using DSG/GSD rather than LNG/NET pills (NB *smokers present* in both groups).

All this is compatible with the hypothesis that the DSG/GSD pills have a relatively lower arterial disease risk, almost certainly focused among the women with risk factors like smoking. But this is just one study, numbers of cases are very small, and direct comparison of the products only just shows a significant difference. More studies are needed to confirm these findings.

4.112 HOW WOULD YOU PUT THE VTE RISKS IN PERSPECTIVE?

See Table 4.8, page 170 at Q 4.96 and Figure 4.11 (Q 4.98). The new studies confirm that all low dose combined oral contraceptives carry an extremely low risk for healthy women. At the time of writing, the latest advice in a Press Release (7 April, 1999) from the UK Department of Health (DoH) – issued after the 1998 review by the Medicines Commission of the VTE issue – 'found no new safety concerns' about 3rd generation desogestrel (DSG) or gestodene (GSD) products.

'An increased risk of venous thromboembolic disease (VTE) associated with the use of oral contraceptives is well established but is smaller than that associated with pregnancy; which has been estimated at 60 cases per 100 000 pregnancies. Some epidemiological studies have reported a greater risk of VTE for women using combined oral contraceptives containing desogestrel or gestodene (the so-called third generation pills) than for women using pills containing levonorgestrel (LNG) – the so-called second generation pills' **[sic: category also includes norethisterone (NET) pills].**
'The spontaneous incidence of VTE in healthy non-pregnant women (not taking any oral contraceptive) is about 5 cases per 100 000 women per year. The incidence in users of second generation pills is about 15 per 100 000 women per year of use. The incidence in users of third generation

pills is about 25 cases per 100 000 women per year of use: this excess incidence has not been satisfactorily explained by bias or confounding. The level of all of these risks of VTE increases with age and is likely to be increased in women with other known risk factors for VTE such as obesity.'

'Women must be fully informed of these very small risks. ... Provided they are, the type of pill is for the woman together with her doctor or other family planning professionals jointly to decide in the light of her individual medical history.'
                                                                    (My emphasis)

Note in the above DoH quotation that even though they accept a real difference between the two 'generations' of COCs – and as we have seen this is hotly disputed by some authorities – the estimated risk for DSG/GSD pills has been reduced to 25 cases per 100 000. Therefore the *attributable number of cases* (10 per 100 000) through using DSG/GSD brands rather than one of the others is small. Using the rates given and taking the estimated 1–2% mortality for VTE, there is only a 1–2 per million difference in annual VTE mortality between DSG/GSD products and LNG/NET products. It has been estimated that there is a one in a million risk in each hour of travel by car. Even if the whole difference is accepted as real, therefore:

> *This mortality difference equates at the worst to choosing, on a Sunday afternoon, to risk a 2-hour drive in the country rather than sitting in one's garden! And that difference relates to a whole year of use of the two kinds of product. ...*

Such a difference in risk is small enough, in comparison with the risks (Figure 4.11) which are taken in everyday life, for a well-informed woman to take if she so chooses: for example, because she finds a DSG/GSD brand preferable for her quality of life and reduction in so-called minor side-effects such as acne, headaches, depression, weight gain, or breast symptoms.

4.113 IS INTOLERANCE OF THE LNG/NET PILL BRANDS THROUGH NON-LIFE-ENDANGERING BUT NEVERTHELESS 'ANNOYING' SIDE-EFFECTS ACCEPTABLE AS SUFFICIENT GROUNDS FOR A WOMAN TO USE A DSG/GSD BRAND?

Yes, this is clear in the above DoH quote, indeed it was accepted from the outset, in the original letter circulated by the British CSM – *provided* she understood and accepted the tiny excess risk of VTE. In my experience as a counsellor of pill-takers, the difference in risk compared with an LNG/NET brand is easily seen by many women as unimportant compared with the risks of life generally. Moreover the real difference is probably even less than the 10 per 100 000 (cases) or 2 deaths per million assumed in the above discussion – for all the reasons given at Q 4.103 above.

SELECTION OF USERS AND FORMULATIONS: CHOOSING THE 'SAFER WOMEN', AND THE 'SAFER PILLS'

4.114 WHAT IS YOUR RECOMMENDED FRAMEWORK FOR GOOD PILL MANAGEMENT?

We want *safer pills* for what I call the '*safer women*', maximum safety as well as efficacy. But what the *safer pills* actually are will vary somewhat, depending on research data as it is received, and on characteristics of the woman herself. We need a framework for choice of users as well as choice of pills:

1 *What are the facts, about benefits versus the risks?* Given the evidence, or the best assessment of biological plausibility when the evidence is not there:
2 *Who should never take the pill?* (the *absolute* contraindications)
3 *Who should usually or often not take the pill?* – maybe, but then with special advice and monitoring (the *relative* contraindications now classified by WHO as described at Q 4.130).

[All these contraindications will be described in detail later (Qs 4.130–4.135), since they take so much space that they would hamper this discussion.]

These crucial questions 2 and 3 are expanded in the next Question and help to identify:

4 *Which is the appropriate pill?*
5 *Which second choice of pill?*

This means taking account of:

- biological variation in the pharmacology of contraceptive steroids (Qs 4.155 and 4.156);
- endometrial bleeding as a possible biological measure of their blood levels (Qs 4.157–163);
- what is known about their side-effect profile (Q 4.245 and 4.246).

Finally,

6 *What is necessary for monitoring during follow-up?* including

(a) the implications of the pill-free interval (Qs 4.15–4.32);
(b) blood pressure (Qs 4.183–4.186);
(c) headaches, especially migraines (Qs 4.147–4.154);
(d) management of important new risk factors or diseases
    (Qs 4.180–4.196, 4.199–4.244);
(e) management of minor side-effects (Qs 4.197 and 4.198, 4.245
    and 4.246).

The answers to the next Questions re prescribing are based on my leading article (*BMJ* 1995;311:1111–12) and the statement from the Clinical and Scientific Committee of the Faculty of Family Planning, UK, issued in December 1995, and later published in shortened form (BMJ 1996;312:121), and the above statement by the Deputy Chief Medical Officer for the DoH in April 1999. See also Q 4.96 above and the article on evidence-guided prescribing of COCs by Hannaford and Webb (*Contraception* 1996;54:125–29.) The papers cited give all the most important references.

TABLE 4.10 RISK FACTORS FOR VENOUS THROMBOEMBOLISM

	Absolute contraindication	*Relative contraindication*
Family history (parent or sibling under 45)	Clotting abnormality or tests not done	Clotting factors done, normal
Overweight (high body mass index)	BMI > 39	BMI 30–39
Immobility	Confined to bed	Wheelchair life
Varicose veins	Past thrombosis	Extensive VVs

Notes:
1. A single risk factor in relative contraindication column indicates use of LNG/NET pill, if any COC used.
2. N.B. Synergism: more than one factor in the relative contraindication column means COC method is absolutely contraindicated, also if a definite risk factor is combined with age >35.
3. The literature on the association of smoking with venous thromboembolic disease is mostly negative but see page 160 (Farmer).
4. There are also important acute VTE risk factors which need to be considered in individual cases: notably long-haul aeroplane flights, dehydration through any cause and recent SCUBA diving.
5. See also Q 4.110 re antiphospholipid antibodies (acquired thrombophilia) = WHO 4.

NB This table is to be used in conjunction with Table 4.11, page 185.

4.115 IF FOR THE TIME BEING WE ACCEPT THAT LNG/NET PILLS ARE LESS LIKELY TO LEAD TO VTE (HOW MUCH LESS LIKELY BEING UNCERTAIN) HOW SHOULD THIS AFFECT OUR PRESCRIBING IN CONTEXT WITH RATHER MORE IMPORTANT FACTS?

1 As just stated, prescribers should first take a comprehensive personal and family history to exclude the established *absolute and relative contraindications* to the use of combined oral contraceptives. A personal history of definite venous thromboembolism remains an absolute contraindication to any COC containing EE combined with any progestogen.

2 The risk factors for venous thromboembolism (VTE) and arterial wall disease must be assessed, separately and most carefully. See Tables 4.10 and 4.11. Alone, one risk factor from either table is a relative contraindication (second column of each table) unless it is particularly severe (first column).

3 Multiple risk factors, or any risk factor in Tables 4.10 and 4.11 when combined with age above 35 years, always have the same significance: that the COC should be avoided (absolutely contraindicated). BMI being above 30 is important because it features in both tables: *see the remarks and footnotes, in these Tables which are fundamental to modern pill-prescribing.*

4.116 WHICH PILL FOR ORDINARY FIRST-TIME USERS OF COMBINED ORAL CONTRACEPTIVES?

[A listing of all the actual pill formulations available and related issues comes later, Qs 4.121–4.127].

1 **All marketed pills may now be considered 'first line'.** See the section in bold of DoH statement (Q 4.112). Given the tiny, not yet finally established difference in VTE mortality between the two 'generations', the woman's own choice of a DSG or GSD product after (well-documented) discussion must be respected: even if based on no more than the presence of acne, or a friend's recommendation, or the need for better cycle control, indeed her perception of any issue of quality of life. *'The informed user should be the chooser'.*

2 **Young first-time users:** despite what just said, an LNG or NET product should in my view remain the usual first choice. As a rule one should prescribe intially a low dose LNG/NET pill, containing no more than

TABLE 4.11 RISK FACTORS FOR ARTERIAL CARDIOVASCULAR SYSTEM DISEASE

Risk factor	Absolute contraindication	Relative contraindication	Remarks
Family history of arterial CVS disease in parent or sibling <45	Known atherogenic lipid profile – or tests not available	Acceptable blood lipid profile or first attack in relative >45 (see text)	POP is usually a better choice oral method for all relative contraindications + consider LNG-IUS
Cigarette smoking	? 40+ cigarettes/day	5–40 cigarettes/day	
Diabetes mellitus (DM)	Severe, or diabetic complications present (e.g. retinopathy, renal damage)	Not severe/labile, and no complications, young patient with short duration of DM	See Q 4.143
Hypertension	BP >160/100 mmHg on repeated testing	BP 140–159/90–99	See Qs 4.183–4.184
Overweight	BMI >39	BMI 30–39	
Migraine	Focal aura symptoms; severe, or ergotamine treated migraine	Migraine without focal aura, sumatriptan treatment. If there is also another risk factor, or age is above 35 see Q 4.152.	Relates to thrombotic stroke risk – see Qs 4.147–4.153. If headaches without focal aura mainly in the pill-free interval, consider tricycling

Notes:
1. Synergism: if more than one relative contraindication applies, or if woman now above aged 35, do not use COC.
2. Smoking: The risk at a given age among smokers is not reached until 10 years later by non-smokers, implying that smoking 'ages the arteries'. See page 170.
3. Note overweight appears in both Tables 4.10 and 4.11 – if that is the sole risk factor it indicates use of an LNG/NET pill (i.e. Table 4.10 takes precedence). Best choices: Loestrin 20 or the new 20 μg EE+LNG pill.
4. Some of the numbers selected are arbitrary and perhaps too strict if they are the sole problem (for example the COC might actually be allowed, reluctantly, to a currently healthy 25 year old admitting to two packs of cigarettes a day). They also relate to use for contraception. Use of COCs for medical indications often entails a different risk/benefit analysis, i.e. the extra therapeutic benefits may outweigh expected extra risks.

NB This table is to be used in conjunction with Table 4.10, page 183.

35 µg ethinyloestradiol and no more than 150 µg levonorgestrel or 1 mg norethisterone. Yet preparations containing desogestrel or gestodene may have an additional therapeutic role in women with specific medical conditions, such as acne and hirsutism.

Reasons: first-timers include an unknown subgroup who are VTE-predisposed + VTE is a more relevant consideration than arterial disease at this age + the pills are cheaper.

3 **Single risk factor for venous thrombosis**: LNG or NET product preferred, if COC used at all.
4 **Single risk factor for arterial disease**: see Q4.118.

4.117 WHICH PILL FOR A WOMAN WHO FINDS SHE DOES NOT TOLERATE A LNG/NET COC – BECAUSE OF PERSISTENT BREAKTHROUGH BLEEDING OR ANDROGENIC OR OTHER 'MINOR' SIDE-EFFECTS – OR WHO JUST WANTS A CHANGE?

As already stated, the differential risk between pill types is small compared with other ordinary risks in life, and the pill difference may even be smaller than the 1995 estimates (see above). If a woman actually or *predictably* will not tolerate an LNG or NET COC, because of persistent breakthrough bleeding or 'minor' side-effects such as acne, headaches, depression, weight gain, or breast symptoms, or wants a change for personal reasons, use of a DSG or GSD product is medicolegally very secure.

To quote the Faculty of Family Planning, 'the prescriber should respect the user's informed choice' if she chooses to (continue to) take any marketed pill, 'even if only because she is satisfied with it'. *The informed user should be the chooser.*

4.118 WHICH PILL FOR A WOMAN WITH A SINGLE DEFINITE ARTERIAL RISK FACTOR (FROM TABLE 4.11)? OR HEALTHY AND RISK-FACTOR-FREE BUT ABOVE AGE 35?

All the studies, including the RCGP study, the Oxford/FPA study, the American Nurses study, WHO (1998) and MICA (1999), have been *unable* to detect any increased risk of acute myocardial infarction (AMI) in non-smokers, whether they were current or past pill-takers. This means the arterial event risk of using *all* the modern low-oestrogen brands must be very small, if not absent, for women free of arterial risk factors. But it is high when they are present (the RCGP's relative risk estimate is 20.8 for

COMBINED ORAL CONTRACEPTION

smoking pill-takers), the risk increases with age and the case-fatality rate for AMI is also much higher (Q 4.99).

Therefore I do not feel the suggestive data that DSG/GSD pills *might* have relative advantages for arterial wall disease in higher risk women should be discounted.

Switching to a low oestrogen DSG or GSD pill should logically be at least mooted with smokers (and others with an arterial risk factor) *as they get older* (late 20s to early 30s) – for the two reasons:

1 That it is only in the older age group that arterial disease becomes common enough to be relevant to prescribing policy.
2 If she has already been on *any* COC (EE combined with any progestogen) for some years without a VTE she is relatively unlikely to be one of the individuals with a hereditary (or acquired) predisposition to venous thrombosis. Those women would be likely to suffer a VTE event relatively early during pill use (or during any full-term pregnancy) and so leave the population of long-term users. Yet this previous uncomplicated use does not entirely exclude the risk of VTE in future, especially as, regardless of using any pill, VTE risk goes up with *age*.

Until we have the option of a 20 µg GSD product, Mercilon 20 may often be the most logical choice for these women (no later than age 35 though!!); and also for arterial risk-factor-free women from 35 to 50 years of age. (Loestrin 20 would currently be a better product if there were any additional concern about VTE risk.)

4.119 PRESUMABLY THE VERBAL CONSENT OF WOMEN NOT USING THE PILL BRANDS RECOMMENDED BY THE CSM MUST BE WELL RECORDED?

Yes: if a DSG/GSD pill is chosen (whether for this arterial risk factor indication or just because the woman prefers it on quality of life grounds) there must, for medicolegal security, always be a full contemporaneous record:

• of the risk factor history;
• that the woman accepts a possibly increased risk of VTE – amounting at most to 10 cases (or 0.2 deaths) per 100 000 per year, relative to other formulations.

This counselling must also be backed always by a user-friendly leaflet, such as the COC leaflet produced by the UK FPA, and it is prudent to note down the date of issue of the leaflet that was given.

There remains considerable uncertainty here, through lack of epidemiological data. Intriguingly, one of the main metabolites of norgestimate (NGM) is biologically active (levo)norgestrel (22% by weight, equivalent to about 55 μg of the 250 μg in each tablet). As we saw above this is a relatively anti-oestrogenic progestagen. So one might expect some counteraction of the oestrogenicity, and maybe therefore the VTE thrombogenicity, of the 35 μg of ethinyloestradiol which Cilest contains.

At present we cannot be certain whether the same argument would mean that norgestimate – plus its metabolite levonorgestrel 55 μg in conjunction with its other active metabolites (especially 17-deacetyl-NGM) acting together – in combination with 35 μg EE would be relatively better *for the arterial walls* than levonorgestrel 150 μg in Microgynon 30?

We need more data. In practice, we can continue to use Cilest without the medicolegal anxieties raised by the CSM letter of 18/10/95. Cilest seems to be working out as not specially to be favoured when one has a strong concern *either* about VTE *or* about the arterial walls; but it remains a valuable choice for many women.

[Another progestagenic substance used in UK combination pills is cyproterone acetate, which is an anti-androgen used in the formulation Dianette and considered later, Q 4.237, in relation to treatment for acne and hirsutes. This is clearly an oestrogen-dominant product, and its VTE risk is unlikely in my view to differ significantly from DSG or GSD containing pills.]

MORE ABOUT THE AVAILABLE PILL FORMULATIONS

It is much easier to say what they are not! The doses in the first brands marketed in the 1960s, on which indeed much of the early epidemiology was based, were clearly too high. On the market then was a brand which gave more of the same oestrogen in a day than is now given in a week; and

TABLE 4.12 REDUCTION IN DOSES SINCE COMBINED PILLS WERE FIRST INTRODUCED

	Dose of sex steroid per tablet in 1962	Minimum of same as used in 1992
Ethinyloestradiol (EE)	150 µg in Enovid 10	20 µg in Mercilon 20, Loestrin 20
Norethisterone (NET)	10 000 µg in Ortho-Novum 10	500 µg in Ovysmen/Brevinor

Note: 15 µg EE pills are now marketed in continental Europe (and expected in the UK).

virtually the same daily dose of a progestagen as now covers a complete cycle! See Table 4.12.

In short, safer pills seem generally to be 'smaller pills'. Both the constituent hormones are capable of unwanted metabolic effects and their epidemiological consequences. After saying that the question is still, after all these years, impossible to answer more specifically. And anyway it will depend on whether one is considering arterial or venous disease.

Above all we must retain a *range* of formulations so as to have flexibility in prescribing when 'minor' side-effects occur (Qs 4.197 and 4.198, 4.245 and 4.246).

A policy based on preferring 'smaller' pills should reduce the risk of *major side-effects*. Clinical experience with the lowest doses also shows that, with one exception, *minor side-effects* (see Q 4.198) are less frequent and less severe.

What is the exception? The obvious one is cycle control: but that can be handled, as part of the follow-up prescribing scheme to be described (Q 4.155–4.172).

4.122 WHAT ARE THE FUNDAMENTAL PROBLEMS IN APPLYING A 'SAFER PILLS' POLICY?

1. The first is *knowing what they really are*. There are almost no RCTs and too few cohort studies comparing formulations, with large enough numbers and relevant epidemiological end-points. And if the VTE versus arterial disease story which led to the 'pill-scare' of October 1995 is eventually confirmed beyond doubt, it will be clear that we all had our hands burnt by relying on (the more easily obtainable) metabolic surrogate markers like HDL-cholesterol. ...

2 Then there is *individual variation*. A medium-dose pill for one woman could be in its biological effect a low-dose pill for another, or a high-dose pill for a third.

It is thus a false expectation that any single pill will suit all women. We return to this point below, see Figure 4.14 and Qs 4.155–4.172.

4.123 WHAT ARE THE PILL BRANDS AVAILABLE, AND HOW MAY THEY BE CLASSIFIED?

The practitioner is faced with a variety of formulations (Table 4.13; Figure 4.12). As first proposed by Dr Barbara Law, former Chairman of the Joint Committee on Contraception, they may be grouped in ladders according to the particular progestagen they contain, each lower rung representing a lower hormone content than those above (Fig. 4.12). The philosophy behind this display is that the lower down a ladder one is, the less likely is injury if one falls off! The POPs are shown as being the least likely to cause side-effects – on ground level.

4.124 WHY ARE THERE ONLY FIVE LADDERS IN FIGURE 4.12, AND HOW DO THEY DIFFER FROM EACH OTHER?

1 Since norethisterone acetate is converted in vivo with better than 90% efficiency to norethisterone, all formulations using it are part of the norethisterone group.
2 Cyproterone acetate is considered later (Q 4.237)

4.125 WHY IS D-NORGESTREL CALLED LEVONORGESTREL? PLEASE EXPLAIN.

Norgestrel is a racemic mixture of a *d*-isomer and *l*-isomer. It is given the prefix '*d*' because it shares the same special orientation as other molecules which by the conventions of stereochemistry are all called the *d*-forms. However, when in solution it deviates light in the opposite direction (i.e. to the left) and is therefore known as levonorgestrel.

The opposite applies to *l*-norgestrel which rotates light to the right. It is also biologically inactive. Yet it has to be metabolized. Hence where there exists a choice (e.g. see Table 5.1) it is preferable to use the nearest equivalent brand which uses pure levonorgestrel.

TABLE 4.13 FORMULATIONS OF CURRENTLY MARKETED COMBINED ORAL CONTRACEPTIVES

Pill type	Preparation	Oestrogen (μg)	Progestagen (μg)
Monophasic			
Ethinyloestradiol/ norethisterone type	Loestrin 20	20	1000 Norethisterone acetate*
	Loestrin 30	30	1500 Norethisterone acetate*
	Brevinor	35	500 Norethisterone
	Ovysmen	35	500 Norethisterone
	Norimin	35	1000 Norethisterone
Ethinyloestradiol/ levonorgestrel	Microgynon 30 (also ED)	30	150
	Ovranette	30	150
	Eugynon 30	30	250
	Ovran 30	30	250
	Ovran	50	250
Ethinyloestradiol/ desogestrel	Mercilon	20	150
	Marvelon	30	150
Ethinyloestradiol/ gestodene	Femodene (also ED)	30	75
	Minulet	30	75
Ethinyloestradiol/ norgestimate	Cilest	35	250
Mestranol/ norethisterone	Norinyl-1	50	1000
Bi/triphasic			
Ethinyloestradiol/ norethisterone	BiNovum	35	500 } 833† (7 tabs)
		35	1000 } (14 tabs)
	Synphase	35	500 (7 tabs)
		35	1000 } 714 (9 tabs)
		35	500 (5 tabs)
	TriNovum	35	500 (7 tabs)
		35	750 } 750 (7 tabs)
		35	1000 (7 tabs)

TABLE 4.13 (cont'd)

Pill type	Preparation	Oestrogen (μg)	Progestogen (μg)	
Bi/triphasic (cont'd)				
Ethinyloestradiol/ levonorgestrel	Logynon (also ED)	30 } 40 } 32† 30 }	50 } 75 } 92† 125 }	(6 tabs) (5 tabs) (10 tabs)
	Trinordiol	30 } 40 } 32 30 }	50 } 75 } 92 125 }	(6 tabs) (5 tabs) (10 tabs)
Ethinyloestradiol/ gestodene	Tri-Minulet	30 } 40 } 32 30 }	50 } 70 } 79 100 }	(6 tabs) (5 tabs) (10 tabs)
	Triadene	30 } 40 } 32 30 }	50 } 70 } 79 100 }	(6 tabs) (5 tabs) (10 tabs)
New monophasic brand‡				
Ethinyloestradiol/ levonorgestrel	Microgynon 20	20	100	

*Converted to norethisterone as the active metabolite.
†Equivalent daily doses for comparison with monophasic brands.
‡This brand is not available at time of writing, but is expected.

See also Q 4.127 for new products awaited.

4.126 WHICH COC BRANDS ARE NORMALLY UNACCEPTABLE FOR ROUTINE PRESCRIBING?

1 The 50-μg oestrogen brands, since the aim of effective contraception is achievable with less oestrogen in most cases. *However, there are very definite exceptions* (Qs 4.166 and 4.203).
2 The brands giving 250 μg of levonorgestrel (*Eugynon 30, Ovran 30*) do markedly lower HDL-cholesterol, which seems to be worth avoiding. Their use should be restricted to gynaecological indications, such as the maintenance treatment of endometriosis (see Q 4.129), though I prefer initially to tricycle Microgynon 30.

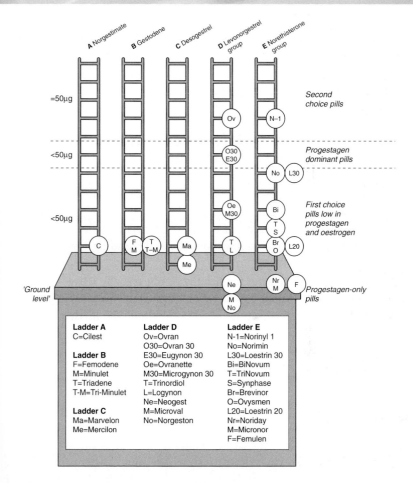

Figure 4.12   Pill ladders – arranged by progestagen. Q 4.123 and following.

4.127 WHAT NEW FORMULATIONS ARE ON THE HORIZON?

Gracial – a 22-day biphasic, giving desogestrel 25 µg + EE 40 µg for 7 days, then desogestrel 125 µg + EE 30 µg for 15 days – was expected years ago, is licensed in continental Europe but is still (1999) not marketed in the UK.

There are potentially very useful 20 µg or even 15 µg EE products combined with gestodene, some with the recommended shortened pill-free interval (Q 4.27), also available abroad. But their marketing in the UK is likewise still delayed, I understand by medicolegal considerations arising out of the CSM's 1995 letter.

'*Microgynon 20*' is the working name for a useful 20 μg EE + 100 μg levonorgestrel product, still awaited in the UK.

INDICATIONS AND CONTRAINDICATIONS FOR THE COC METHOD, IN DEPTH

4.128 FOR WHOM IS THE COC METHOD PARTICULARLY INDICATED?

The patient who decides that maximum protection from pregnancy and independence from intercourse are the most important features *in her own view*. But she may also use it without currently needing contraception (Q 4.129).

It is particularly valuable for the healthy young sexually active non-smoking woman who is sufficiently motivated to be a reliable pill-taker. If and when she is at risk of STIs she should be advised to use condoms as well.

4.129 FOR WHAT DISORDERS AND DISEASES IS THE COMBINED PILL PRESCRIBED?

Because the extra requirement for treatment increases the benefit side of the benefit–risk equation, it may sometimes be acceptable to prescribe higher-dose pills or to give the COC to women with one or more relative contraindications. A specialist's advice should be sought where appropriate.

The COC can be invaluable therapy to:

1 relieve spasmodic dysmenorrhoea;
2 'regulate' menstrual cycles, in cases of prolonged bleeding with no demonstrable pathology, but also for secondary amenorrhoea once characterized. Indeed, the reason for any cycle irregularity or secondary amenorrhoea should always be determined first: but then the pill may well be the most appropriate treatment, especially for hypo-oestrogenic states (see Qs 4.64–4.66);
3 relieve premenstrual syndrome. This is not always successful, indeed some women develop similar symptoms when taking the COC.

However, ablating the normal menstrual cycle is well-recognized therapy for PMS. In my experience using a monophasic COC for that purpose but replacing with a 10-week pill cycle through *tricycling* as described at Q 4.31 can be invaluable. Sufferers usually report at least that they now get the PMS symptoms only towards the end of each tricycle (i.e. only five times per year!) – and sometimes that the episodes are milder as well as less frequent;

4 control menorrhagia. If fibroids are present and surgery not indicated a relatively progestagen-dominant pill should be chosen with continued monitoring by the same observer;

5 control endometriosis as maintenance after first-line treatment (progestagen-dominant brand, best to start with Microgynon 30 using the tricycle regimen (see Qs 4.31 and 4.227));

6 control functional ovarian cysts (see Q 4.59), and ovulation pain if severe;

7 relieve oestrogen deficiency, e.g. in athletes with amenorrhoea (Qs 4.64) and to control gynaecological/menstrual cyclical symptoms in healthy non-smoking peri-menopausal women still requiring contraception – though becoming oestrogen ± progesterone deficient;

8 control the manifestations of the polycystic ovarian syndrome (PCOS), despite this not being a condition of oestrogen deficiency but rather of androgen excess (see Q 4.64). Also useful for acne treatment without PCOS;

9 as prophylaxis against ovarian cancer, for women at high risk (Q 4.56).

NOTE: Triphasic pills are usually not appropriate for these indications, since the intention is often to abolish the normal cycle, and they may too closely simulate it.

4.130 WHAT IS THE WHO SYSTEM FOR CLASSIFYING CONTRAINDICATIONS?

This system, which I had a hand in devising at a WHO meeting in Atlanta early in 1994, is described in a WHO document WHO/FRH/FPP96.9. There are four categories, as shown in the Box below. Numbers 1 and 4 are unchanged when compared to what we are used to (i.e. when the method is *always* or *never* usable). The useful new feature of the classification is separation into two categories of *relative* contraindication:

WHO classification of Contraindications
[with amplifications by J. Guillebaud]

1 A condition for which there is no restriction for the use of the contraceptive method

'A' is for ALWAYS USABLE

2 A condition where the advantages of the method generally outweigh the theoretical or proven risks

'B' is for BROADLY USABLE

3 A condition where the theoretical or proven risks usually outweigh the advantages. But – respecting the patient/client's autonomy – if she accepts the risks and rejects or should not use relevant alternatives, the method can be used with caution/additional care

'C' is for CAUTION/COUNSELLING, if used at all

4 A condition which represents an unacceptable health risk

'D' is for DO NOT USE, at all

Notes:
1 Although the A–B–C–D scheme is a helpful aide-memoire to what each category signifies, I shall stick with the WHO's 1–2–3–4 classification in this book to avoid any confusion. So wherever WHO 3 is mentioned below 'Caution, extra counselling' is intended.
2 Clinical judgement is required in consultation with the contraceptive user, especially:
   (a) in all category 3 conditions – would another method be an even better choice?
   (b) If more than one condition applies. As a working rule, two category 2 conditions moves the situation to category 3; and if any category 3 condition applies the addition of either a 2 or a 3 condition normally amounts to category 4 (DO NOT USE).

NOTE: We must not lose sight of the purpose of this WHO initiative, which is to remove 'medical barriers' to contraceptive use: i.e. wrong or misclassified contraindications, which end by depriving people of what would be the best method for them and may lead to avoidable pregnancies!

4.131 WHAT ARE THE ABSOLUTE CONTRAINDICATIONS TO COCs (ALL FORMULATIONS)? – i.e. WHO 4. ...

Any compilation of contraindications reflects the judgement of the compiler, as much as the available science at the relevant date. The answers to this and the next two questions are as assessed by me in 1999!

- Many important diseases are considered in considerably more detail elsewhere – **please see Index.**
- NB: very few of the contraindications to the COC (whether absolute or relative) apply to the LNG-IUS, Q 6.143–6.144, which can be a most useful choice.

A. Past or present circulatory disease

- Any past proven *arterial or venous thrombosis.*
- *Ischaemic heart disease* or angina, all *cardiomyopathies, Kawasaki disease* (maybe WHO 3 after full recovery).
- *Severe or combined risk factors for venous or arterial disease* **(see Tables 4.10, 4.11, pages 183 and 185). Includes**: if the family or personal history strongly suggests testing for a thrombophilia or lipid disorder and the tests cannot be done.
- Known *atherogenic lipid disorders*: COC usually avoided while total cholesterol is above 8 mmol/l. Check with physician – may be or become WHO 3 situation.
- Specific *prothrombotic abnormalities* of coagulation/fibrinolysis – including the *congenital thrombophilias* with abnormal levels of individual factors; presence of any *acquired thrombophilia* especially the *antiphospholipid syndrome.*
- Other conditions known to predispose to thrombosis including: severe primary or secondary *polycythaemia; Klippel–Trenaunay syndrome; blood dyscrasias; some autoimmune and rheumatoid disorders* with this risk, including *polyarteritis nodosa, scleroderma* and *severe SLE;* and *postsplenectomy* for any indication if the *platelet count is above $500 \times 10^9/l$* (WHO 3 if lower platelet count).
- *Elective major or leg surgery* – from 2 but preferably 4 weeks before, until 2 weeks after full mobilization (do not demand that the COC be stopped for minor surgery such as laparoscopy); during *leg immobilization* e.g. after a fracture, or *varicose vein treatments*; and during exposure to *high altitude* (above 4500 m);

- *Severe inflammatory bowel disease*, including *Crohn's disease* also comes into this category during attacks, or WHO 3 in remissions.
- *Migraine with focal aura, and severe migraine* ('status migrainosus'); migraine *requiring ergotamine treatment*.
- *Transient ischaemic attacks* even without headache.
- *Past cerebral haemorrhage*, especially if secondary to *cerebral venous thrombosis*. But can otherwise be WHO 3 following surgery.
- Most types of *structural* or *uncorrected valvular heart disease* (discuss with cardiologist, could be WHO 3); intermittent or sustained *arrhythmias; atrial septal defect* (risk of paradoxical embolism); *pulmonary hypertension*.

B. Disease of the liver

- *Active liver disease* (whenever liver function tests currently abnormal, including infiltrations and cirrhosis);
- *Cholestatic jaundice*, if pill-related, or history of cholestatic jaundice in pregnancy (check with physician, may be WHO 3); Dubin-Johnson and Rotor syndromes which are congenital deficiencies of hepatic excretion. (But Gilbert's disease is WHO 1–2).

> **NOTE:** After any viral hepatitis, severe infectious mononucleosis or other reversible hepatocellular damage; COC-taking may be resumed 3 months after liver function tests have returned to normal.

- *Liver adenoma, carcinoma. FNH* (Q 4.91) is WHO 4, but could be WHO 3 with careful imaging during follow-up.
- *Gallstones* (but COCs may be resumed after cholecystectomy (WHO 2) – take surgeon's advice).
- The *acute porphyrias* (other porphyrias are in WHO 2 or 3 – Qs 4.218–219).

C. History of serious condition affected by sex steroids or related to previous COC use

- *Acute porphyrias, SLE, cholestatic jaundice*, already mentioned.
- *Chorea.*
- *COC-induced hypertension.*
- *Pancreatitis due to hypertriglyceridaemia.*
- *Pemphigoid gestationis* (formerly called herpes gestationis).
- Stevens–Johnson syndrome (*erythema multiforme*), if COC-associated.

- *Trophoblastic disease* but only until hCG levels are undetectable. (In the USA this is considered a relative contraindication even when hCG present, partly because chemotherapy is given to almost all cases of trophoblastic disease anyway).
- This is not necessarily a complete list of relevant diseases – **see Q 4.134 for how to assess any new condition affecting your patient.**

D. Existing or possible pregnancy

E. Undiagnosed genital tract bleeding

F. Oestrogen-dependent neoplasms
- *Breast cancer* (some oncologists permit COCs in selected cases in prolonged remission – but always WHO 3).
- Past breast biopsy showing premalignant *epithelial atypia* (see Q 4.87).
- All other cancers are normally relative contraindications (WHO 2, rarely 3), supervised use being permitted.

G Miscellaneous
- *Allergy* to a constituent of the tablets.
- *Haemolytic uraemic syndrome/thrombotic thrombocytopenic purpura.*

These poorly understood, related thrombotic syndromes may relapse repeatedly (hence WHO 4).

- Past *benign intracranial hypertension* (BICH).
- *Amaurosis fugax*: this transient complete loss of vision usually signifies transient retinal ischaemia, so obviously contraindicates the COC (WHO 4).

H. Woman's own continuing anxiety *re* COC safety, unrelieved after counselling

Several of the above (e.g. D, E, F and H) are not necessarily permanent contraindications.

4.132 RELATIVE CONTRAINDICATIONS – HOW ASSESSED AND HOW APPLIED?

Here we have the impact not just of my judgement as compiler, but yours as prescriber! The art of medicine is nowhere better shown than in assessing how strong each of the contraindications at Q 4.133 is (and that differs within the list – hence my use of the new WHO scheme of Q 4.130 above – as well as in different individuals), and then:

- balancing the risk of each against the benefits to each pill-taker;
- with allowance for synergism between risk factors and the general teaching that two or more relative contraindications equal one absolute contraindication (see also Q 4.130, Note 2(b));
- all in the light of everything relevant like her probable fertility and her other contraceptive choices;
- and *all, most emphatically, being discussed openly with the woman, so that she makes the final decision.* ...

Now see Q 4.133.

4.133 WHAT ARE THE RELATIVE CONTRAINDICATIONS TO THE COC?

1 First see Tables 4.10 (page 183) and 4.11 (page 185), i.e. risk factors for circulatory disease are all relative contraindications, mostly WHO 3: provided normally that only one is present, and not to so marked a degree that it alone would absolutely contraindicate this method. This category includes *essential hypertension* controlled by treatment; also past *toxaemia of pregnancy* which seems greatly to increase the risk of myocardial infarction in smokers (RCGP and MICA studies).

2 Long-term *partial immobilization* (e.g. in a wheelchair). *Complete* paralysis of the lower limbs is viewed by some as an absolute contraindication, especially if the BMI is >30.

3 *Sex steroid-dependent cancers in remission.* Seek the specialist's advice: most will (appropriately in my view) permit COC use for *melanoma* in remission after treatment (whether or not diagnosed during pill-taking). But the history of *breast cancer* is almost invariably considered an absolute contraindication (WHO 4) to the COC (Q 4.131).

4 *Oligo-/amenorrhoea* should be investigated but the pill may subsequently be prescribed – WHO 2 – or even positively indicated (WHO 1; see Qs 4.60–4.65)

5 *Hyperprolactinaemia*: this is now considered only a relative contraindication for patients under specialist supervision (WHO 3).

6 Very *severe depression*, if likely to be exacerbated by COCs (WHO 3). But unwanted pregnancies can be very depressing!

7 *Chronic systemic diseases.* These are discussed further below (see Qs 4.134–4.142). In general they are *weak* relative contraindications, category WHO 2, mainly signifying extra counselling and above average monitoring. Examples in the stronger WHO 3 category are: *porphyria*

cutanea tarda (see (Q 4.219); *Crohn's disease* in remission (see Q 4.141); *diabetes* (see Q 4.143); *chronic renal disease*; and mild (not steroid-treated, in remission) *systemic lupus erythematosis* (SLE), though the presence of antiphospholipid antibody absolutely contraindicates the COC (see Qs 4.131 and 4.142). In these the common reason for special caution is that the condition may lead in various ways to an increased risk of circulatory disease. If that risk became established, as in a diabetic with evidence of arteriopathy, it would be an absolute contraindication, see Q 4.143. In the case of SLE and Crohn's there is also the risk of sex hormones causing deterioration of the condition.

Splenectomy, for whatever reason performed (e.g. in the treatment of sickle-cell disease), is only a relative contraindication, WHO 2). However *the platelets should be monitored*, initially at least annually, and a count rising to above 500×10^9 per litre would absolutely contraindicate the oestrogen of the COC (WHO 4).

8 Diseases requiring long-term treatment with *enzyme-inducing drugs* which might reduce the efficacy of the pill (see Qs 4.34 and 4.36): provided the recommended regimen is followed, this is only WHO 2.

9 New relative contraindications now include:
 (a) if a young (< 40 years) *first-degree relative has had breast cancer* (WHO 3);
 (b) the presence of *BBD* (WHO 2) but WHO 4 (?3) if atypia, see Q 4.87;
 (c) during the monitoring of *abnormal cervical smears* (WHO 2);
 (d) during and after definitive *treatment for CIN* (WHO 2);
 Women in groups (a) and (b) need recounselling after about 4–5 years' use. CIN follow-up (i.e. groups (c) plus (d)) amounts to only a very *weak* relative contraindication, due to the data suggesting the COC is a co-factor for CIN, so it would be standard practice to continue the COC, with monitoring as advised by the laboratory.

4.134 ON WHAT CRITERIA CAN ONE DECIDE WHETHER THE COC MAY BE USED FOR PATIENTS WITH INTERCURRENT DISEASE?

First, there are some conditions which are positively benefited (see Qs 4.55 and 4.129) or at least not affected. There are persistent medical myths (see Q 4.252), and it is unfortunate that women continue to be unnecessarily deprived of the COC for the wrong reasons, like thrush, uncomplicated varicose veins, past amenorrhoea, current hypo-oestrogenic amenorrhoea (e.g. weight-related) or fibroids.

It is impossible to list every known disease or state which might have a bearing on pill-prescribing, but here are some useful criteria:

In general, discover first what the disease does in relation to known risks or effects of the COC. Does it cause *changes which summate with adverse effects of the COC*? Does it:

1 Increase the risk of arterial or venous thrombosis, anywhere? This includes consideration of restricted mobility.
2 Predispose to arterial wall disease?
3 Adversely affect liver function?
4 Show a tendency to an important degree of sex hormone dependency, either by medical reputation (usually then a relative contraindication), or in that individual (absolute contraindication). If there was deterioration with previous administration of steroid hormones or during pregnancy, it means enough to be an absolute contraindication if the condition is serious.
5 Require treatment with an enzyme-inducing drug?

If 5 is true the pill can still be an option, but special conditions apply (see Q 4.36). If 1–4 apply there is the real problem of deciding whether the COC should be absolutely or (as at Q 4.133) relatively contraindicated (meaning not WHO 4 but WHO 3).

NB, *The added risk obtaining in pregnancy may fully justify some increased risk due to the COC*, at least in young and hence more fertile women, primarily because it is so effective. Its other benefits may also be highly relevant in some conditions. This is not so, however, for the list at Q 4.131 (WHO 4, absolute contraindications). For them, remember injectables and IUDs/IUSs!

If none of the above criteria apply, then the condition could normally be added to the following list in Q 4.135.

4.135 CAN YOU LIST THOSE MEDICAL CONDITIONS IN WHICH THE COC IS BROADLY USABLE SINCE THERE IS NO CONVINCING EVIDENCE THAT DETERIORATION MAY BE CAUSED?

According to current information, the following diseases all come into this 'Broadly usable' category (WHO 2):

AIDS/HIV (see Q 4.243), asthma, Gilbert's disease, treated Hodgkin's disease (if fertility preserved), hereditary lymphoedema, multiple sclerosis, myasthenia gravis, Raynaud's disease (unless the phenomenon proves to be symptomatic of a contraindicating condition), renal dialysis, retinitis pigmentosa, rheumatoid arthritis, sarcoidosis, spherocytosis, thalassaemia major, thyrotoxicosis and Wolff–Parkinson–White syndrome. Also most cancers under treatment, if hormone dependency or an increase in the risk of thrombosis are not suspected.

In individual cases the prescriber should, nevertheless, first review the checklist at Q 4.134 above and, normally, consult with the hospital specialist(s) supervising treatment for the main disorder: to obtain their support and also to guard against unforeseen drug interactions, etc. Such women need extra supervision within primary care as well (shared care). NB reliable protection from pregnancy is often particularly important when chronic diseases are present.

NOTE: There are of course many other illnesses in the textbooks, too numerous to mention here: the solution to prescribing queries is to evaluate each condition as described in Q 4.134 above.

4.136 IS THE COMBINED PILL BEST AVOIDED AT HIGH ALTITUDE?

There is certainly an issue to discuss with the woman concerned. Acute mountain sickness can kill, through hypoxia leading to acute pulmonary oedema and cerebral oedema, and blood clots in the small arteries are a feature *post-mortem*. In milder attacks well short of that, when unacclimatized people climb above about 3000 m (*c.* 10 000 ft), there is an increasing risk of venous or arterial thromboembolism, including strokes. Increased capillary permeability leads to shifts in body fluids, tissue oedema and haemoconcentration, leading to raised blood viscosity in the short term. Although fibrinolysis is increased at altitude and during exercise, other circumstances in climbing are thrombogenic: fluid loss or inadequate intake, trauma, immobility in tents when the weather closes in.

Acetazolamide (Diamox), which has been shown to improve climbing performance and prevent acute mountain sickness, acts as a mild diuretic and might exacerbate the thrombotic risk. There is also pulmonary hypertension in the more severe cases.

From the practical point of view, the COC is very useful to control menstrual bleeding, especially if tricycled. Yet BTB is a common problem for some women at altitude.

Autonomy is an important principle here: rock-climbing is orders of magnitude more dangerous than any risks modifiable by choice of contraceptive! The woman must have freedom to take an added risk, but the prescriber has autonomy too if s/he thinks the risk of COC unacceptable (WHO 4).

The Newsletter of the International Society for Mountain Medicine discussed the issue in April 1998. Table 4.14 summarizes the consensus reached concerning COC use.

4.137 IS THERE A CONTINUING PROBLEM FOR THOSE WHO LIVE LONG TERM AT HIGH ALTITUDE?

In residents, after prolonged acclimatization there is a physiological polycythaemia which slightly increases blood viscosity; but this alone would be only a weak relative contraindication (WHO 2) to EE in the combined pill.

TABLE 4.14 USE OF THE COC AT HIGH ALTITUDE

Circumstances	Advice based on WHO categories
If altitude to be >4500 metres for more than 1 week	WHO 4 DO NOT USE (Could be WHO 3, cautious use if she is aware of risks, is sure in her mind and no other risk factors)
Never reaching 4500 metres, or for less time	WHO 3 CAUTION (Could be WHO 4, however, if any risk factor for venous or arterial disease. If more than one risk factor, should not use COC even at sea level!)
All others, including most trekkers	WHO 2 BROADLY USABLE, again after assessing other risks/risk factors. (But woman should be fully informed of small added risk of venous/arterial thrombosis inevitable at altitude)

NB. Always reassess in the light of new factors developing, e.g. immobilization, trauma, dehydration
Alternatives: all other methods OK, including any progestagen-only method (e.g. injectable or the POP). Emergency contraception is also usable (any form).

4.138 WHAT ABOUT LONG-HAUL AEROPLANE FLIGHTS AND THROMBOSIS RISK?

As the sole risk factor this is WHO 2 – the COC is broadly usable and need not, indeed should not be stopped (the risks of pregnancy would be far greater!). However, although all commercial flights are pressurized to the equivalent of about 2000 m, there are now numerous case reports of pulmonary embolism and some deaths (with or without the pill). As at high altitude, some extracellular to interstitial fluid shift is common; mild ankle oedema results, but more important is the likelihood of intravascular volume depletion and haemoconcentration. Other important factors are the maintained sedentary position, coupled with a diuresis due to alcohol and caffeine, all perhaps superimposed on dehydration due to prolonged sunbathing on a Far Eastern beach just before boarding!

Evaluation of risk factors especially for VTE (Table 4.10, page 183) is again essential. If the woman has a high BMI she should forget glamour and wear support hose. She also might consider stopping HRT just to cover the intercontinental flight. But as far as the pill itself is concerned,

To quote my book *The Pill*:

There is no necessity to come off the pill – many flight attendants use it all the time. But follow their example and take some exercise during the flight: such as a brief walk around the plane every hour or so.

4.139 MAY THE COMBINED PILL BE PRESCRIBED TO PATIENTS WITH SICKLE-CELL DISORDERS?

Yes is the answer for those with sickle-cell trait. The situation with regard to homozygous sickle-cell disease (SS and SC genes) is more uncertain. There is an increased risk of thromboembolic disease especially strokes in such women, and pregnancy may precipitate a crisis. The COC imitates pregnancy, and the oestrogen of the pill might in theory lead to superimposed thrombosis during the arterial stasis of a crisis. Therefore, until recently most manufacturers and many authorities have included the frank sickling diseases among absolute contraindications to the COC. However studies in the West Indies and West Africa have shown that the COC ought now to be considered only a relative contraindication (WHO 2, especially when balanced against the great risks of pregnancy in sicklers). Injectables especially DMPA, are usually an even better choice (see Q 5.95).

4.140 MAY A WOMAN WHO HAS MADE A COMPLETE RECOVERY FROM A SUBARACHNOID HAEMORRHAGE, AND HAD HER INTRACRANIAL LESION TREATED, USE THE COMBINED PILL?

The COC is relatively contraindicated (WHO 3) if there is a close subsequent watch for hypertension, but the POP or an injectable would be preferable. This is because almost all women on the combined pill have a detectable slight increase in systolic and diastolic blood pressure, and one can never be certain that such a woman would not have some other weakness of a cerebral artery or angiomatous malformation.

4.141 WHY ARE THE INFLAMMATORY BOWEL DISEASES (CROHN'S OR ULCERATIVE COLITIS (UC)) RELATIVE CONTRAINDICATIONS?

1   Both occur more commonly in COC-takers in some studies. Crohn's (but not UC) is also strongly linked with smoking.
2   Non-granulomatous colonic Crohn's may improve if the COC is stopped (see Q 4.216). But 300 pill takers with stable disease had no more flare-ups over time than non-takers (*Gut* 1999; 45: 218–22).
3   In exacerbations of either illness there is a high risk of thrombosis, especially venous thromboembolism. Therefore if the COC is used it should be only in cases not prone to severe hospitalized exacerbations, and if such occur the pill should be stopped at once, and would be absolutely contraindicated so long as the disease remained severe (WHO 4).

Malabsorption. Since contraceptive steroids are so well absorbed, mainly in the jejunum which is unaffected, malabsorption of the COC is usually not a problem in either condition.

4.142 MAY THE COC BE USED BY WOMEN WITH SYSTEMIC LUPUS ERYTHEMATOSUS (SLE)?

Increasingly, this is being seen as an *absolute contraindication* (WHO 4) *except in the mildest very stable fully investigated cases not on steroids, with close supervision* (WHO 3 – but a progestagen-only method would be preferable). This is because of the following:

1   There are now numerous case reports and some comparative studies describing the onset or flaring up of symptomatic SLE when oestrogen was given, either in the COC or even, interestingly, as hormone

replacement therapy postmenopausally. SLE may deteriorate seriously with renal involvement for the first time during use of COCs, but not with progestagen-only therapy.

2 There is a recurring theme of recovery or improvement once the artificial oestrogen was discontinued.

3 Cases may develop the lupus anticoagulant/antiphospholipid antibody and once detected the COC is definitely contraindicated for fear of thrombosis.

Obviously each patient has to be taken on her own merits. But since progestagen-only pills and injections have been tried in SLE women with no significant increase in episodes of active disease, these are usually *preferred to the COC.*

4.143 MAY THE COMBINED PILL BE USED BY PATIENTS WITH ESTABLISHED DIABETES MELLITUS (DM)?

Arterial disease is a major hazard for diabetics; hence ideally they should avoid oestrogen with its prothrombotic risks. A barrier method, or the POP (see Q 5.45), or Implanon™, or an IUD/IUS, are all to be preferred.

In practice, however, some young diabetics are permitted use of an ultra-low-oestrogen combined pill using a 'lipid friendly' progestagen. Mercilon with only 20 μg oestrogen would be a good choice. Necessary criteria are:

1 Young, ideally under age 25, and preferably having had DM for a short time.

2 Free of *any* signs of complications of the disease, affecting arteries, nerves, kidneys or retina.

3 Free of the other conditions in Table 4.11, page 185. It is vital that such a patient is not also a smoker, hypertensive or with a BMI above 30.

4 Perceived to need maximum protection against pregnancy and there is no satisfactory alternative. In short: WHO 3 at best, otherwise WHO 4.

Diabetics occasionally then need an increased dose of insulin, not in itself a problem. They should be on the COC for the shortest possible time, encouraged to have their family as young as their circumstances allow, and then be transferred to another long-term method – ideally IUD/IUS or possibly sterilization.

4.144 MAY POTENTIAL OR LATENT DIABETICS TAKE THE COC?

Yes: caution used to be advised, because the early pills did impair glucose tolerance and create hyperinsulinism. However the RCGP study and others have shown absolutely no increase in the incidence of late-onset-type DM among current or ex-pill-users. Moreover, the more recent lowest-dose COCs do not even raise plasma insulins significantly. None of the following need therefore be considered as contraindications: a strong family history of DM (maturity onset); gestational diabetes; birth of a baby weighing more than 4.5 kg (10 lb).

Such women are just supervised a little more closely than usual and need particular advice to avoid obesity.

4.145 IF A YOUNG WOMAN SUFFERS A THROMBOSIS IN AN ARM VEIN AFTER AN INTRAVENOUS INJECTION, DOES THIS MEAN A PREDISPOSITION TO THROMBOSIS? SHOULD SHE AVOID THE COC (WHO 4), IN FUTURE?

The answer is no. The episode would be due to a chemical thrombophlebitis. This is not associated with any tendency to venous thrombosis elsewhere in the body.

4.146 IN WHAT WAY DOES THE POSSESSION OF BLOOD GROUP O INFLUENCE PRESCRIBING POLICY?

Women possessing blood group O have been shown to have a lower risk of thrombosis than those with other blood groups. The protective effect probably applies to arterial as well as venous disease. Knowledge of her blood group may therefore be helpful in a positive way, when prescribing to a woman who is otherwise not an ideal pill-user. For example, one would be happier to prescribe the COC to a 34-year-old smoker if she were known to be blood group O rather than A.

MIGRAINE HEADACHES, WITH AND WITHOUT AURA

4.147 WHAT IS A WORKING DEFINITION OF MIGRAINE AND WHY IS IT SO IMPORTANT IN PILL PRESCRIBING?

Whole chapters have been written just on this definition, and please read the article by Anne MacGregor and myself in the *British Journal of Family Planning* 1998;24:53–60. Migraines are here simply defined as unpleasant one-sided headaches with nausea, often but not always with a pulsating quality and photophobia/phonophobia.

Studies have shown an increased risk of ischaemic stroke in COC-users. There is evidence that this risk is further increased in migraine sufferers, especially with other arterial risk factors like smoking. Less well evidence-based but probably important (so prescribers need to be cautious, pending further data): certain features of the women or of the headaches may help to focus the risk of this rare catastrophe in a pill-taker. While trying to 'catch' such women, the recommendations below have been devised (and should be interpreted) in such a way as not to exclude unnecessarily too many women from a useful contraceptive, thereby adding in the risks of pregnancy. ...

4.148 WHAT ARE THE CLINICALLY SIGNIFICANT SYMPTOMS?

The symptoms to be carefully enquired about are those occurring during *migraine with aura* (formerly 'classical migraine'), evolving over several minutes and starting before the headache itself, resolving well within one hour. They are termed *focal neurological symptoms*:

- Visual symptoms (occur in 99% of true auras):
  - loss of sight, or of part or whole of the FIELD of vision, on one side (homonymous hemianopia). NB: complete loss of vision (amaurosis) in one eye is different. As it might be due to retinal artery or vein thrombosis it would require urgent attention including stopping the COC forthwith;
  - Teichopsia/fortification spectra, in which a bright scintillating angulated line enlarges from a bright centre on one side to form a C-shape surrounding the area of lost vision (*bright* scotoma).
- Other unilateral sensory disturbance (marked paraesthesia spreading up from fingers of one arm, or one side of the tongue); leg is rarely affected.
- Disturbance of speech (nominal dysphasia, paraphasia or dysarthria)
- Motor disturbance (unusual, e.g. weakness of a limb).

Note the absence of photophobia or *symmetrical* blurring or 'flashing lights': the main feature that the relevant symptoms share is asymmetry, meaning that they are 'focal' or interpretable as due to (transient) cerebral ischaemia.

4.149 WHAT IMPORTANT SYMPTOMS OR FEATURES ARE NOT TYPICAL OF MIGRAINE WITH AURA, AND HOW SHOULD THEY BE MANAGED?

These are:

- *sudden* onset or longer duration of the SAME symptoms as in Q 4.148;
- a *black* scotoma;
- sensory or motor loss affecting the whole of one side of the body or lower limb only.

These suggest possible cerebral thromboembolism or a transient ischaemic attack (TIA) and still mean the COC should immediately be stopped. But as with loss of consciousness or epilepsy they (unlike a straightforward history of migraine with focal aura) also signify *urgent referral* to a neurologist.

- It is reported also that it is possible in SCUBA divers to confuse with migraine the symptoms of compression sickness (which of course requires urgent transfer to a decompression chamber).

4.150 SO WHAT ARE THE ABSOLUTE CONTRAINDICATIONS? (TO COMMENCING OR CONTINUING THE COC, I.E. WHO CATEGORY 4)

1 *Migraine with aura during which there are the focal neurological symptoms of* Q 4.148. They are usually asymmetrical and typically preceding the headache itself. Should they occur, the *artificial oestrogen* of the COC should normally be stopped and thereafter avoided to minimize the risk of superimposed thrombosis causing permanent ischaemia – i.e. a thrombotic stroke.

2 *All other migraines even without aura which are unusually frequent/severe.* 'Status migrainosus' describes attacks lasting more than 72 hours, which contraindicate the COC absolutely – *unless* they resolve completely after treatment for medication misuse (see below).

3 *All migraines treated with ergot derivatives,* due to their vasoconstrictor actions.

4 *Moderately severe migraines without aura* PLUS additional arterial risk factors or relevant interacting diseases (e.g. connective tissue diseases linked with stroke risk).

See Figure 4.13 which comes from our article already quoted.

The additional risk factors are from Table 4.11 (page 185) above and they do include age above 35 (see Footnote 1 therein). They usually need to be more than one in number for migraines without aura to enter the category WHO 4, but one added risk factor could suffice if it was 'strong' (WHO 3) e.g. essential hypertension requiring treatment (Q 4.187).

4.151 WHAT ACTION SHOULD BE TAKEN APART FROM STOPPING THE COC?

Above all, organize with the woman an acceptable effective alternative contraceptive method! It is not a 'pill or nothing situation'.

In all the above circumstances any of the *progestagen-only, oestrogen-free* hormonal methods may be offered, immediately: similar headaches may continue, but now without the potential added risk from prothrombotic effects of the ethinyloestradiol. Particularly useful choices are DMPA (Q 5.82) and the LNG-IUS (Q 6.143), or a modern copper IUD.

4.152 SO WHEN IS MIGRAINE A 'STRONG' RELATIVE CONTRAINDICATION TO THE COMBINED PILL (WHO CATEGORY 3)?

See Figure 4.13. This means primarily migraine without focal aura where one (not 'severe') risk factor for ischaemic stroke is present. A good example of this is age above 35, even as the only risk factor. The reason for caution comes from considering how the attributable risk rises with age. According to Lidegaard's Danish data (in which women with aura were not excluded but most subjects had migraine without aura, occurring at least once per month):

The background annual risk of thrombotic stroke for women at age 20 is 2 in 100 000. Even with migraine > once per month, plus taking COC, this rises to 10 in 100 000. But at age 40, background risk is 20 in 100 000, rising to 56 in migraineurs (same attack frequency) and, with the same risk ratio (1.8) as for younger women, adding the COC makes 100 in 100 000 total incidence. And that is without being able to quantify the extra risk of focal aura.

Another WHO 3 example would be a 20-plus cigarette smoker in her 20s with moderately frequent/severe migraines without aura – because the (low) background incidence at 20 would have to be multiplied by a relative risk of 5 or 6 through having migraine and also taking the COC.

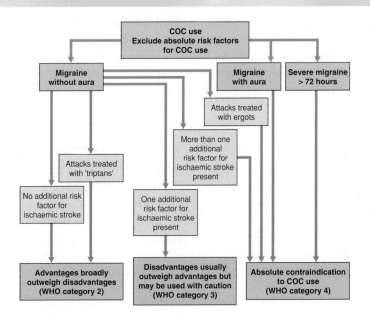

Figure 4.13 Flow diagram for COC use and migraine.

WHO category 3 always means caution/counselling. Along with general advice about controlling/watching for new risk factors, and the specific advice below about important possible future changes in her headache symptoms (see Q 4.148), the opportunity should be taken to discuss alternatives to the COC: particularly new options like modern IUDs and IUSs.

Q 4.153 WHEN WOULD MIGRAINE BE ONLY A WHO 2 RISK, AND HOW WOULD YOU COUNSEL SUCH WOMEN?

In my opinion the COC is 'Broadly usable' in all the following cases:

1 *Migraine without focal aura*, and also without any arterial risk factor from Table 4.11 and still under age 35.

   If these or other 'ordinary' headaches occur particularly in the pill-free interval, tricycling the COC may help (see Q 4.31).

2 *Use of a triptan (e.g. sumatriptan)* in the absence of any other contraindicating factors.

3 *Distant past history (at least 5 years earlier) during adolescence of migraine with focal aura*, before commencing the COC and no recurrences.

The COC may be given a trial with detailed forewarning about focal symptoms (see below)..

4   *The occurrence of a woman's first-ever attack of migraine without aura while on the COC.* It should be stopped if she is seen during the attack, but provided there were none of the features listed at Q 4.149, the COC can be later restarted with the usual counselling/caveats below.

> **NOTE:** The counselling of all such women (WHO category 3 and 2) must include specific instruction to the woman regarding those changes in the character or severity of her headache symptoms which mean she should stop the method and take urgent medical advice. These symptoms are at Q 4.148, and in more lay terms also appear – for all pill-takers to read (as is ideal) – in the Box on page 5 of the FPA's current Combined Pill leaflet.

4.154 WHICH COC BRANDS OR REGIMENS ARE BEST FOR HEADACHES AND NON-FOCAL 'COMMON' MIGRAINES?

Monophasic pills are generally preferred to triphasic pills (fully described below Q 4.174–4.179). The latter are not good for women with a tendency to any variety of headaches, since the extra fluctuations of the hormone levels may act as a trigger. In addition, in any woman whose headaches tend to happen in the PFI, it can be enormously helpful to prescribe the tricycle regimen, but again with a monophasic pill (see Q 4.31). *Note:* this is provided such migraine headaches never have focal symptoms.

INDIVIDUAL VARIATION IN BLOOD LEVELS OF SEX STEROIDS: THE IMPLICATIONS FOR TREATMENT OF THE SYMPTOM OF BREAKTHROUGH BLEEDING (BTB)

4.155 SINCE WOMEN VARY, IF THE FIRST PILL BRAND DOES NOT SUIT WHAT GUIDELINES ARE THERE TO HELP TO INDIVIDUALIZE THE SECOND OR SUBSEQUENT PILL PRESCRIPTION?

Some women do react unpredictably and several brands may have to be tried before a suitable one is found. Some are never suited. This is hardly surprising. Individual variation in motivation and tolerance of minor side-effects is well recognized, and the management is fully discussed later in this chapter. But as we shall see there is *also* marked individual variation in blood levels of the exogenous hormones and in responses at the end-organs, especially the endometrium.

To give a brief summary of what follows, prescribers should try to identify early in the use of the COC method, if necessary over a series of visits, the lowest dose for each woman which does not cause the annoying symptom of BTB. This should minimise adverse side-effects (both serious and minor) and also reduce the measurable metabolic changes. This approach does not impair effectiveness.

4.156 WHAT ARE THE IMPLICATIONS OF INDIVIDUAL VARIATION IN ABSORPTION AND METABOLISM FOR THE BLOOD LEVELS OF THE EXOGENOUS STEROIDS IN THE AVERAGE PILL-USER?

1 Blood levels, whether of EE or of all the progestagens which have been studied, vary at least ten-fold between women who are apparently similar, taking the same formulations and sampled exactly 12 hours after their last tablet was swallowed (see Fig. 4.14). The pharmacokinetic area under the curve (AUC) varies less, but still about threefold.

This is due to individual variation:
(a) in absorption;
(b) in metabolism, in the gut wall and in the liver, see Qs 4.33 and 4.34;
(c) in degree of binding to transport proteins especially SHBG in the blood plasma, which themselves are variably altered by different pills;
(d) in the efficiency with which normal EE is reformed and reabsorbed by the activity of the large bowel flora (see Q 4.34).

2 In addition to variable blood levels between women, there is a superimposed variation in target organ sensitivity. This is very difficult to assess and complicates matters further (see Q 4.170).

3 Then there is a further five- to tenfold fluctuation in any woman between the peaks after absorption and the troughs when the next daily tablet is taken. This saw-tooth pattern is shown in Figures 4.2 and 5.3 (see Q 5.85). Figure 5.3 also conveys one of the presumed advantages of slow-release systems of administration: relatively constant daily blood levels.

Titration of COC dose

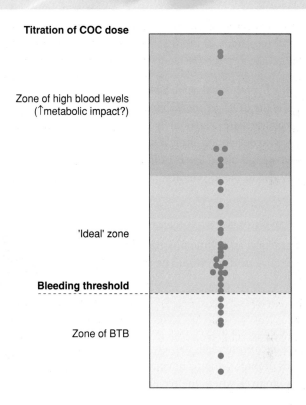

Zone of high blood levels
(↑metabolic impact?)

'Ideal' zone

Bleeding threshold

Zone of BTB

Figure 4.14 Schematic representation of the approximately 10-fold variability in peak blood levels of both contraceptive steroids, and the rationale of suggested 'titration' against the bleeding threshold. Q 4.156 and following.

4.157 WHAT IS THE RELEVANCE TO PILL-PRESCRIBING OF THIS GREAT VARIATION IN BLOOD LEVELS AND AUC BETWEEN DIFFERENT WOMEN TAKING THE SAME FORMULATION, AS IN FIGURE 4.14?

First, as already discussed fully above (see Q 4.38), there is pretty good evidence from research on enzyme inducers that women whose blood levels are low tend to suffer problems with endometrial stability (chiefly BTB). They may even conceive (especially if they ever lengthen the PFI).

4.158 WHAT ABOUT THOSE WOMEN WITH RELATIVELY HIGH CIRCULATING BLOOD LEVELS OF ARTIFICIAL STEROIDS? WHAT EVIDENCE IS THERE THAT SIDE-EFFECTS CAN BE CORRELATED?

It is a very tenable hypothesis that *metabolic changes and both major and minor side-effects of the COC are more common and more marked in those women whose blood levels are exceptionally high.* In support, pill-takers in an American study who developed clinical hypertension were statistically more likely to have high blood levels of EE, than control takers of similar pills without any rise in blood pressure.

4.159 IS IT FEASIBLE TO MEASURE THE LEVELS OF EITHER THE OESTROGEN OR PROGESTAGEN IN BODY FLUIDS?

This is not yet practical as a clinic procedure, though a simple testing kit for levels in the saliva or urine would be useful.

4.160 WITHOUT BLOOD LEVEL MEASUREMENTS, HOW MIGHT ONE ATTEMPT TO 'TAILOR' THE PILL TO THE INDIVIDUAL WOMAN?

I believe that one can, to a degree (see below). But not by the approach which used to be recommended, namely attempting to base the choice on assessed features of that woman's normal menstrual cycle. This was, in my view, always illogical, when one recalls that all COCs remove the normal cycle and replace it with an artificial one. That being so it is surely preferable to make the replacement cycle as good as it can be for all. The aim is that it should, after adjustments during follow-up (see Qs 4.245 and 4.246, and Tables 4.17 and 4.18), eventually be 'better' than each woman's normal cycle, rather than a slavish imitation of it.

I therefore promote the 'tailoring' approach which follows, designed to discover with the woman's cooperation the 'smallest' pill which gives her adequate control of her cycle.

4.161 IN FIGURE 4.14, WHAT DOES ABSENCE OF BTB MEAN?

On the hypothesis of Q 4.158, it could mean two very different things. Absence of BTB means either that the woman has ideal blood levels of the artificial hormones, or that they are *higher than necessary* for the desired effect of contraception – with plausibly a greater risk than necessary of causing unwanted effects.

4.162 HOW THEN MIGHT WE AVOID GIVING THE WOMEN WHO TEND TO THE HIGHER BLOOD LEVELS (OR LARGER AUC) A STRONGER PILL THAN THEY REALLY NEED?

By attempting during follow-up to give each woman the 'smallest' (lowest dose) pill her uterus will allow, without bleeding. This may mean titrating downwards, trying a pill lower in the same ladder – if not already tried and found to cause BTB.

4.163 WHAT IF BTB DOES OCCUR? DOES SHE NEED A HIGHER DOSE OR DIFFERENT FORMULATION?

Maybe! A higher dose pill (or a phasic or gestodene variety, see Qs 4.173 and 4.174) might be appropriate. But first and foremost, *important alternative causes of the bleeding must first be excluded* (see Table 4.15). I am aware of a young woman who was seen by a number of different doctors and nurses during 1991, complaining of BTB. They kept trying different brands without success until someone passed a speculum and, tragically, found an inoperable (adeno)-carcinoma of the cervix. She had had a reportedly negative cervical smear 1 year previously, but this was no excuse for the failure to examine. Note carefully also *all* the other possibilities in the Table; also Q 4.31 *re* tricycling.

4.164 WHAT OTHER 'Ds' MIGHT BE ADDED TO THOSE IN TABLE 4.15?

Since the last edition, during my lectures around the world a number of others have been suggested with varying degrees of seriousness, from the floor.

More causes of Breakthrough bleeding:

D for **D**octor-caused (poor instruction/advice)

D for **D**ud pills: iatrogenic causes (which have really happened) include wrong prescriptions for POPs and HRT products instead of the COC. Overdue **D**ate (time-expired product) or other cause of **D**amaged product is another possibility!

D for **D**iathesis/**D**yscrasia: a coincidental bleeding disease could first manifest itself this way.

A *note of caution*: first eliminate other possible causes!

The following checklist is modified from the book by Sapire (see Further Reading):

Disease – EXAMINE the cervix. It is not unknown for bleeding from an invasive cancer to be wrongly attributed to BTB. *Chlamydia* often causes a blood-stained discharge due to endometritis

Disorder of pregnancy causing bleeding (e.g. because of recent abortion, trophoblastic tumour)

Default – missed pill(s). Remember that the BTB may start 2 or 3 days later and be very persistent thereafter

Drugs – especially enzyme-inducers, see Qs 4.34 and Q 4.38 – cigarettes also relevant (Q 4.164). ...

Diarrhoea with VOMITING – diarrhoea alone has to be very severe to impair absorption significantly, see Q 4.25

Disturbance of absorption – likewise has to be very marked to be relevant, e.g. after *massive* gut resection.

Diet – gut flora involved in recycling EE may be reduced in vegetarians. Could sometimes be a factor in BTB, but not usually an important effect

Duration too short – minimal BTB which is tolerable may resolve after 2–3 months, see Qs 4.167, 4.266. See also Q 4.32 *re* BTB during tricycling (possible need to 'bicycle' instead)

Finally, after the above have been excluded:

Dose – if she is taking a monophasic, try a phasic pill
- increase the progestagen or oestrogen component
- try a different progestagen
- consider using a 50 µg pill or combination (see Qs 4.167, 4.168)

D for **D**rink: alcohol and other non-therapeutic substances; i.e. **D**rugs, chiefly because their abuse is a likely cause of **D**efault. (Liver enzyme induction by alcohol is not thought to be important.) Cigarettes are also now clearly linked (Oxford/FPA and Rosenberg studies, Am J Obs Gynecol 1996; 174: 628–32) to breakthrough bleeding, both in the pill cycle and in the normal cycle. This is thought to be the effect of increased catabolism of oestrogen induced by constituents of tobacco smoke)

INITIAL CHOICE OF PREPARATION, AND EARLY FOLLOW-UP

We are now in a position to consider how best to put the above facts and principles into practice. The objective is that each woman receives the *least long-term metabolic impact that her uterus will allow*, i.e. the lowest dose of contraceptive steroids which is just, but only just, above her own bleeding threshold.

4.165 WHAT IS THE NORMAL CHOICE FOR THE FIRST PILL PRESCRIPTION?

As previously stated there is no proven 'best buy'.

In general one does not choose the more complicated triphasics (see Qs 4.174–4.179) or 20 μg pills when future compliance is suspect. Pills known to have a relatively high rate of BTB are also best kept for trial later, when a new user is better able to cope (but all users must be advised about BTB should it occur, since forewarned is forearmed; see Q 4.266).

4.166 WHICH WOMEN MAY NEED CONSIDERATION OF A STRONGER FORMULATION (50 μg) FROM THE OUTSET?

Those women who are known to have reduced bioavailability of the COC:

1 Women on long-term enzyme-inducing drugs (see Qs 4.34–4.36 and 4.203).
2 Rarely, women with established malabsorption problems (e.g. massive small bowel resection).

In addition:

3 Some women who have had a previous contraceptive failure with the COC, yet claiming perfect compliance or having missed no more than one tablet. But unlike 1 and 2, most of these should be given a standard formulation or the same (monophasic) as they previously had, only now tricycling the packets plus a shortened PFI after every third pack (see Q 4.27).

4.167 WHAT PILL SHOULD FOLLOW IF BTB IS UNACCEPTABLE AFTER 2–3 MONTHS' TRIAL AND THERE IS NO OTHER EXPLANATION?

Provided that the other causes in the list in Table 4.15 have been carefully excluded, if BTB occurs and is unacceptable early on, or persists beyond about three cycles, the next strongest brand up the 'ladder' in Figure 4.12

219

may be tried. In general, gestodene-containing COCs have a good reputation for cycle control. Phasic pills may come into their own here, especially if the cycle control problem includes absent WTB. But the excessively progestagen dominant (less 'lipid friendly') brands Eugynon 30/Ovran 30 are best avoided unless indicated for special medical/therapeutic reasons.

If after trying lower dose options BTB can only be prevented by a 50 µg oestrogen pill, for that particular woman the latter need not be considered a 'strong' brand. I explain this to women as at Q 4.39.

The answer to Q 4.167 is different for BTB late in a sequence of tricycling: if this applies, see Q 4.32.

4.168 IF CYCLE CONTROL IS A BIG PROBLEM, MAY ONE PRESCRIBE TWO PILLS, FOR EXAMPLE ONE 'MARVELON' PLUS ONE 'MERCILON 20' DAILY, TO CONSTRUCT A 50 µg DESOGESTREL PRODUCT?

Yes, I would support this, but in selected cases with due caution as for other situations outside the strict terms of the Data Sheet. Whenever more than one tablet is swallowed per day, this is an unlicensed use of a licensed product, and the 'named patient' criteria must be fulfilled – see Appendix 1, page 507.

Though evidence-based, this could be a little more difficult to justify than with long-term users of enzyme-inducer drugs, who have been proved regularly to have lower bioavailability of the COC. If, remotely, in these circumstances a thrombotic or other serious CVS event occurred it might be more difficult to establish that there had not been another cause for the bleeding problem – perhaps at the end-organ (see Q 4.170) – and hence that 'too much' oestrogen was not being given by the two pills a day regimen.

4.169 LATER ON, IF THERE IS GOOD CYCLE CONTROL, AMONG ESTABLISHED ASYMPTOMATIC COC-USERS, SHOULD ONE TRY MOVING DOWN THE LADDER?

At the time of repeat prescription, the possibility of trying a lower-dose brand (if available) should always be considered. Otherwise one will never know whether they might not be equally suited to a lower and probably safer dose. If no lower dose exists, both prescriber and taker of the pill can have the satisfaction of knowing that metabolic risks and hence probable risk of side-effects have been minimized within the context of marketed products.

4.170 LOW BLOOD LEVELS OF THE ARTIFICIAL HORMONES USUALLY CAUSE BTB – BUT IS ALL BTB CAUSED BY LOW BLOOD LEVELS?

No. It is true that BTB is not a totally accurate marker of blood levels, and indeed variability in BTB or WTB with the same blood level could be caused by variation at the end-organ (the endometrium). This is indubitably true, and probably explains much of the light BTB common in the first one or two cycles and the late tricycle bleeding discussed at Q 4.32.

But women find BTB annoying in any event. Why give more drug than the minimum to prevent the annoying symptom? The dose administered should be only just above (and not enormously above) the bleeding threshold: whether mediated by low blood level or an unusually susceptible end organ. Hence titration downwards in those *without* BTB is still logical. But caution is essential in the reverse situation, as stressed already at Q 4.163 and Table 4.15 – *remember particularly to check for Chlamydia!*

4.171 SHOULD WOMEN WITH BTB BE ADVISED TO TAKE ADDITIONAL PRECAUTIONS? CAN THEY RELY ON THEIR COC?

It has been suggested that attempting to find the best choice of pill by titrating downwards at follow-up, in the way described above, will lead to breakthrough conceptions. Yet pill-takers who conceive rarely report having had BTB beforehand. That conceptions rarely occur unless pills are (also) missed is, I believe, for the following reasons:

1 First, it is a tribute to the fact that even the current low-dose pills are amazingly effective, with back-up contraceptive mechanisms (notably the progestagen 'block' to cervical mucus penetration by sperm) operating even if breakthrough ovulation should occur.
2 Second, it seems that (fortunately) BTB is an early warning – usually occurring when there is more circulating artificial steroid than the minimum to permit conception – in compliant women. (It may well be true, though, that BTB implies a reduced *margin for error*, so these women ought to be more careful than usual about not lengthening the PFI, Qs 4.15–4.18.)

3   Third, it is likely that the bleeding from the uterus itself temporarily enhances the anti-implantation contraceptive mechanism.
4   Fourth, while present, BTB probably reduces coital frequency!

4.172 HOW WOULD YOU SUMMARIZE THIS POLICY?

All we want to do is give the lowest metabolic impact to the woman that her endometrium will allow. I would stress however that this prescribing system is based on the hypothesis of Figure 4.14, which is only now being rigorously tested. I would ask the reader to judge its plausibility and my view that it should be followed, pending the discovery of any better scheme.

4.173 WHAT SHOULD BE THE SECOND CHOICE OF PILL IF THERE ARE NON-BLEEDING SIDE-EFFECTS?

See below, Qs 4.245 and 4.246 and Tables 4.17 and 4.18

THE PROS AND CONS OF PHASIC PILLS

4.174 WHAT ARE PHASIC PILLS AND WHAT ARE THEIR ADVANTAGES?

Their main claimed advantage is that they tend to give a better bleeding pattern for a given (low) dose of hormones, using the given progestagen. For example, Logynon/Trinordiol gives an average daily dose of 92 μg of LNG (combined with 32.4 μg of EE). If this low dose of progestagen were used in a daily fixed-dose regimen, the incidence of BTB would be unacceptable.

Unexpectedly, the same has *not* been demonstrated for the gestodene-containing triphasics (Table 4.13), when compared with their actually slightly lower-dose monophasic equivalents! However all the gestodene combined pills are reported to give better cycle control than the levonorgestrel- or norethisterone-containing triphasics, particularly in the early months of use.

All except one triphasic (Synphase) imitate the normal menstrual cycle to some extent, in particular by there being a higher proportion of the progestagen to the oestrogen in the second half of the pill-taking cycle. Histologically, this leads to the production of an endometrium which appears more like the normal secretory phase, with more gland formation and the presence of spiral arterioles. This improved histology probably lies behind the good WTB which occurs (some patients complain it is too good!).

4.175 WHAT ABOUT THE OTHER POSTULATED ADVANTAGE, THAT THE APPROXIMATION TO THE NORMAL CYCLE WILL ITSELF LEAD TO A REDUCTION IN LONG-TERM SIDE-EFFECTS?

That is unlikely I think, though not impossible. On the contrary, some of the beneficial effects – which seem to relate to the very fact that the pill-cycle produces more stable hormone levels and is *not* the same as the normal cycle (see Q 4.57) – might also be reduced. As yet, we just do not know.

4.176 WHAT ARE THE DISADVANTAGES OF PHASIC OCS?

These can be listed as follows:

1 An increase in the time required to explain the pill packet to the user.
2 An increase in the risk of pill-taking errors, maybe particularly by teenagers – though some companies have made the newer packaging much more 'user-friendly'.
3 A reduction in the margin for such errors (particularly in view of the low dose being taken in the very first phase right after the 'contraceptively dangerous' pill-free time – see Qs 4.15, 4.24).
4 Some women complain of symptoms which imitate the premenstrual syndrome, such as breast tenderness, in the last phase of pill-taking before the withdrawal bleed.
5 They are obviously not a good choice for women with (non-focal) migraines or anyone prone to headaches or mood changes or any symptom which tends to be precipitated by hormone fluctuations.
6 In the UK they are extra expensive to the Health Service, since the pharmacist or dispensing doctor is paid a separate dispensing fee for each of the three phases – and even for the *placebo* phase of Logynon ED!
7 A small problem with postponing withdrawal bleeds (see Q 4.179), and for the same reason they are not suitable for tricycling (see Q 4.31).
8 Studies in Holland, Australia and New Zealand have all found that triphasics are definitely over-represented, among the COCs reportedly in use, by pill-takers presenting with unwanted 'breakthrough' conceptions. The reasons may include compliance problems due to complexity of the packaging and also relatively lower innate efficacy – see answer (3) above.

4.177 SO FOR WHOM MIGHT PHASIC OCS BE CHOSEN?

1 The main indication is for cycle control with low dose, especially to get a good withdrawal bleed. (*Note* however that in both the norethisterone and gestodene pill ladders the phasics are not actually quite the lowest dose products.)
2 Upon request, if the woman likes the idea of 'imitating the menstrual cycle'; they usefully increase choice if side-effects occur with monophasic products.

4.178 WHAT ARE YOUR VIEWS SPECIFICALLY ABOUT BINOVUM AND SYNPHASE?

1 *BiNovum* in my view is a brand which has almost no place now that TriNovum is available. TriNovum gives a lower mean daily progestagen dose (750 µg instead of 833 µg), gives at least as good cycle control, and has much better packaging.
2 *Synphase*. This may be useful for women experiencing BTB in the middle of the packet of a fixed-dose brand, especially Ovysmen/Brevinor. It is the only triphasic pill which has the highest progestagen to oestrogen ratio in the middle phase. However in comparison with Trinovum there is a negligible reduction in mean daily progestagen (714 µg rather than 750 µg).

4.179 HOW MAY A WOMAN POSTPONE THE WITHDRAWAL BLEED ON A PHASIC PILL?

There is no problem with Synphase. As with fixed-dose pills, see Q 4.255, two packets may simply be taken in a row without the usual 7-day break. But if this is tried with one of the other phasic brands, BTB is likely (not certainly) to occur early in the new packet, because of the abrupt drop in progestagen from the higher level in the last phase of the previous packet.

There are two possible solutions, as in Figure 4.15.

Contraceptive efficacy will be maintained throughout either scheme.

1 Tablets from the last phase of a 'spare' packet may be taken, thereby giving 7, 10 or 14 days' postponement according to the phasic brand in question.
2 Alternatively, the woman may follow immediately with a packet of the 'nearest' fixed dose brand up the same ladder in Figure 4.12 and

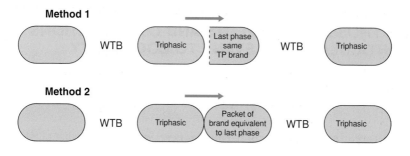

Figure 4.15 How to postpone periods with triphasic pills. Q 4.179. *Note*: for Synphase just run on packets.

Table 4.13 (i.e. the nearest equivalent to the final phase of her phasic pill). To be specific, this means using one of the brands listed in Table 4.16.

NB: to clear up possible confusion, this procedure of Figure 4.15 is not in the least necessary if the women has missed pills late in her packet. In that case the advice in Q 4.19 is all that is required to maintain efficacy. If she has a bleed early in the new pack she was expecting that anyway.

TABLE 4.16 POSTPONING 'PERIODS' WITH PHASICS

Name of phasic*	Brand to follow* to delay WTB using method 2 of Figure 4.15
Logynon	Microgynon
Tri-Minulet	Minulet[†]
TriNovum	Norimin
Binovum	Norimin
Synphase	Synphase

*Or the identical equivalent by another manufacturer from Table 4.13 – the alternatives are Trinordiol, Ovranette, Triadene and Femodene

[†]There would be a small risk of a BTB episode here since Minulet has 25 µg less gestodene than phase 3 of Tri-Minulet

FOLLOW-UP ARRANGEMENTS: THE MONITORING OF THOSE SIDE-EFFECTS AND COMPLICATIONS PARTICULARLY RELEVANT TO COC SAFETY

4.180 WHAT ARE THE MAIN ASPECTS OF PILL MONITORING, ONCE (SO FAR AS IS POSSIBLE) THE 'SAFEST' PILL BRAND HAS BEEN IDENTIFIED FOR THE INDIVIDUAL?

After careful selection and counselling as described above, the list of what can (and should) be done during long-term monitoring is short – but important.

In summary, good practice would be to:

1 Ask at each visit about *headaches* and particularly about any change in associated symptoms (Q 4.148). Advise in advance about all the warning symptoms in Q 4.191 below, including those relevant to migraine.

2 Look for the onset of any new cardiovascular risk factors – or intercurrent disease with the same implications (Q 4.134) – especially if one is already present (e.g. arrival of age 35 in all smokers).

3 Look for the warning signs, primarily a rise in blood pressure (see Q 4.185), or the onset of or change in character or worsening of migraines (see Qs 4.147–4.154). The migraine sufferer needs to be prospectively advised (i.e. more specifically than just the list at Q 4.191)

4 Arrange 3-yearly routine cervical cytology, with a bimanual examination only when clinically indicated (see Q 4.182).

5 Advise on breast awareness (*without it becoming a nerve-racking ritual*) along with a good leaflet. The pill-taker should know that you will be prepared to examine her on clinical grounds, i.e. if she ever notices some change in her breasts, but *routine professional breast examination has no evidence-base.*

6 Advise *re* special situations, notably immobilization, long haul air flights, high altitude holidays, major surgery and the treatment for varicose veins (see Qs 4.192 and 4.193).

4.181 HOW OFTEN SHOULD PILL-TAKERS BE SEEN, AND BY WHOM?

In my opinion, everything depends on whether the pill-taker is one of the 'safer' women or not (see Qs 4.133–134). The prescriber should mentally classify the pill-taker into one of the two categories – a form of triage really – on which follow-up arrangements depend.

1   Women with any of the recognised relative contraindications (primarily WHO 3) or with any important chronic illness should normally be seen by the doctor: with a low threshold for more frequent visits, perhaps 1–3 months after the first prescription; and it would be unlikely that the gap between checks would increase to more than 6-monthly thereafter. The reason is simple, they are the ones in whom the cardiovascular risks are focused: the heavy smokers have an inbuilt times ten or more greater risk of having a heart attack than any risk-factor-free women (see Q 4.96 and Table 4.8, page 170).

Even so the COC is such a safe product that it could be entirely appropriate for a family planning trained nurse to care for many women in this category: i.e. as described immediately below, just more frequently, following an agreed protocol.

2   The ordinary 'safer' women are still seen 3 months after the first pill prescription, or any change of brand, for BP check and symptom assessment, as well as to answer any queries. Subsequent visits are usually 6-monthly, but the frequency in this low-risk group can be further reduced: I advise that if the BP is stable after 2 years, annual checks are sufficient. IPPF even suggests this annual check policy starts after just one year.

It is good practice and an appropriate use of scarce resources for the follow-up checks to be regularly delegated to the practice nurse, so long as she is family planning-trained (ENB Course 901 or equivalent). There must be an agreed protocol specifying when (e.g. at what blood pressure level) she should call in the doctor.

Both nurses and doctors should recognize that pill-takers in this category 2 are 'very different animals!' from the first group, very unlikely indeed to suffer a serious adverse effect – after the first year in which the majority of the rare idiopathic VTEs may occur.

4.182 IDEALLY, SHOULDN'T ALL PILL-TAKERS HAVE A FULL PELVIC EXAMINATION AT LEAST ANNUALLY?

No, I consider this part of medical mythology. Please turn to Q 4.68. Though most of the disorders listed there can be picked up by a careful bimanual examination, it is useless as a screening procedure. It should be reserved for cases where there are relevant symptoms, i.e. on clinical grounds.

Moreover, everything listed is less likely to happen in pill-takers anyway, compared with, for example, the partners of intermittent condom-users! Those are the ones at increased risk of ovarian cysts (benign or malignant), fibroids, endometriosis, ectopics, etc.; better to persuade them to come in, and be examined this way, if you can, rather than the pill-takers!

4.183 HOW FREQUENTLY SHOULD THE BLOOD PRESSURE (BP) BE MEASURED, AND WHY IS IT SO IMPORTANT?

BP should be measured pretreatment and thereafter at 3 months; then 6 monthly; and then if it is entirely stable after 21–24 months at least annually in category 2 women (see Q 4.181). Studies have shown that the COC causes a measurable increase in both systolic and diastolic BP, a small increase in most women and a large increase in a few (estimated at up to 1% with modern pills):

1 *Moderate hypertension* – defined now as above 160/100 – increases the risks of most varieties of arterial disease and can even become irreversible. (Malignant hypertension has rarely been attributed to the COC.). If pill-induced it is fully reversible if the pill is discontinued promptly.

2 *Mild hypertension* – BP 140–159/90–99 – even this should be taken seriously especially if there are other circulatory risk factors (see Q 4.185).

4.184 AT WHAT LEVELS OF BP SHOULD THE PILL BE STOPPED?

Previously, it was agreed in the UK that *repeated* readings above 160/95 would be too high both for starting and continuing with the COC. However, WHO is slightly more permissive, stating that a level on repeated testing which does not exceed 159 systolic or 99 diastolic is WHO 3 for the COC, but that 160/100 or above is WHO 4. Therefore, I now use these internationally agreed levels.

4.185 WHEN SHOULD A RATHER SMALL RISE IN BP, PERHAPS NOT OUT OF THE NORMOTENSIVE RANGE, NEVERTHELESS LEAD TO A CONSIDERATION OF CHANGE OF METHOD?

Behind this question are the studies which show that hypertension acts as a marker for an increased risk of arterial disease. Studies by the life insurance companies, of large populations, have shown that raised BP is associated with a small but measurable reduction in life expectancy, even in women. While it is not certain that pill-induced mild hypertension has the same significance as the idiopathic variety, it would be prudent to assume that it does. Faced therefore with a 33-year-old, heavy-smoking woman with a BP repeatedly around 135/85 – knowing that before pill-taking it was, say, 110/70 – one would prefer she switched to another method of birth control right away rather than continuing to the upper limit of 35 years.

4.186 SO CAN THE BP BE USED AS AN ONGOING TEST OF LIABILITY TO ARTERIAL DISEASE?

This is what I am suggesting. In other words, for years pill-prescribers have longed for a simple clinical test, for example, a reagent which could be added to a woman's urine in the clinic and would turn it green if she could safely continue with the COC and red if she should discontinue. It is my view that we have that test already – not perfect, but usable in the same kind of way. A rise in BP is like a red or at least pink test, implying that the woman (especially if she already has a risk factor) has now entered a category at increased risk of arterial disease.

4.187 CAN PATIENTS ON HYPOTENSIVE TREATMENT BE LEGITIMATELY GIVEN THE COC?

This is WHO 3 in my view, and the POP or an injectable would be better choices among hormonal methods. But the COC may be acceptable in a young, non-smoking woman who accepts the extra risk, will use no other method of birth control, and after full consultation with the physician supervising control of her hypertension.

NOTE: This presupposes that the woman's hypertension is not pill related (which would be WHO 4). It would not be acceptable for a woman whose hypertension was induced by the COC (and readily reversible by simply stopping it in favour say of the POP), then to be given antihypertensive drugs in order to enable her to stay on it. There can be few occasions when treating the side-effects of one drug by other powerful drugs can be anything but bad medicine.

4.188 WHAT TYPES OF MIGRAINE INDICATE THAT THE COMBINED PILL SHOULD BE STOPPED?

Please reread Qs 4.147–4.153. To recap, these are:

- any change in the character of migraine to include focal neurological symptoms in the aura (Q 4.148), symptoms which are usually asymmetrical and explicable by transient cerebral ischaemia;
- migraines which are exceptionally severe;
- migraine without aura plus more than one additional risk factor for stroke;
- concurrent treatment with an ergot alkaloid.

In these categories the *oestrogen* of the combined pill should be stopped forthwith, and usually for ever. This is for fear that the transient ischaemia might become permanent by a thrombotic stroke. But all other contraceptives are options: the POP and injectables may be started right away.

4.189 WHAT ABOUT THE OCCURRENCE OF THE WOMAN'S FIRST EVER MIGRAINE ATTACK WHILE TAKING THE COC? SHOULD SHE STOP THE METHOD?

Yes, at the time it occurs, this is also an indication to stop the COC. But if it had no serious sequelae on that first occasion and no attack features focal symptoms, I consider that subsequent cautious COC use is acceptable (WHO 2: Q 4.153). However she must be warned in simple terms about the important symptoms to watch out for in future (see Q 4.148).

4.190 WHAT ABOUT 'ORDINARY' HEADACHES OCCURRING ON THE COC?

These are not a contraindication, more in the nature of a common, more or less tolerable, side-effect and one for which the woman may or may not ask help. If so, it is well worth ascertaining whether the headaches tend to occur in the pill-free week. If they do, the tricycle regimen, using the lowest acceptable fixed-dose formulation, leads, at worst, to the woman experiencing only five headaches a year instead of 13! (see Q 4.31).

4.191 WHAT SYMPTOMS SHOULD LEAD PILL-USERS TO TAKE URGENT MEDICAL ADVICE (POTENTIAL MAJOR PROBLEMS)?

Pill-users should be told to (a) transfer at once to another effective method of birth control and (b) come under medical care without delay, pending diagnosis and treatment, if any of the following should occur (this list is a form of revision of the chapter so far!):

1 Severe pain in the calf of one leg (possible deep venous thrombosis).
2 Severe central pain in the chest or sharp pains on either side of the chest aggravated by breathing – could be myocardial infarction or pulmonary embolism.
3 Unexplained breathlessness with or without the coughing up of blood-stained sputum – could be pulmonary embolism.
4 Severe pain in the abdomen (see Q 4.217).
5 Any unusually severe, prolonged headache, especially if it is the first ever attack or gets progressively worse, or is associated with the symptoms at 6–9 below (see Qs 4.147–4.153).
6 A bad fainting attack or collapse, with or without focal epilepsy.
7 Weakness or paraesthesia suddenly or gradually affecting one side or one part of the body.
8 Marked asymmetrical disturbance of vision, especially loss of a visual field or teichopsia.
9 Disturbance of the ability to speak normally (nominal aphasia).
10 A severe and generalized skin rash (which could be erythema multiforme).

Most of the above are potentially thrombotic or embolic catastrophes in the making; but often there is a non-pill-related explanation.

Clinical signs which may not be complaints but still demand urgent action (including stopping the COC) are:

11 The onset of jaundice (see Qs 4.211 and 4.212).
12 High blood pressure (i.e. above 160/100, see Qs 4.183 and 4.184).

The pill should also normally be discontinued forthwith if immobilization is necessary after an accident, or emergency major or leg surgery is required (see Qs 4.192–4.196 below).

IMPLICATIONS OF SURGERY

4.192 SHOULD A COMBINED PILL-USER DISCONTINUE TREATMENT BEFORE ELECTIVE MAJOR SURGERY?

This is WHO 3–4. It all depends on the nature of the surgery. My opinion on this is a little more cautious than some pronouncements (e.g. the

THRIFT Consensus Group, *BMJ* 1992;305:567–74). If it is major surgery, lasting more than 30 minutes and involving immobilization thereafter, i.e. mainly in bed for at least 48 hours, *or* less major but associated with hypotension or prolonged immobilization thereafter, or any surgery involving the legs:

1 The COC should be discontinued at least 2 (preferably 4) weeks before the operation. Many coagulation factors are back to normal by 2 weeks, in fact, but there is insufficient evidence to state that 2 weeks' discontinuation would always suffice.

2 The COC should also not be recommenced until the first menstrual period which is at least 2 weeks after full mobilization.

The reason for this advice is the well-established increased risk of deep venous thrombosis (DVT) postoperatively, and the potential for this to be increased by the prothrombotic changes caused by oestrogens. Vessey *et al.* (*BMJ* 1986;292:526–28) estimated the risk of clinical VTE post-operatively as 0.96% on low-dose pills and 0.5% for non-takers. Given these figures a policy of stopping the COC has the potential to prevent about 500 VTEs and up to 10 deaths in every 100 000 major operations.

> **NOTE:** For the reason that they are oestrogen-free, the above rule does not apply to the POP nor to progestagen-only injectables/implants which may be continued without a break during major surgery. Indeed they may be appropriately chosen to cover the time on a waiting-list (see Q 4.195)

4.193 SHOULD THE COC BE STOPPED FOR A MINOR OPERATION SUCH AS LAPAROSCOPIC STERILIZATION?

This is definitely unnecessary (WHO 2), since the risk of postoperative DVT is vanishingly small after such minor surgery. The same applies to dental extraction. 'Iatrogenic' pregnancies seem frequently to be caused this way.

However, since thromboembolism occurred after 3 of 438 laparoscopic cholecystectomies in a 1993 report from Sydney (one was fatal), it would be best to avoid COC use prior to *complex* laparoscopies.

4.194 WHAT ABOUT MINOR LEG SURGERY, SUCH AS OPERATIVE ARTHROSCOPY, OR LIGATION OF VARICOSE VEINS? OR INJECTION TREATMENT FOR LEG VEINS?

These are quite another matter. Oestrogen-containing therapy should be discontinued 4 weeks before either such surgery or sclerotherapy, and avoided for the duration of leg bandaging thereafter.

4.195 WHAT CONTRACEPTION IS SUITABLE BEFORE AND AFTER SURGERY WHILE THE COC IS CONTRAINDICATED?

Progestagen-only methods are all appropriate. A good choice might be DMPA (see Q 4.192). The first injection may be given at any time in the woman's pill-taking cycle, after which she just finishes the current packet. If irregular bleeding is a problem, a new packet of her usual pill may be started as early as 2 weeks after full mobilization, without waiting for the expiry of the 12 week's duration of the injection. After all, DMPA and the COC are quite often given together to control irregular bleeding (Q 5.128).

4.196 WHAT SHOULD BE DONE IF A PATIENT WHO IS A PILL-TAKER IS ADMITTED AS AN EMERGENCY FOR MAJOR SURGERY OR ORTHOPAEDIC (FRACTURE) TREATMENT WITH IMMOBILIZATION?

In these circumstances the risk of DVT is high, especially if she is overweight. The COC should be discontinued at once and careful consideration given to the use of subcutaneous heparin prophylaxis. This would be particularly important for gynaecological, orthopaedic and cancer surgery.

Do not forget to ask the young girl on traction, after falling from her boyfriend's motor bike, to stop taking her (combined) pills. Indeed, the immobilization involved in treating a leg fracture after a skiing accident even as an outpatient can be sufficient for many continental orthopaedic surgeons to recommend heparin prophylaxis. I would term this a WHO 3 situation: depending on the case, switching to a progestagen-only contraceptive might well be preferable while the leg is in plaster.

DEALING WITH OTHER SIDE-EFFECTS AND EVENTS DURING PILL-USE

4.197 WHAT GENERAL POINTS CAN BE MADE ABOUT THE SO-CALLED 'MINOR' SIDE-EFFECTS?

1 First and foremost they frequently do not seem minor to the woman affected!
2 Many of them are common in the general population, hence it is difficult to be sure that the COC is to blame in an individual case.
3 The frequency of complaint depends on many factors, including anxiety about possible harm due to the therapy.
4 Many can be classified under two main headings:
   (a) those related to cycle control (see Qs 4.165–4.172);
   (b) those which are also common in pregnancy.

4.198 WHICH ARE THE COMMON, OFTEN PREGNANCY-MIMICKING MINOR SIDE-EFFECTS?

The order below is *alphabetical*. Not all are also commoner in pregnancy, and in some cases the link with the COC may well not be causal.

Common:
1 acne (usually benefited, but may worsen with levonorgestrel pills);
2 breast enlargement and bloatedness with fluid retention;
3 cramps and pains in the legs;
4 cystitis and other urinary infections;
5 depression and loss of libido;
6 gingivitis;
7 hair loss (or gain) – Q 4.239;
8 headaches;
9 nausea;
10 vaginal discharge (non-specific) and cervical 'erosion'/ectopy
11 weight gain.

Less common;
1 breast pain (see Qs 4.230 and 4.246);
2 chloasma (see Q 4.239);
3 galactorrhoea (see Q 4.230);
4 superficial thrombophlebitis.

There are also some more serious conditions which are similarly commoner in pregnancy. For example, some immune disorders (see Q 4.242); chorea, cardiomyopathy, pemphigoid gestationis, haemolytic uraemic syndrome and cholestatic jaundice; not to mention hypertension and venous and arterial thrombosis.

Subsequent questions consider the management of side-effects, considered by systems – excluding the circulatory system (already dealt with in some detail).

CENTRAL NERVOUS SYSTEM

4.199 IS DEPRESSION COMMONER AMONG PILL-TAKERS THAN CONTROLS, AND HOW CAN IT BE MANAGED?

In the RCGP study it was shown that for every 130 depressed pill-users there were 100 who were non-OC-using controls. This implies that only 30 of the 130 could really blame the COC, even in the much higher doses then given. But there are some who are free from depression when off treatment, with recurrence when rechallenged. In a proportion, altered tryptophan metabolism leads to lowered pyridoxine levels. In these pyridoxine may be beneficial (use less than 100 mg daily to avoid reversible peripheral neuropathy): in the study from Wynn's unit, 50 mg daily was given, taking up to 2 months to be effective. Others may require a change of progestagen or change of method, with or without antidepressant therapy.

Depression could also be secondary to other pill side-effects (e.g. headaches, or loss of libido). But the Oxford/FPA Study (1985) ruled out any link between the COC and 'serious' psychiatric illness, which includes severe depression needing hospital referral.

4.200 HOW DOES THE COC AFFECT LIBIDO?

Loss of libido is reported particularly among those who are also depressed. Many extrinsic factors may explain this, including placebo reaction to the COC or frustrated desire for a child. However, there are certainly some cases where there is a real physiological effect of the hormones. Contrariwise, in some women libido is actually increased because the method is so reliable, non-intercourse-related, and often reduces premenstrual tension. This makes female-initiated sexual activity late in the pill cycle more common than it is late in the normal cycle.

4.201 HOW SHOULD ONE MANAGE THE COMPLAINT OF LOSS OF LIBIDO?

1 First, the pill may be irrelevant to the problem. Discuss fully psychosexual aspects of the relationship, and the marital and family circumstances, and offer referral for counselling as appropriate.
2 Second, check whether part of the problem is soreness or dryness – which could be caused locally by thrush, or a vulval skin eruption, or suturing following delivery.
3 Use of a water-soluble lubricant may help.
4 Finally, consider changing to a more oestrogen-dominant pill (see Q 4.246 and Table 4.18).

4.202 HOW MAY THE COC AFFECT EPILEPSY?

The condition is not initiated by the COC. The attack rate is often reduced, though rarely it may be increased. Avoid *triphasic* COCs (see Q 4.176). Liver enzyme-inducer antiepileptic therapy is one of the few indications for at least a 50-µg oestrogen COC with *tricycling* (see Qs 4.36–4.39). Moreover, regardless of therapy, if fits are commonly initiated around the pill-free time tricycling a monophasic may reduce their frequency. Injectables are another good option (see Q 5.93 (12)).

4.203 IF EPILEPTICS AND OTHERS ON CHRONIC ENZYME-INDUCING TREATMENTS ARE ON THE PILL, HOW SHOULD THEY BE MANAGED?

First, please read Qs 4.15–37 before this answer.
I used to advise as well as the increased dose, *shortening* the PFIs. But pending the marketing of the active 24 + 4 placebo packs mentioned at Q 4.8, it simplifies compliance to eliminate most of them instead: by using the *tricycle regimen* (see Q 4.31). This also appears to improve epilepsy control, though no comparative trial has been published. After three consecutive packets the woman should still shorten the PFI, arbitrarily to just 4 days. Diary cards may be helpful.

If subsequently the woman complains of BTB, exclude another cause (see Q 4.163) and consider bicycling (Q 4.32).

The next step is to try two tablets a day, e.g. of 30- or 35-µg fixed-dose pills. If necessary the combined oestrogen content of the two pills per day can be increased to 90 μg (maximum), titrated against the BTB. In this way the usual policy of giving the minimum dose of both hormones to be just above the threshold for bleeding (see Qs 4.163 and 4.165) can be followed. The epileptic can be reassured that she is 'climbing a down escalator' (see Q 4.39).

Caution is necessary when enzyme inducers are withdrawn, since it takes some weeks for the liver's level of excretory function to revert to normal. See Q 4.40 for the details.

4.204 WHAT ABOUT HEADACHES AND MIGRAINES?

These very important subjects have already been covered, under 'risk factors' (see Qs 4.147–4.154) and 'monitoring' (see Qs 4.188–4.190)

4.205 HOW CAN THE PILL AFFECT THE EYES?

If any acute visual disturbance occurs the woman should be told to stop the pill at once, pending further investigation.

1. At worst, acute loss of vision in one eye (black scotoma) could be caused by retinal artery or vein thrombosis or haemorrhage. *Amaurosis fugax* is the term given to temporary blindness in one eye usually attributed to retinal ischaemia. The COC should be stopped and avoided thereafter (WHO 4).

2. Loss of a field of vision (bright scotoma) may signify transient cerebral ischaemia. This also must be taken seriously, see Q 4.148, though not caused by an eye problem.

3. *Benign intracranial hypertension (BICH)*. This is a rare condition of unknown aetiology causing raised intracranial pressure and papilloedema with impairment of visual acuity and headache – usually in young women with significantly raised BMI. Hospital admission is essential for imaging to exclude a tumour and then sometimes for repeated lumbar puncture to reduce intracranial pressure.

The weak association with the COC and with contraceptive hormones (e.g. Norplant) is probably coincidental. However as the condition is certainly not that 'benign' with regard to the eyesight – there is a risk of permanent optic atrophy if it is recurrent/persistent – it is considered an absolute contraindication to starting or continuing the COC.

This would of course also be the true if the eventual diagnosis was cerebral vein thrombosis, as applies in some cases.

4   Blurring of vision with photophobia may be a normal manifestation of diffuse 'common' migraine without aura. If it occurs completely unassociated with headaches, fundoscopy should be performed to exclude retinal vein thrombosis.

4.206 WHAT ABOUT THE PILL AND CONTACT LENSES?

An increased likelihood of discomfort or rarely corneal damage among contact lens users taking the COC was reported with the old hard lenses (and stronger pills). It is believed to be explained by a slight degree of corneal oedema. With modern soft lenses and low-dose pills this problem is now uncommon. If it occurs, the woman should see her optician, and a brand containing the lowest possible dose of both steroids should be tried. Rarely, women have to make a straight choice between their contact lenses and this contraceptive method.

4.207 DOES THE PILL CAUSE OR AGGRAVATE GLAUCOMA?

There is no evidence of any effect even among those with a family history: though of course intraocular pressure rarely rises significantly during the peak childbearing years.

GASTROINTESTINAL SYSTEM

4.208 DOES THE COC CAUSE NAUSEA OR VOMITING?

Nausea may occur particularly in the first cycle. The symptom is commonest in underweight women. They can usually be reassured, though it may recur after the PFI with the first pills of the next packet; nausea usually affects fewer or none of the first pills in each subsequent pack. Changing to a more progestagen-dominant pill may help (Q 4.246). Vomiting is most unusual, but if within 2 hours it could interfere with absorption of a tablet and hence affect cycle control and efficacy (see Q 4.25).

Both symptoms are oestrogen-related and are thus not so frequent with modern pills. They are commoner in very under-weight women, and in them may be intolerable, starting with the very first tablet and with every COC tried. More usually perseverance is rewarded. Use tablets with 30 or only 20 µg of oestrogen – or oestrogen-free (i.e. the POP). Nausea may also be helped by taking the pill at night rather than in the morning.

Vomiting starting for the first time after several months of trouble-free pill-taking should not be attributed to the pill. Consider pregnancy for one thing.

4.209 HOW OFTEN IS WEIGHT GAIN ON THE COC TRULY DUE TO IT, AND HOW MAY IT BE MINIMIZED?

The fear of this is one of the things that most puts young women off the pill. Yet clearly not all weight gain is caused by the pill; it is often blamed unfairly. It can help to inform a prospective user that most studies of modern pills show weight changes roughly as follows in the first year of use:

- weight gain of more than 2 kg in 20–25%;
- unchanged or within ± 2 kg, 60%;
- actual loss of more than 2 kg in 15–20% (and they do not complain!)

Also very relevant is that if women start the pill while still in their teens, a steady increase of weight during adolescence is common normally, without pills.

There is also a kind of cyclical weight gain which is oestrogen linked (see Q 4.246) and due to fluid retention. This is more noticeable in some than others, tending to be shed with a diuresis in the pill-free week.

Sustained weight gain can be marked in some individual women due mainly to an increase in appetite. Major change may imply unusual metabolic disturbance by steroid hormones, as also with injectables (see Q. 5.96) – or an eating disorder.

Apart from appropriate advice about diet and (often more relevantly) exercise, lower-dose brands of different progestagens may be tried; before perhaps transferring to a different method such as the POP.

4.210 HOW SHOULD JAUNDICE IN A COC-USER BE MANAGED?

First, the pill should be stopped immediately, since it has additive effects on liver metabolism. If some form of infectious hepatitis is diagnosed the COC is normally not restarted until at least 3 months after the liver function tests have returned to normal.

Abnormal liver function tests caused by any other mechanism (e.g. cirrhosis) contraindicate the method (WHO 3–4 according to severity), though the POP is usable (see Q 5.53).

4.211 HOW OFTEN IS JAUNDICE CAUSED BY THE PILL?

Rarely. Cholestatic jaundice is commoner among COC-users and also in pregnancy. Either past history normally contraindicates the pill, though if *only* a pregnancy history it could be discussed as WHO 3 (with appropriate forewarning). Gilbert's disease is incidental and benign (WHO 2).

4.212 DOES THE COC CAUSE GALLSTONES?

The increased risk of this condition among COC-users is significant only during the early years of pill-taking. This suggests that the risk applies primarily to predisposed women. Studies of bile biochemistry have shown that contraceptive steroids can accelerate cholelithiasis.

4.213 IF A WOMAN HAS HAD DEFINITIVE TREATMENT FOR GALLSTONES MAY SHE USE THE COC?

If the treatment was medical, the COC would be best avoided (WHO 3) because of the risk of recurrence. If the woman has had definitive surgical treatment by cholecystectomy, many surgeons will permit use of the COC if no other method is acceptable (WHO 2).

4.214 IS ACUTE PANCREATITIS LINKED WITH THE COC?

Yes, in part perhaps through the link with gall-bladder disease. Most of the sporadic cases had cofactors like obesity, alcohol abuse, hypertriglyceridaemia, or lipid problems, and there have been few reports since the advent of sub-50-μg pills.

If a woman suffers an attack of this condition on the COC artificial oestrogen is contraindicated (WHO 4) if triglyceride levels are high (above 5.6 mmol/l), or perhaps WHO 3 if they are not. Otherwise she could transfer to any progestagen-only method.

4.215 WHAT ARE THE PRESENTATION AND MANAGEMENT OF COC-RELATED BENIGN LIVER TUMOURS (SEE Q 4.91)?

They present with abdominal pain and an upper abdominal mass, and sometimes with a life-threatening haemoperitoneum. The treatment is surgical removal. Subsequently both the COC and progestagen-only methods should be avoided (see Qs 4.91, 4.131, 5.52).

4.216 IS THE COC, LIKE CIGARETTES, LINKED WITH CROHN'S DISEASE?

This example of inflammatory bowel disease is discussed in Q 4.141. In case-control studies pill-use was commoner only among women with colonic Crohn's of the non-granulomatous variety. The condition often resolved if the COCs were discontinued. It would be logical if the woman could give up cigarettes as well!

In severe cases of any inflammatory bowel disease the risk of thromboembolism during exacerbations generally puts the COC into WHO category 4.

4.217 WHAT IS THE DIFFERENTIAL DIAGNOSIS OF ABDOMINAL PAIN WHICH COULD BE RELATED TO COC USE?

1 Thrombosis of major intra-abdominal vessels such as the hepatic veins or a mesenteric artery or vein;
2 gallstones (see Q 4.212);
3 pancreatitis (see Q 4.214);
4 liver adenoma (see Q 4.215);
5 Crohn's disease (see Q 4.216);
6 acute porphyria (Q 4.218).

Much more commonly the pain will have an *unrelated* aetiology!

INBORN ERRORS OF METABOLISM

4.218 WHY IS THE COC CONTRAINDICATED IN THE ACUTE PORPHYRIAS, AND WHAT ADVICE SHOULD BE GIVEN TO THOSE WITH LATENT PORPHYRIA (IN THEIR GENOME) BUT WHO HAVE NOT SUFFERED AN ATTACK?

Both combined pills *and* (NB) progestagens alone may provoke attacks of acute porphyria. All who have had an acute attack – especially if that was itself triggered by either of these hormones – are therefore in category WHO 4 for both hormones.

Those who are asymptomatic but have the inherited enzyme defect and excrete excess porphobilinogen in their urine are also in WHO 4 for the COC. But the progestagen-only method of emergency contraception (Q 7.5) may be cautiously used provided the risks are fully explained and accepted

(WHO 3): special caution is necessary if the woman is in her teens or early 20s since these are the ages at which first attacks of acute porphyria are commonest.

The POP may also be tried with considerable caution in latent cases if no other contraceptive is acceptable (WHO 3). Anecdotally, I have treated a latent acute porphyria case successfully with the POP after she had twice had no symptoms with the levonorgestrel-only emergency method. But injections (and arguably implants) should never be used, since they cannot be rapidly stopped like tablets if a first attack actually is provoked.

4.219 SHOULD THE COC BE AVOIDED BY WOMEN WITH NON-ACUTE PORPHYRIAS?

This is a complex subject and further advice for individual cases can be obtained from the Porphyria Service of the Department of Medical Biochemistry at the University Hospital of Wales in Cardiff, CF4 4XW.

They stress that the acute hepatic porphyrias are the main problem, and the other porphyrias are not in WHO category 4 for synthetic oestrogens and progestagens. Generally they would be in WHO 2. However oestrogens have been blamed for the pathogenesis of *porphyria cutanea tarda*, and patients who have been treated should be warned that they might relapse and need further treatment if the COC were used (i.e. it is in category WHO 3).

RESPIRATORY SYSTEM

NOTE: Beware of the label 'pleurisy' which Vessey showed was twice as likely to be given to a COC-taker as to a non-user. ... If unexplained pleuritic chest pain or dyspnoea occurs (especially in a COC-taker recently returned from holiday after a long haul flight!) this is pulmonary embolism until proved otherwise (see Q 4.191).

4.220 DOES THE COC PROMOTE ALLERGIC RHINITIS OR ASTHMA?

There is some tenuous evidence of a causal association between COC use and these conditions, particularly the former (see Q 4.242). But many with both complaints continue to use modern COCs with apparent impunity.

Professor Farmer in his GP database study (1999) showed – unexpectedly – a doubled risk of VTE in patients with asthma. This may not be completely explicable by diagnostic bias and needs further study.

URINARY SYSTEM

4.221 WHAT IS THE LINK BETWEEN COC USE AND URINARY TRACT INFECTIONS?

Several studies have shown that such infections are commoner in COC-users than in controls. Women on the pill may have more frequent intercourse, thus increasing their risk of so-called 'honeymoon cystitis'. But some studies have also shown an increased incidence of symptomless bacteriuria in COC-users, resolving when the pill is stopped. This suggests a causal link, so it may sometimes be worth transferring to another method (but the choice of an occlusive cap needs to be carefully made – see Q 3.51).

REPRODUCTIVE SYSTEM – OBSTETRICS

4.222 WHAT ARE THE RISKS TO THE FETUS IF THE WOMAN CONTINUES TO TAKE THE COC DURING EARLY PREGNANCY?

In animal research, sex steroids can certainly be teratogens. Diethylstilboestrol is a non-steroidal oestrogen which can harm the human fetus, often with very delayed manifestations; and the complex literature about deliberate hormone use (e.g. the former hormone pregnancy tests) in early pregnancy includes some studies which suggest an increased incidence of rare congenital abnormalities.

The copious literature is largely reassuring about the COC. The rate of birth defects in the Oxford/FPA and RCGP studies following COC exposure in pregnancy was no higher than expected in any group of women having a planned baby. In a major Connecticut study of 1370 abnormal babies there was no increase in COC use during the pregnancies compared with the mothers of normal infants. Studies of national birth defect registers in Hungary and Finland also strongly suggest that pill use in pregnancy has no effect on visible malformations, though multiple births are commoner.

The rule that a pregnant woman should avoid all drugs, especially in the first trimester, remains the ideal. But the situation envisaged by the question is not uncommon – can the woman be given any kind of risk estimate? She can certainly not be promised a normal baby. Quite apart from the uncertainty about rare anomalies, at least 2% of all babies show an important abnormality. Bracken (1990) found a relative risk from COC use of 0.99 (i.e. no detectable change) for all important malformations, in a meta-analysis of 12 prospective studies. This agrees with the large population-based case-control studies.

Note that there should be no added risk at all after failed postcoital hormone treatment, which is given before implantation (see Q 7.19).

4.223 IS THERE ANY RESIDUAL FETAL RISK FOR EX-PILL-USERS?

Here the balance of the published work is heavily tilted towards absence of risk. In 1981 an expert scientific group of the WHO declared categorically that there was no evidence of any adverse effects on the fetus of pill use prior to conception. The only residual anxiety relates to the fact that alterations in mineral and vitamin levels have been observed in OC-users (see Q 4.93; Table 4.7). These may take a few weeks to revert to normal; and supplementation with vitamins (most importantly folic acid) at and after conception has been shown to reduce the risk of neural tube defects in women with a previously affected baby.

4.224 SHOULD WOMEN STOP THE COC WELL AHEAD OF CONCEPTION?

Some authorities advise that they should discontinue the pill and use a mechanical method of contraception for two to three cycles. This has not been proved to help, though it should certainly do no harm. Ultrasound scanning has lessened the importance of this for dating of the pregnancy. Although most authorities do not consider them important, some couples do find it reassuring that there are no detectable changes from normal in vitamin and mineral metabolism by about 2 months post pill. The FPA pill leaflet no longer recommends waiting for one or more natural periods before trying to get pregnant.

A woman who conceives sooner than any arbitrary time should, in the light of Q 4.223, be very strongly reassured. Avoiding drugs and cigarettes is far more important! Along with an adequate, balanced diet, the Chief Medical Officer recommends a daily dose of 0.4 mg folic acid as routine prophylaxis against neural tube defects, starting before conception.

Specialist advice should be obtained *before conception*, if a woman on anti-epileptic therapy plans a baby.

For trophoblastic disease, see Q 4.75.

REPRODUCTIVE SYSTEM – GYNAECOLOGY

4.225 HOW DOES THE COC AFFECT THE SYMPTOMS ASSOCIATED WITH THE MENSTRUAL CYCLE?

Beneficially in most respects (see the summary list at Q 4.55). *Premenstrual syndrome* was less common overall in the RCGP study. But any prescriber knows that some individual pill-takers do complain of a similar symptom-complex towards the end of each packet, with fluid retention, breast tenderness and depression/irritability predominating. These symptoms seem to be commoner on phasic pills. However, overall they remain more frequent in (so-called) normal cycles than in monophasic pill-taking cycles, especially if two or more packets are taken in succession (Qs 4.31 and 4.129).

Similarly, most women notice the menstrual flow to be both lighter and less painful, but a minority who normally have light menses actually report the reverse.

BTB, absent WTB on the COC and secondary amenorrhoea after COC use are cycle symptoms considered elsewhere (see Qs 4.10, 4.60–4.66 and 4.155–4.172). *Remember all the non-pill causes of BTB* (Qs 4.163 and 4.164, Table 4.15)!

4.226 WHAT IS THE EFFECT OF COCs ON PELVIC INFECTION, FUNCTIONAL OVARIAN CYSTS AND FIBROIDS?

See Qs 4.58, 4.59 and 4.129.

4.227 WHAT EFFECT DOES THE COMBINED PILL HAVE ON ENDOMETRIOSIS?

This condition is sometimes treated but more often maintained in suppression by a progestagen-dominant COC such as Eugynon 30 or Microgynon 30, best on a tricycle basis (see Q 4.31).

There is also a strong clinical impression that it is less common among users of combined OCs, and this has received confirmation by the RCGP and Oxford/FPA but not by all studies.

The most significant gynaecological effect of the COC is a benefit: protection against cancers of the ovary and endometrium, discussed at Qs 4.56, 4.73–4.74.

4.228 DOES THE COC CAUSE VAGINAL DISCHARGE?

Do not attribute this to the pill without first eliminating other causes.

1 *Cervical erosion* (now better known as ectopy). This was definitely commoner in the prospective studies based on COCs containing 50 µg or more of oestrogen. It still occurs, though less frequently, on modern pills and requires treatment only if the woman complains.
2 On the other hand, some women especially if taking progestagen-dominant pills complain of vaginal dryness.
3 It is still generally believed that *thrush (candidiasis)* is more frequent in COC-users. Yet a paper with the title 'The pill does not cause 'thrush' ' was published in the *British Journal of Obstetrics and Gynaecology* in 1985. The journal would never have allowed such a title if this study of over 1300 women attending three departments of genitourinary medicine in England had been the slightest bit equivocal! Other recent studies are confirmatory.

    This is perhaps because current low-oestrogen pills have less pregnancy-mimicking effect on the glycogen content of vaginal cells. In practice it should certainly not be assumed that modern pills are to blame in any case of recurrent thrush. Genitourinary medicine experts currently recommend for such cases the daily application of any standard imidazole cream to the anogenital skin, continuing for many weeks if not indefinitely.
4 *Trichomonas vaginitis.* COCs seem to provide some (as yet unexplained) protection against this, but none against the transmission of other STIs.

4.229 DOES THE COC AFFECT OTHER VAGINAL CONDITIONS?

1 There is a suggestion from research in the USA that the COC protects against the rare *toxic shock syndrome.*
2 No effect of the pill either way has been reported on the incidence of *bacterial vaginosis.*

THE BREASTS

4.230 WHAT EFFECTS DOES THE COC HAVE ON THE BREASTS?

For *benign breast disease* see Q 4.91, and for *breast cancer* see Qs 4.79–4.88. Most women notice an increase in size of their breasts and some change in texture. These effects may be acceptable, but breast tenderness is not. The latter may occur with any pill formulation but seems particularly associated with the last phase of phasic brands.

Galactorrhoea among pill-takers is rare and needs investigation (plasma prolactin). A pituitary adenoma or microadenoma should be definitely excluded before dismissing this as a minor side-effect.

4.231 SHOULD THE COMBINED PILL BE USED DURING LACTATION?

In my view the answer is a definite no, on several counts. First it is an 'overkill' since practically 100% contraception can be obtained by the combination of lactation with the POP (see Q 5.15). Second, the COC frequently reduces the volume and quality of milk, and third a larger dose of hormone is being given to the breast-fed infant than would be the case with the POP.

MUSCULOSKELETAL SYSTEM

4.232 IF GIVEN TO YOUNG, POSTPUBERTAL GIRLS, WILL THE COC CAUSE STUNTING OF GROWTH? INDEED, ARE ANY OTHER ADVERSE EFFECTS MORE LIKELY IN VERY YOUNG TEENAGERS THAN IN THE OLDER YOUNG WOMAN?

Given in high dose to young female animals, oestrogen alone can lead to premature closure of the epiphyses. However there is no evidence that a daily dose of 30 µg or even 50 µg of EE, especially when taken with progestagen, has this effect in postpubertal girls. Menstruation normally starts when adult weight and height have mostly been achieved. Pill taking should always be delayed until menstruation is established.

Young teenagers need good counselling, if the COC is to be prescribed at all. The risks they run are great, affecting so many aspects of emotional development, their future ability to have stable relationships, their total sexual and reproductive health (Q 8.3, 8.10–8.11). But they are the risks of early sexual activity. There are no proven risks specific to the COC which are known to be greater when it is started at 13 than at 23. So the strictly pharmacological considerations are not different from those for a woman in her early 20s.

4.233 IS THE COC ASSOCIATED WITH CARPAL-TUNNEL SYNDROME, PRIMARY RAYNAUD'S DISEASE, CHILBLAINS, AND CRAMPS IN THE LEGS?

All these associations have been described, and some are probably causal, especially the first in the list. Raynaud's phenomenon may be a manifestation of a contraindicating condition (such as a connective tissue disorder which might itself promote arterial disease), so the symptom must be investigated.

Otherwise if these problems are troublesome it is worth a trial of discontinuation of the COC; but it may also be continued if the patient so desires.

4.234 HOW SHOULD ONE ASSESS THE COMPLAINT OF LEG PAINS AND CRAMPS?

Careful assessment and examination are important. If bilateral the symptom is less likely to be significant but look for water retention, varicose veins, chilblains or associated Raynaud's phenomenon.

If unilateral, deep venous thrombosis must be excluded. If in doubt the pill should be stopped and the patient referred for further investigation. Her contraceptive future depends on an accurate diagnosis being made.

4.235 HOW MAY THE COC AFFECT ARTHRITIS AND RELATED DISORDERS?

A reduction in rheumatoid arthritis risk has emerged in some studies but not others. A 1990 meta-analysis suggested COCs may slow progression of the disease. More recently, Jorgensen *et al.* in *Annals of Rheumatic Diseases* 1996;55:94–98 were confident that the observed benefit is real.

Tenosynovitis and a form of allergic polyarthritis may occur, but causation has not been proved. (*Re SLE*, see Q 4.142).

CUTANEOUS SYSTEM

4.236 WHICH SKIN CONDITIONS MAY BE IMPROVED BY COCs – AND WHICH COCs?

Acne, seborrhoea and sometimes hirsutism may all be benefited by oestrogen-dominant COCs (and indeed all may be exacerbated by the reverse – see Qs 4.245–4.246).

4.237 SHOULD DIANETTE BE CONSIDERED AS A COMBINED PILL, OR PRIMARILY AS AN EFFECTIVE TREATMENT FOR ACNE AND HIRSUTISM?

It should be considered primarily as the latter, especially useful (after full investigation) in the polycystic ovary syndrome (Q 4.64).

It is an anti-androgen/synthetic oestrogen combination (cyproterone acetate (CPA) 2 mg with ethinyloestradiol (EE) 35 µg), for the oral treatment of moderately severe acne and mild hirsutism in women.

These are its indications; but it is also a reliable anovulant like other COCs and usually gives good cycle control as well. It has similar rules for missed tablets, interactions with drugs including antibiotics, absolute and relative contraindications, and requirements for monitoring. It can be free of charge to the woman if the prescription is marked 'for contraception', or with the female *symbol* for 'female' (♀).

Although practically everything about the COC applies also to Dianette, it is certainly an oestrogen-dominant product with a higher VTE risk in the 1996 WHO report than LNG products. Since it permits EE to raise SHBG and HDL-cholesterol, it must have the potential also to allow the oestrogen to have relatively greater effects in a prothrombotic direction than a levonorgestrel product would (see Q 4.106). Although there are no clear epidemiological data, my own current working hypothesis is therefore to put it in the same category as a 'third generation' desogestrel/gestodene product and follow the prescribing guidelines at Q 4.114–4.120 above.

Caution is necessary because so many prospective users have high BMIs; though an added factor allowing a little more latitude in decision-making is that the product is being used for the added benefit of *therapy*, not just for contraception.

4.238 WHAT SHOULD BE THE MAXIMUM DURATION OF TREATMENT WITH DIANETTE?

This needs to be individualized. In the Data sheet it is 'recommended that treatment is withdrawn when the acne or hirsutism is completely resolved', but 'repeat courses may be given if the condition recurs'.

There are some concerns related to hepatic effects including benign and malignant liver tumour risk in long-term use – mostly based on animal work and much higher doses of the cyproterone acetate. So it is usual to encourage patients to switch to another oestrogen-dominant product (Q 4.245) when their condition is controlled – usually after 1 to 3 years, but sometimes much longer, especially if symptoms recur when off Dianette. This assumes that they fully accept the possible hepatic and prothrombotic risks.

Incidentally, switching to Marvelon or Mercilon as the follow-on oestrogen-dominant pill would be entirely logical since, despite the absence of any 'edict' against it, Dianette must be in the same safety category.

4.239 WHICH SKIN CONDITIONS ARE MORE COMMON IN COC-USERS?

1 *Chloasma/melasma.* This 'pregnancy mask' may develop in women on the COC after exposure to sunlight, just as in pregnancy. The condition may be very slow to fade after the pill is stopped. Mild degrees may be masked by careful use of cosmetics and tolerated if exposure to sun can be reduced. A progestagen-only contraceptive may help, but the condition can also recur with the POP. A non-hormonal method may have to be chosen.

2 *Photosensitivity.* This is more common in COC-takers. Very rarely it may be the first manifestation of one of the porphyrias (usually non-acute type, Q 4.219). Once acquired, like chloasma it tends to be permanent even if the pill is discontinued.

3 *Pemphigoid (herpes) gestationis.* If this serious skin condition occurs it absolutely contraindicates the COC.

4 *Hirsutism* is unlikely to be truly caused by the COC, but may be helped by an oestrogen-dominant product, especially Dianette.

5 *Loss of scalp hair.* There may be a true link, but not a long-term pill-related problem. Head hair density is always the resultant of the *telogen* (resting) and *anagen* (growth) phases. In pregnancy, and similarly in some women on the COC, a greater proportion than usual of the hair is synchronized into the growth phase. This is fine at the time, but can lead to a noticeable synchronized loss some time later – as is often reported in the puerperium.

6 *Telangiectasia, rosacea, neurodermatitis, spider naevi, erythema multiforme, erythema nodosum, eczema,* and possibly other skin disorders – all these have been described but not established, as possibly causally associated or exacerbated by COCs, in a minority of women. *Melanoma* is discussed at Q 4.133.

4.240 WHAT ACTION SHOULD BE TAKEN IF SUCH SKIN PROBLEMS PRESENT IN A COC-TAKER?

First, consider discontinuing the COC. Severe conditions such as *erythema multiforme* or *pemphigoid gestationis* would normally mean future avoidance of this method. If the condition has an immune/allergic basis it is usually unclear whether the COC steroids are the actual allergens (see Q 4.244). According to the views of the woman herself, therefore, and any dermatologist involved, if the condition is mild she may be cautiously rechallenged with a low-dose COC perhaps containing a different progestagen, or with the POP. Recurrence would suggest another method.

4.241 DOES THE COC CAUSE GINGIVITIS? ANY OTHER ORAL PROBLEMS?

Hypertrophic gingivitis is a rare but well-recognized complication of COC use. Lesser degrees are more common, as in pregnancy. Symptoms are minimized by good oral hygiene.

'Dry socket', a painful state after tooth extraction, is also said to be commoner in COC-users.

ALLERGIES AND INFLAMMATIONS

4.242 WHAT EFFECT DOES THE COC HAVE ON IMMUNE MECHANISMS?

Several studies on immunoglobulins have suggested that artificial sex steroids can modify immune mechanisms. The effects are of a similar nature to, but less marked than, those associated with pregnancy. A study from France, however, in which antibodies to EE were reported in patients suffering from venous thrombosis, has not been confirmed.

The RCGP Study in particular among the prospective studies showed an increase in inflammations and some disorders which are believed to have an immune basis. However, as shown in Figure 4.16 these are partly balanced by a well-established protective effect against thyroid over- and under-activity, and probably rheumatoid arthritis (see Q 4.235). Once again, as with both malignant and benign tumours (Figs 4.8 and 4.9), combination OCs seem to be capable of causing both beneficial and adverse effects within the same medical field. Causative associations are not all proven by any means and the magnitude of the effects described in Figure 4.16 is mostly small; but we badly need more information.

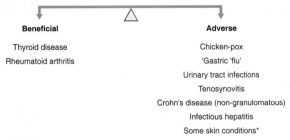

Figure 4.16 Immune disorders/inflammations and the pill. Q 4.242

4.243 DOES USE OF THE COC PROMOTE TRANSMISSION OF HIV INFECTION? OR MAKE AIDS MORE OR LESS LIKELY AFTER INFECTION?

To cut a long story short, 'no' seems the current best answer to both questions – though this field of research is notoriously difficult. Effective contraception is obviously important for any woman known to be HIV positive, so the COC is a useful option to be able to use as well as the condom. The LNG-IUS and DMPA may be even better choices. They do not appear to worsen the prognosis.

Studies among prostitutes in Nairobi were the first to suggest an increase in the likelihood of seroconversion to HIV positive if the COC were used; but a causative link has not yet been established.

4.244 DO WOMEN SOMETIMES BECOME ALLERGIC TO THE COC HORMONES, OR IN COC-USERS IS THERE AN INCREASED TENDENCY TO REACT TO OTHER ALLERGENS?

Anecdotal data exist to suggest that either may occur. For example, in vitro studies of blood lymphocytes suggested hypersensitivity to mestranol in two cases (one of erythema multiforme, one of erythema nodosum). On the other hand I have had a case of erythema nodosum who was able to go back on the same brand of COC without suffering any recurrence.

4.245 ARE THERE ANY GUIDELINES FOR SELECTING THE NEXT PILL IF A PATIENT COMPLAINS OF ANY MINOR SIDE-EFFECT AND WISHES TO CONTINUE THE METHOD?

NOTE: Never forget there may be another, non-pill-related, explanation for any side-effect, and that a side-effect may be caused or highlighted because of anxiety or a psychosexual problem. See the Preface. This applies particularly to this and the next question, and the linked Tables 4.17 and 4.18.

With modern COCs, an emotional or psychosexual explanation becomes more probable (though *not* invariable) if a woman keeps on returning with a wide assortment of side-effects after only taking a few tablets, and nothing ever seems to suit.

TABLE 4.17 WHICH SECOND CHOICE OF PILL? A: RELATIVE OESTROGEN EXCESS

Symptoms	Conditions
Nausea	Benign breast disease
Dizziness	Fibroids
Cyclical weight gain (fluid)	Endometriosis
'Bloating'	
Vaginal discharge (no infection)	
Some cases of breast fullness/pain	

Treat with progestagen-dominant COC, such as Loestrin 30, Microgynon 30, Eugynon 30 (but with caution regarding lipids)

On first principles, first take a history and, as appropriate, then examine. After that, if the side-effect relates to BTB or absent WTB she should either be switched to a *phasic pill* or moved 'higher up the ladder' (see Q 4.167).

TABLE 4.18 WHICH SECOND CHOICE OF PILL? B: RELATIVE PROGESTAGEN EXCESS

Symptoms	Conditions
Dryness of vagina	Acne/seborrhoea
Some cases of:	Hirsutism
Sustained weight gain	
Depression	
Loss of libido	
Lassitude	
Breast tenderness	

Treat with oestrogen-dominant COC, such as Ovysmen/Brevinor or Marvelon; or Dianette (an acne treatment which is also contraceptive, containing 35 µg of EE combined with 2 mg cyproterone acetate). Caution necessary, in that oestrogen-dominance may link with a slightly higher risk of VTE, see Q. 4.106.

Phasic pills may be worth changing *from*, however, if the symptoms are showing cyclical variation – e.g. breast tenderness, PMS-like symptoms (cyclical irritability, etc.). Monophasic pills, perhaps sustained for more than one packet consecutively (tricycling), can be of real benefit here.

For all other minor side-effects there are two empirical rules and two more specific ones. The empirical rules are:

1 Reduce the dose where possible (this will normally be the dose of the progestagen, as nearly all pill-takers should be on 30–35 µg of the oestrogen).

2 Alternatively, switch to another progestagen ladder (Fig. 4.12). For the more specific rules, see Q 4.246.

4.246 WHAT ARE THE MORE SPECIFIC RULES?

1 For side-effects or conditions which have become associated (through clinical experience, and sometimes by formal research) with a relative excess of the oestrogen, prescribe a more progestagen-dominant COC.

2 Conversely, for symptoms which have become associated with the progestagen, prescribe an oestrogen-dominant COC. This policy is summarized in Tables 4.17 and 4.18.

SPECIAL CONSIDERATIONS:
WHEN TO COME OFF THE PILL?

4.247 ARE THERE BENEFITS TO BE GAINED FROM TAKING BREAKS FROM COC USE? IS DURATION OF USE OF ANY RELEVANCE?

From the point of view of *preservation of fertility*, the answer is a categorical no on both counts (see Qs 4.67–4.68). In relation to all the examples of *circulatory disease*, duration of use has now been found to have no effect (see Q 4.96).

Even if intuitively it is still felt best to limit total duration of use, breaks will be of no value; *unless the breaks are so long as to have a real influence on total accumulated duration of use* (Fig. 4.17).

It is worth reminding any woman with this concern that during 10 years she has in fact taken 130 breaks! Moreover, there is increasing evidence that the body tends to restore metabolic changes towards normal during each PFI (see Qs 4.29–30).

Metabolic risk markers show no apparent progression beyond 2 years' continuous use. It could even be argued that repeated restarting of the COC might be more harmful than the relatively steady-state situation that is maintained during sustained use.

The main problem with breaks of several months at a time was well shown in a study in which during a planned break of just 6 months one quarter of young women had unwanted pregnancies.

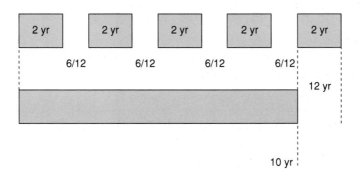

Figure 4.17 Breaks and accumulated duration of use of the COC. Q 4.247. The blocks represent segments of pill-taking duration (in which the only breaks taken are the pill-free weeks). Note how a woman who takes 6-monthly breaks every 2 years still accumulates 10 years of total duration in 12 years

4.248 WHAT IF SHE IS HARD TO CONVINCE THAT A BREAK WILL NOT BENEFIT HER

Of course we should *never* force anyone to continue: if they want to make a break then what matters most is to arrange an effective and satisfactory alternative. But so often the notion is not hers at all, it comes from a friend or a magazine, and if so Q 4.247 may help to reassure her about continuing.

4.249 WHAT ABOUT DURATION OF USE AND CANCER RISK? (Qs 4.70–4.90)

There are studies which show beneficial effects on cancer of the ovary and endometrium, and others showing possible harmful effects on cancer of the liver, cervix and breast. In each of these opposite categories both the beneficial and the adverse effects described are usually found to be greater with increasing duration of use! (The exception is breast cancer, where age and recency of use are the important factors, Q 4.82).

So the advantages of increased duration of use would help to balance the disadvantages. Short breaks are again unlikely to be relevant, see Figure 4.17.

Since at present it is impossible to state with certainty whether the good effects of pill use outweigh the adverse effects on cancer overall (see Q 4.72), though they may do so, it is equally impossible to assess accurately the changes on both sides of the equation caused by increased duration of use. See below, Q 4.250 and Table 4.19. The pros and cons seem roughly in balance.

4.250 HOW MUCH SHOULD AGE *PER SE* INFLUENCE PRESCRIBING, WITH REGARD TO BOTH CARDIOVASCULAR SYSTEM (CVS) RISK AND CANCER?

CVS RISKS AND AGE

Here opinions have changed since the first edition of this book, triggered by the landmark decision of the US FDA's Fertility and Maternal Health Drugs Advisory Committee in October 1989. Their recommendation, subsequently endorsed by the FDA itself, was for:

The removal of all age limits on the use of (combined) oral contraceptives by healthy non-smoking women – i.e. free of all risk factors.

TABLE 4.19 MANAGEMENT BY AGE, SMOKING AND DURATION OF COC USE

A: Age and COC use

	Age (years)				
	30	35	40	45	50
Smoker	Review	Change method	(COC contraindicated for contraception) (POP and HRT usable)		
Non-smoker	–	Review	Review	Review	Change method, or no method now if post menopause

B: Accumulated duration of use

	Duration (years)				
	4–5	10	15	20	25+
Smoker	Review	Second review	?Change method	Change method	–
Non-smoker	–	Review	Review	Review	Review

Both smokers and non-smokers with a relevant family history of breast cancer (or other risk factor) should review use carefully every 5 years (see Q 4.87).

Was this a cavalier decision, flying in the face of previously agreed practice? I think not, because:

1 non-smoking pill-takers are actually much 'safer' than we used to think;
2 modern prescribing and monitoring are more structured and careful;
3 the pills themselves are believed to be safer;
4 above all, we now have a much better appreciation of the benefits of the COC to gynaecological and some aspects of general health for women, most particularly older women (see Qs 8.38–8.39).

In short, even though the CVS risks (and breast cancer risks, see below) climb somewhat with age, the benefits increase at least as much and the risk/benefit ratio until the average age of the menopause is therefore probably unchanged. But only at their own request for healthy non-smokers!

After age 50 fertility is so low that I recommend using a less strong contraceptive than the COC anyway (see Q 8.53).

NOTE: The important issue of how to diagnose the menopause when it is masked by the COC or other hormones is discussed at Qs 5.63–5.65, 5.127, 8.43–8.47.

CANCER RISKS WITH AGE

These show a general increase with age; and the new 1996 CGHFBC 'model' for breast cancer risk shows that the pill-attributable 24% increment applied to an increasing background risk means proportionally more cases as the pill is used by older women (Q 4.86). But the COC protects against cancer of the ovary and endometrium whose incidence rises particularly above age 40. The extent of this balancing of the risk is difficult to quantify.

This new uncertainty about breast cancer risk is somewhat of a deterrent to older women, but fortunately there are several equally effective new choices for them (new IUDs, IUSs, implants).

4.251 IF A SMOKER REALLY DOES GIVE UP CIGARETTES AT AGE 35, MAY SHE CONTINUE TO TAKE THE COC? AND IF SO, UNTIL WHAT AGE?

There are no good data about this important question, for both practical and ethical reasons. Ex-smokers are a rare breed and their CVS morbidity would need examining prospectively with and without continuing to take the pill. We can extrapolate to some extent from the British Regional Heart Study of 7735 *men*, which reported that in ex-smokers of up to 20 cigarettes a day no excess risk of ischaemic heart disease (IHD) was observed in those who had quit 6–10 years prior to the screening, compared with never-smokers. However heavy ex-smokers (20 per day) still had a significantly higher risk after 11–20 years.

Other studies show a marked early decline in risk of IHD, due to loss of the acute metabolic effects of smoking; but they suggest in men that it takes 10 years to return to the levels seen in never-smokers. If this delay is due to early coronary atheroma generated by years of smoking, one must be concerned about the prothrombotic effects of ethinyloestradiol in any COC (Q 8.41).

In a 1990 report from the US in *women* ex-smokers, 'the increase in risk of a first myocardial infarction dissipated after 2–3 years'. This is more rapid than among the British men, but it does not establish safety if COCs had been taken and continued to be taken. The ex-heavy-smoker cannot be reassured like the risk-factor free woman about continuing with the pill until her menopause (Q 4.250); though in my view this is WHO 3, not absolutely contraindicated.

SOME REVISION QUESTIONS

4.252 WHAT ARE THE MEDICAL MYTHS ABOUT PRESCRIBING THE PILL?

Table 4.20 list is not exhaustive, but includes some important examples currently believed by some health care professionals.

TABLE 4.20 PILL MYTHS

Myth – Do not prescribe the COC in the following circumstances:	Actuality – The COC is:
Wish to optimize fertility	Beneficial (Q 4.68)
Fibroids	Beneficial (Q 4.91)
Current amenorrhoea, after investigation	Beneficial (Q 4.64) (sometimes)
Past amenorrhoea, resolved	Neutral (Q 4.66)
Recent menarche (if cycling)	Neutral (Q 4.232)
History of gestational diabetes (watch weight)	Neutral (Q 4. 144)
Thrush	Neutral (Q 4.228)
Recent trophoblastic disease (hCG now normal)	Neutral (Q 4.75)
Sickle cell trait	Neutral (Q 4.139)
Thalassaemia	Neutral (Q 4.135)
Epilepsy (allowing for drug interactions)	Neutral (sometimes beneficial) (Q 4. 202)
Sickle cell anaemia	Relative contraindication (Q 4.139)
Migraine (non-focal, tolerable, no change)	Relative contraindication (Q 4.154)
Cervical neoplasia (preinvasive)	Relative contraindication (Q 4.78)
Hyperprolactinaemia	Relative contraindication (Q 4.64)
Wish to minimize overall cancer risk	Unknown (but avoiding COC might even increase this risk) (Q 4.73)

4.253 WHAT ARE THE PILL MYTHS RELATING TO CONTINUING USE OF THE METHOD?

TABLE 4.21 PILL MYTHS (continued)

Myth	Actuality
1 There should be a break from pill use every few years	False (Q 4.247)
2 Duration of pill use should never be more than 5 (or 10) years at a time	False (Qs 4.247–4.249)
3 The pill should be stopped in all women reaching 35 years	Smokers (or if risk factors) (Q 4.250)
4 The COC should be stopped before all surgery	Only for major or leg surgery (Q 4.192)
5 Stop COC if there is prolonged absence of withdrawal bleeds (to preserve fertility)	Irrelevant (Q 4.10)

There are also myths which many doctors share with pill-takers about 'missed pills' (see Qs 4.18, 4.259 and 7.23(5)).

4.254 IN WHAT IMPORTANT SITUATIONS DO DOCTORS COMMONLY FORGET TO ENQUIRE WHETHER THE PATIENT IS ON AN OESTROGEN-CONTAINING PILL?

1 Emergencies, involving surgery, immobilization of a leg for fracture, or confinement to bed.
2 When elective arrangements are made for a major operation, or for surgery or sclerotherapy for varicose veins.
3 When any potentially interacting drugs are prescribed – especially rifampicin and griseofulvin.
4 When arranging any laboratory test, especially of the blood. Results of many tests may be modified by the COC (see Table 4.7, pages 155–6).

SOME QUESTIONS ASKED BY USERS ABOUT THE COC

4.255 I AM TOLD THROMBOSIS HAS TO DO WITH CLOTS – I HAVE CLOTS WITH MY PERIODS SO DOES THIS MEAN THAT I CAN'T USE THE PILL?

Far from it! Clots with the periods just means that they are heavy, and could well improve dramatically if you went on the pill – the COC would be better than the POP.

4.256 CAN I POSTPONE HAVING A PERIOD?

Certainly. The bleeding you get between packets of pills is actually entirely caused by you when you take a 7-day break between packets. It is really a 'withdrawal bleed' rather than a proper period, and there is no reason why from time to time you should not run two packets on to each other so there is no break and therefore no bleeding. The rules are a little different, however, for so-called phasic pills (see Q 4.179). Also it is not recommended that you simply take pill packets endlessly without any breaks – unless there is a special reason and then we recommend the so-called tricycle regimen (see Q 4.31, Fig. 4.4).

4.257 DO I ALWAYS HAVE TO SEE PERIODS AT WEEKENDS?

Certainly not. If it happens to have worked out that your periods are tending to come at weekends on the COC, all you need to do is to take some extra pills one month to move your withdrawal bleeding to a more convenient time (Q 4.50). Discuss with your doctor which pills to take if it happens to be a phased type (see Q 4.179).

4.258 MY 'PERIOD' IS MUCH LIGHTER THAN NORMAL, ALMOST ABSENT IN FACT AND A DIFFERENT COLOUR – DOES THIS MATTER?

No, anything from quite average sort of bleeding through to nothing at all can be normal for the response of an individual woman's womb to the stopping of the pill's hormones. Should you have no periods at all 2 months in a row, you should take prompt advice to eliminate the possibility of pregnancy and also to discuss whether you should start the next packet. This action should be taken even if you have only missed one withdrawal bleed, when you missed pills – or if there was earlier vomiting, severe diarrhoea or treatment with an interacting drug.

(Many other questions are asked about issues related to bleeding on the COC, whether normal, abnormal, or absent. These can be answered by reference to Qs 4.10, 4.32, 4.38, 4.50, 4.61–4.66, 4.165–4.179, 8.17 (18–26).

4.259 IS IT SAFE TO MAKE LOVE IN THE 7 DAYS BETWEEN PILL PACKETS?

Yes: but only if no pills have been missed (by forgetting, stomach upset or drug interaction) towards the end of the previous packet, and also only if you do in fact start another packet after the pill-free week (see Qs 4.15–4.24 and 8.17(16)). *Beware*, particularly when you come off the pill for any reason, including because of being sterilized.

4.260 WHICH ARE THE MOST 'DANGEROUS' PILLS TO BE MISSED – PRESUMABLY IN THE MIDDLE OF THE MONTH?

Not so, the middle of the month is the least bad time to miss pills, though you should not make a habit of missing any. ... The worst pills to be missed are any that result in lengthening of the pill-free time (see Qs 4.15, 4.18, 4.24). Never be late starting your next packet! This is something lots of people don't even consider as missing a pill.

4.261 ARE THERE ANY PROBLEMS IN PILL TAKING FOR FLIGHT CREWS?

It is easy for them, or other air-travellers, to become confused about regular pill-taking because of passing through different time zones. The effectiveness problem is greatest when flying due West, since the new bed-time pill might be late, many hours more than a day later than the preceding one. One solution is a watch which gives the time at their home base as well as local time. If in doubt on arrival at a new destination or if deciding to switch to morning rather than evening pill taking with a new pack, air-travellers should err on the side of taking a pill too early rather than late: especially leaving only 6.5 rather than 7.5 days between packets.

4.262 MY SKIN HAS GOT WORSE ON THE PILL, YET I WAS TOLD IT SHOULD GET BETTER – WHY IS THIS?

It all depends on the severity of your acne and which pill you have been given. The recommended ones are at Q 4.246 (Table 4.18).

4.263 DOES USING EITHER THE COC OR THE POP DELAY THE MENOPAUSE?

No. This occurs as a result of an inexorable process of egg loss which seems to be unaffected by anything, including never having babies and pill-taking. It even occurs at the same time as it otherwise would in women who as a result of surgery have been left with only one ovary. But it can be brought on earlier by a hysterectomy.

4.264 CAN I TAKE ANTIHISTAMINES FOR HAYFEVER AND THE PILL?

The ones given by your GP, or which you may purchase in the chemist, seem to cause no important change in the effectiveness of your pill. Other medicines may do, however (see Qs 4.33 and 4.34, Table 4.3), and the warning sign of an interaction can be bleeding during tablet-taking. Always tell any doctor, dentist or hospital that you take the pill.

4.265 IS IT TRUE THAT YOU ARE MORE LIKELY TO GET DRUNK IF YOU ARE ON THE PILL?

Some research published in 1984 suggested this, since it showed that alcohol leaves the body more slowly in pill-users than in non-pill-users. Subsequently, other researchers in Australia found the opposite, that pill-takers recovered from the effect of alcohol more quickly than non-takers! But the take-home message about which there is no argument is that *all* women should be extra careful about alcohol. This is because their smaller livers make it have a bigger effect than in men, both short term and long term (meaning that the risk of liver damage is greater in women).

4.266 WHAT ARE THE TAKE-HOME MESSAGES FOR ANY NEW PILL-TAKER?

1 Your FPA leaflet: this is not to be read and thrown away, it is something to keep safely in a drawer somewhere for ongoing reference. ...
2 The pill only works if you take it correctly: if you do, each new pack will always start on the same day of the week.
3 Even if bleeding like a 'period' occurs (breakthrough bleeding), carry on pill-taking. Ring for advice if necessary. But it usually settles in 8–12 weeks.
4 Lovemaking during the 7 days after any packet is only safe if you do go on to the next one: otherwise (if you are stopping the pill for any reason) start using condoms after the last pill in the pack.

5 Even if your 'period' has not stopped yet, never start your next packet late. This is because the pill-free time is obviously a time when your ovaries are not getting the contraceptive, so might anyway be beginning to escape from its actions.

6 For what to do if any pill(s) are more than 12 hours late, see Q 4.17.

7 Other things that may stop the pill from working include vomiting and some drugs (Qs 4.25, 4.33–4.42).

8 See a doctor at once if the things at Q 4.191 occur

9 As a one-off manoeuvre you can take extra pills or shorten one pill-free gap to make sure your withdrawal bleeds avoid weekends.

10 Good though it is as a contraceptive, the pill does not give adequate protection against sexually transmitted infections. Whenever in doubt, especially with a new partner, use a condom *as well*.

Finally, and crucially, always feel free to telephone or come back (maybe to the practice nurse) for advice at any time.

5

Oestrogen-free hormonal contraception

PROGESTAGEN-ONLY PILL (POP)

BACKGROUND AND MECHANISMS

5.1 WHAT ARE PROGESTAGEN-ONLY PILLS (POPS)?

In the UK these pills contain a microdose of one of three progestagens, either from the norethisterone group (norethisterone and ethynodiol diacetate) or levonorgestrel. They are taken on a continuous daily basis.

The first brand of this type contained chlormadinone acetate but it was withdrawn 1 year after introduction in 1969 when toxicity tests using the Beagle bitch showed that this progestagen tended to cause breast nodules, which could become malignant. As with Depo-Provera (see Q 5.110), it is now realized that this breed of dog is a highly inappropriate animal model.

5.2 WHICH POPS ARE IN CURRENT USE?

See Table 5.1. POPs account for no more than 10% of the UK oral contraceptive market. Yet as we shall see they have much to commend them, especially in the older age group.

5.3 HOW MUCH IS KNOWN ABOUT THE POP METHOD?

The short answer is: still remarkably little. No large cohort studies are in progress, and case-control studies have not been attempted because of the low prevalence of use. Hence we are forced to draw on the few metabolic and clinical studies available; and otherwise to extrapolate from available data on the combined pill (adjusting in an admittedly arbitrary way for absence of artificial oestrogen and presence of a particularly small dose of the progestagen).

TABLE 5.1 PROGESTAGEN-ONLY PILLS IN THE UK

Name	No. of tablets per packet	Progestagen	Dose (µg)
Microval/Norgeston	35	Levonorgestrel	30
Neogest	35	Levonorgestrel	37.5*
Micronor/Noriday	28	Norethisterone	350
Femulen	28	Ethynodiol diacetate	500

*Plus 37.5 µg of inactive isomer
Note: 'Cerazette' a POP with desogestrel 75 µg is expected on the UK market before long.

5.4 WHAT IS THE MODE OF ACTION OF POPS?

This is summarized in Table 5.2. The main action has previously been thought to be the alteration in the cervical mucus. But there is also a considerable effect on ovulation, in most women and in most cycles – at least 60% of the time – and more in older women. Ovulation may be abolished completely leading to amenorrhoea; but even without this there are varying degrees of interference with the ovulatory process as described in Q 5.5

It must therefore be understood at the outset that the hormonal environment of a previously cycling woman on the POP is the result of the *direct effect of the exogenous progestagen* and *an amount of ovarian activity* which varies – both between women and between cycles. This explains the very varied menstrual pattern which is observed, and is also relevant to other side-effects.

5.5 WHAT EFFECTS CAN THE POP HAVE ON OVARIAN FUNCTION?

In individual women, or in the same woman in different menstrual cycles, the effects vary. Although the patterns have been described in four groups, this is for convenience. The situation is better described as a spectrum running from no interference with the ovarian cycle, though to complete quiescence of the ovaries and no follicular or luteal activity.

In a short-term study (1980) of a POP with just 300 µg of norethisterone (i.e. the UK's Micronor/Noriday contains 17% more NET), Swedish workers have described four main groups in this continuum (percentage of cycles in parentheses):

1. Cycles showing almost no change from normal, with apparently normal ovulation, minimal shortening of the luteal phase, and progesterone levels within normal limits (40%).
2. Normal follicular phase but marked shortening of the luteal phase, with lower progesterone levels for a shorter time (21%).
3. Follicular activity with higher peak oestrogen levels than usual; but no ovulation and no progesterone production. Ultrasound scans of the ovaries in POP-users, most probably coming mainly from this group as described by the Swedes, show the formation of abnormal follicles or functional cysts, which may be single or multiple (23%).
4. Diminished follicular activity, low oestrogen levels, no ovulation, corpus luteum formation nor endogenous progesterone production. Ultrasound scanning confirms quiescent ovaries (16%).

TABLE 5.2 VARIOUS PROGESTAGEN DELIVERY SYSTEMS (ALL EXCEPT COC ARE OESTROGEN-FREE)

	Oral		Injectable		Implant
	COC	POP	NET-EN	DMPA	Implanon
Administration					
Frequency	Daily	Daily	2-monthly	3-monthly	3-yearly
Progestagen dose	Low	Ultra-low	High	High	Ultra-low
Blood levels	Rapidly fluctuating		Initial peak then decline		Constant
First pass through liver	Yes	Yes	No	No	No
Major mechanisms					
Ovary: ↓ Ovulation*	+++	+	++	+++	++
Cervical mucus: ↓ sperm penetrability	Yes	Yes	Yes	Yes	Yes
Endometrium: ↓ receptivity to blastocyst	Yes	Yes	Yes	Yes	Yes
Use effectiveness	0.2–3	0.4–4	<2	0–1	0–0.1
Menstrual pattern	Regular	Often irregular	Irregular	Very irregular	Irregular
Amenorrhoea during use	Rare	Occasional	Common	Very common	Common
Reversibility					
Immediate termination possible?	Yes	Yes	No	No	Yes
By woman herself at anytime?	Yes	Yes	No	No	No
Median time to conception from first omitted dose/removal	c. 3 months	c. 2 months	c. 3 months	c. 6 months	c. 2 months

*By two mechanisms – no pre-ovulatory follicles formed, plus no LH surges occur.

> **NOTE:** The POP is often given during lactation (see Q 5.55). The endocrine findings are then as in Group 4, but often shift at the time of weaning variably towards those of Group 1, as expected, with an increasing risk of ovulation.

5.6 HOW DO THE CHANGES DESCRIBED IN THE LAST QUESTIONS SHOW THEMSELVES IN THE MENSTRUAL PATTERN AND AFFECT THE RISK OF CONTRACEPTIVE FAILURE?

1 A majority of the women experiencing cycles of the type in Group 1 above will have regular periods. They are not immune to breakthrough bleeding (BTB), however, probably because of direct effects of the artificial progestagen on the endometrium. Here ovulation is the norm, the pharmacological effects on the pituitary/ovarian axis are minimal; but this means that they are also the group with the highest risk of breakthrough pregnancy. They are relying chiefly on the mucus and perhaps sometimes the endometrial effects for contraception (Fig. 5.1).

2 Groups 2 and 3, which show varying degrees of cycle disturbance, short of complete abolition, merge with each other and are therefore together in the middle column of Figure 5.1. It is from among these women that extra-frequent or erratic, irregular bleeds will be reported: the endometrium no longer receives adequate endogenous progesterone, and many of those in Group 3 also have increased oestrogen stimulation from the increased follicular activity. The bleeding pattern is a *resultant* of this abnormal ovarian activity and the (rather rapid) fluctuations each 24 hours in the level of exogenous progestagen. It would appear that it is in cycles showing the patterns of Group 2 and 3 that symptomatic or asymptomatic functional ovarian cysts may be formed. The risk of breakthrough pregnancy is considerably less than in Group 1, probably almost nil since such a cycle is anovular (though the woman could always have a Group 1-type cycle in another month).

3 In Group 4 at the extreme of the continuum, there is either complete amenorrhoea, or intermittent, very light bleeding. This is caused by irregular shedding of the endometrium, receiving less oestrogen than usual and just the daily exogenous progestagen administration

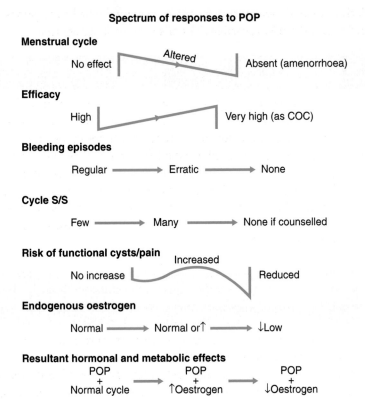

Figure 5.1 Spectrum of responses to the progestagen-only pill. Q 5.5, 5.6, 5.36 and 5.40. *Note* the metabolic effects are minimal anyway in *all* the groups, across the 'spectrum'

(in a saw-tooth pattern, like all oral medications; Q 5.85). The risk of contraceptive failure here is nil. It is of course also the norm for POP-taking during lactation.

5.7 WHAT THEN DOES AMENORRHOEA ON THE POP MEAN?

First, it may certainly be caused by pregnancy, and this must be excluded in the usual way. Once that explanation is ruled out, paradoxically the women experiencing prolonged episodes of amenorrhoea are the ones not ovulating and so actually at least risk of conception. It is from among the Group 1 POP-using women, who are experiencing regular periods and being regularly reassured thereby, that the majority of unplanned conceptions occur. See also Q 5.66 *re* possible risks of sustained amenorrhoea.

5.8 ARE ANY PARTICULAR POPS MORE LIKELY TO CAUSE ERRATIC PERIODS OR AMENORRHOEA?

As has to be said about so many aspects of POP use, the possibility of differences between the POPs has been inadequately studied. The Swedish studies quoted at Q 5.5 were not able to demonstrate any correlation between doses given or measured blood levels of the artificial progestagen and the types of ovarian reaction or the bleeding profile – even though the blood levels also showed wide patient-to-patient variation (see Q 5.9). So it appears that the main factor is the degree to which the end-organs, especially the ovary and the uterus, are susceptible to the effects of the POP in the blood.

5.9 IN POP-TAKERS, IS THERE THE SAME VARIABILITY IN BLOOD LEVELS OF THE STEROIDS AS DESCRIBED FOR THE COC (SEE Q 4.157)?

Yes. There is the same enormous variation between women who are apparently similar, taking the same POP and having their blood levels estimated at the same time after their last tablet was ingested. But variation in target-organ sensitivity appears more important (see Q 5.8) in causing bleeding side-effects.

There is also (as for COC-users) the fact of variation, again about tenfold, between the peak and trough blood levels each day within the same woman. This aspect is discussed at Qs 4.15 and 5.85 (Figs 4.2 and 5.3).

5.10 HOW DOES THE ENTEROHEPATIC CYCLE OPERATE FOR THE POP?

As in Figure 4.5 (see Q 4.14), after the artificial progestagen is absorbed, liver metabolism creates metabolites which re-enter the lumen of the bowel, via the bile. But the action of the bowel flora does not result in reformation of active progestagen. Hence the achieved circulating levels of the POP are normally not dependent on hydrolysis by the intestinal flora and subsequent reabsorption of the progestagen; so antibiotics can have no effect on POP blood levels. However enzyme-inducing drugs may reduce the blood levels and affect efficacy, just as they do with the COC (see Q 5.29).

EFFECTIVENESS

5.11 WHAT IS THE OVERALL EFFECTIVENESS OF THE POP?

As usual, reliability depends greatly on the motivation of the woman. An overall rate of 0.3–4/100 woman-years can be quoted, the higher rate occurring when patient compliance is poor, and particularly at very young ages, as discussed in Q 5.15. The lower rate applies particularly during *lactation* (Q 5.55).

5.12 WHAT IS THE INFLUENCE ON THE EFFECTIVENESS OF AGE, AND OF DURATION OF USE?

In the Oxford/Family Planning Association (FPA) study there was no evidence for the former view that the pregnancy rate increased with duration of use; if anything, the figures are compatible with the reverse (as is found with practically all other methods).

However, there is a marked influence of age (see Table 5.3). The failure rate falls from 3.1/100 woman-years for the age group 25–29 to 0.3 for women above the age of 40. Possible explanations are as follows:

1. The usual influence of declining fertility with age, shown for example also for the IUD (see Q 6.11).
2. Related to (1), it is well known that the prevalence of abnormal menstrual cycles increases with increasing age, and this is likely to predispose to abnormal ovulation (and the woman's POP cycles therefore being in Groups 2–4, as discussed at Q 5.5). Although not reported, it would be expected that the older women in the Oxford/FPA

TABLE 5.3 PROGESTAGEN-ONLY PILL – USER-FAILURE RATES/100 WOMAN-YEARS Oxford/FPA Study (1985 report) – all women married and aged above 25, any duration of use.

| All ages | Age (years) | | | |
	25–29	30–34	35–39	40+
0.9	3.1	2.0	1.0	0.3

NB: These figures are different from those given in Table 0.2, because they are based on nearly twice as many woman-years of observation.

study had a greater incidence of irregular bleeding and amenorrhoea; whereas the younger women would tend to have ovarian cycles which were more 'resistant' to the effect of the exogenous progestagen, and hence more would be ovulating and at greater risk of conception. They would necessarily be relying solely on the other two main effects of the method (on the mucus and endometrium).

3 Older women tend to have less frequent intercourse.

4 It is possibly also true that the younger women were less consistent in their pill taking.

5.13 DO OTHER FACTORS AFFECT THE EFFECTIVENESS OF POPS? WHAT ABOUT BODY WEIGHT?

The Oxford/FPA study was unable to show any statistically significant difference between the failure rate according to which particular POP *brand* was used, though appreciable variation was noted. Cigarette smoking did not appear to be of importance.

Body weight. The Oxford/FPA study did show a trend to higher pregnancy rates with increasing weight. Though not statistically significant, this has to be taken seriously as it is not implausible biologically (see below). Moreover there was significance in similar analyses of data for other progestagen only methods which rely on achieving very similar blood levels.

With both the levonorgestrel-releasing vaginal ring (Qs 5.168) and Norplant (Qs 5.152–5.158), specifically in trials of the higher-silica polymer 373 (an older subcutaneous implant which had a higher failure rate overall), the pregnancy rate was positively correlated to increasing weight. The ring in particular is such a similar method that I feel that the weight effect has to be considered real for the POP also, until a larger POP study or meta-analysis settles the issue. The 'bottom line' for me is:

There is as yet no proof that body mass is *not* important in the effectiveness of the POP.

5.14 WHY DOES THE BODY MASS EFFECT ON EFFICACY SHOW UP WITH SOME LOW-DOSE PROGESTAGEN METHODS AND NOT WITH THE COMBINED PILL AND INJECTABLES?

In reality the interesting observation is the absence of a weight effect with the latter two products. Note the emphasis here on mass or *weight*, *not BMI*. Dilution, of the administered drug in the greater amount of 'water of distribution' (apparent distribution volume) existing in a bigger person – whether they are tall or short – is expected for any drug. It is the basis after all for usually reducing adult doses when giving drugs to children.

My explanation for the absence of an observable effect with the COC and injectables is: that they have too high a safety margin as effective anovulants (coupled with their adjunctive contraceptive effects), in users of whatever weight, for this trend to be detectable in studies of a realistic size. The doses given by the progestagen-only methods of Q 5.13 (the ring and polymer 373 implant) however are nearer the minimum for efficacy, so something like weight can exert a detectable influence on the failure rate.

5.15 WHAT ARE THE IMPLICATIONS OF THE ABOVE FINDINGS WITH REGARD TO EFFICACY?

1   *In lactation*: the combination of full breastfeeding and the POP equates to almost 100% contraception (see Q 1.36). Even the young woman who is overweight would be most unlikely to conceive – until weaning begins anyway. ...

2   *For older women*. The main implication of these findings for them is the remarkable efficacy of the method. Since they are precisely the group who may need to transfer from the COC (see Table 4.10), it is useful to be able to state quite truthfully to a woman over 40: 'Your chances of conceiving if you are a regular taker of the POP are the same as for a 25-year old taking a modern combined pill'. (The Oxford/FPA study gives method-plus-user failure rates of around 0.3 in both instances.)

3   *For the young*. Unfortunately the Oxford/FPA study did not include women under the age of 25. However, extrapolating from Table 5.3, the expected failure rate in teenagers is likely to be quite high, say 4/100 woman-years, especially since compliance tends to be less good in the young.

Some studies which included many women in their twenties have shown acceptable failure rates of 1–2/100 woman-years. So with careful selection and education of users the POP is certainly on the list of options for the young.

4   *For the overweight*. (see Qs 5.13 and 5.14). Pending more data, I personally feel we should warn women weighing above 70 kg (11 stone) of the *possibility* of a higher failure rate than as quoted in Q 5.11. If nothing else is suitable and the woman is *not* breastfeeding, the use of two POPs per day may be considered, particularly in the under 30s. They are after all

compounds with a very safe therapeutic margin. Since this is unlicensed prescribing, it must be done with careful counselling and record-keeping, on the 'named patient' basis (page 507). I usually advise taking both tablets at once for simplicity.

5.16 FOR THOSE USERS WHO ARE STILL OVULATING, HOW LONG DOES THE CONTRACEPTIVE EFFECT ON THE CERVICAL MUCUS LAST, FOLLOWING EACH DOSE?

As illustrated in Figure 5.2, following one tablet the effect appears maximal about 4 hours later, but in this one study there was some return of sperm penetrability around 24 hours. Regular POP-taking seems to abolish this, so one can assume that the cervico-uterine fluid is difficult for sperm to traverse throughout the 24 hours.

Figure 5.2 actually derives from some work in the late 1960s using the POP megestrol acetate (0.5 mg). Similar data are available for levonorgestrel but these studies badly need repeating with more modern investigative techniques.

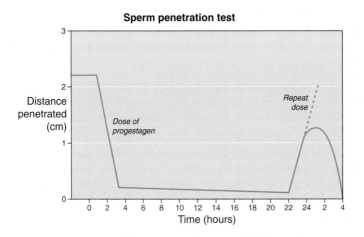

Figure 5.2 Sperm penetration of cervical mucus after progestagen. Q 5.16. *Note* minimum reduction in sperm penetration between 4 hours and 22 hours after a single dose of megestrol acetate (0.5 mg). Unlike the rest of the figure, the effect of a repeat dose is presumed, not experimental. (Redrawn from Cox HJE 1968 The pre-coital use of minidosage progestagens. *Journal of Reproduction and Fertility Supplement* 5: 167–172, Figure 1)

Scanning electron microscope (SEM) studies have shown a characteristic tight mesh of microfibrils in mucus obtained from women using various microdose progestagens – when the progestagenic effect is maximal. However, in cycling women (Group 1 in Q 5.5), if the mucus is sampled at mid-cycle as little as 36 hours after the last tablet was taken the SEM appearances are already nearly back to the normal open mesh of oestrogenic mucus which sperm can readily penetrate. Such studies are prone to artifacts, but others, showing rapid loss of associated cellular and biochemical changes in mucus after discontinuation of progestagens, confirm Figure 5.2. The contraceptive effect of the POP on mucus can be assumed to *disappear* certainly by 12 hours if a woman is late in taking a tablet.

Hence for contraceptive safety a much stricter rule must be observed (see Q 5.20).

5.17 WHAT ENDOMETRIAL EFFECTS HAVE BEEN DESCRIBED IN POP-USERS?

As with other tissues, observations differ according to the variable amount of endogenous ovarian activity superimposed on the direct effect of the progestagen (see Q 5.5 and Fig. 5.1.).

That said, blockade of progesterone receptors occurs, and characteristic changes have been described in the histology of the endometrium on both light and electron microscopy. Uterine glands diminish both in number and in diameter. These and associated biochemical effects are believed to reduce the likelihood of successful implantation.

5.18 HOW IMPORTANT IS THE ENDOMETRIAL EFFECT, HOW LONG DOES IT TAKE TO DEVELOP AND HOW READILY IS IT LOST?

The answers to all these questions are largely unknown. The mucus effect has been more fully studied, but the endometrial effect may well be a useful back-up during long-term POP use, particularly when ovulation is not abolished.

5.19 FOR MAXIMUM EFFICACY OF THE POP, HOW AND WHEN SHOULD IT BE TAKEN?

As implied by Figure 5.2, and the answer to Q 5.16, the answer to 'how?' is: 'extremely regularly'. Indeed I always tell prospective POP-users that the POP is 'a package deal'. In other words 'here is your packet of pills, now get your partner to give you a present – an alarm watch!' Women who are not breastfeeding are encouraged to take their tablets at precisely the same time each day (plus or minus 1 *hour*). There is very much more leeway during full lactation (Qs 5.6, 5.24 and 5.55), since ovulation is then inhibited and the situation is not unlike taking the COC.

Some have concluded from Figure 5.2 that the best regular pill-taking time is in the early evening, if the woman usually has intercourse when she goes to bed. However, that may not be an easy time for good compliance. And the hard data in Figure 5.2 relate to taking only the first tablet in cycling women: it is believed that the mucus effect is thereafter sustained for at least 27 hours with modern POPs.

It is only a minority who have fertile ovulations at all on the POP (at most the 40% in Group 1 of the study reported at Qs 5.5 and 5.6), and would therefore need to rely solely on the mucus effect. For them it might be argued that the worst time for regular pill-taking is just before the commonest time for intercourse: since the woman would then be *regularly* relying on the tablet taken 24 hours earlier. But regular pill-taking is so much the most important thing that if she finds that is her easiest time to remember, so be it. It is often simplest to recommended pill-taking at the time of a main meal (breakfast, lunch or supper) or absolutely *any time* during lactation.

5.20 WHAT RULE DO YOU RECOMMEND FOR MISSED POPS?

It has proved difficult to reach international agreement on the matter of 'missed POP rules'. This is not too surprising in view of: the spectrum of effects of this method on different women and in different cycles (see Q 5.5); the lack of data about the relative importance of the end-organ contraceptive effects in Table 5.2; and the different situation applying during breastfeeding. (Unless otherwise stated the discussion below applies outside of 100% lactation.)

1   There is good agreement among the authorities on one point: since the mucus effect is so quickly lost, *extra precautions should begin if a woman is more than 3 hours late* in taking her POP (27 hours since the last tablet).

2   The difficult part of the advice is: for how long should loss of contraception be assumed? From 1985 to 1992 in the UK the FPA recommended in its instruction leaflets that an additional contraceptive method should be used just for the next 48 hours. But since 1993 the leaflets specify 7 days (see below).

5.21 MOST MANUFACTURERS' DATA SHEETS HAVE SAID FOR YEARS THAT A LATE POP MEANS 14 DAYS' LOSS OF PROTECTION. DOES IT TAKE THAT LONG TO RESTORE THE EFFICACY OF THE POP?

No – most authorities feel that is certainly too long:

1 The pill-free-week problem is non-existent here (cf. Qs 4.15–4.27).
2 The hostile mucus effect seems to be maximal (and sustained) within no more than 48 hours.
3 Even a 2-day rule allows about 5 days for the recommended POP to have its contraceptive effect on the endometrium. (Even if sperm managed to penetrate the mucus before the 2 days of extra contraception started, it would be least 5 days before any blastocyst would start implanting).

5.22 SO WHY ARE 7 DAYS ADDITIONAL PRECAUTIONS NOW RECOMMENDED, IF ONE PILL (OR MORE) IS MISSED FOR MORE THAN 3 HOURS?

1 The main reason initially was pragmatic, faced with the manufacturers' 'over the top' 14-day recommendation.
2 Second, 7 days' extra precautions would, conveniently, be the same duration as in the rule for missed combined pills (see Q 4.17). The 48-hour role did always seem oddly short to women switching from the COC, when the prescriber said it was not quite as effective and stressed how much less margin for error her new pill would have!
3 Third, given the fact that considerably more than half of POP-users actually obtain their main contraception by a block to ovulation (those, especially the older women, whose cycles are in the Groups 2, 3 and 4 of Q 5.5 above): 7 days would allow longer for any lost ovarian suppression to be restored. This may or may not be important in some women: there are no data.

In my opinion it would not be too helpful to change again from this 7-day advice, now we have it in place. It errs on the side of caution and it is more consistent with the COC. But since US authorities and the IPPF recommend only 48 hours added precautions based on the mucus effect, I fear that for some while yet confusion will reign in this matter.

5.23 WHEN SHOULD EMERGENCY POSTCOITAL CONTRACEPTION BE CONSIDERED IN ADDITION, IF POP TABLETS ARE MISSED?

In my opinion, this decision anyway should be based on *the mucus effect*: i.e. emergency pills should be offered for any unprotected intercourse which occurred after the 3 hours delay which might lead to loss of the mucus effect, but before two pills had been taken to restore it (see Q 7.23(6)). The usual 72-hour 'window' from the earliest exposure would apply, and 7 days of extra precautions should then follow, as in the basic UK advice.

5.24 HOW SHOULD THE ADVICE DIFFER IF PROGESTAGEN-ONLY PILLS ARE MISSED DURING LACTATION?

The strict instructions proposed at Qs 5.19–5.23 are designed for women who are not breastfeeding! *During lactation* ovulation is inhibited while there is sustained amenorrhoea; particularly during the first 6 months postpartum when (if the LAM criteria are observed) lactation even without the POP is 98% effective (see Fig. 1.4). Missing a POP is then equivalent to missing a COC in mid-packet (Q 4.22).

The 'leeway' must therefore go up, to at least 12 hours. But because breastfeeding varies in its intensity and to give a consistent message, it is usually wise to keep to the general policy of advising 7 days' added precautions. Some individuals, after discussion, may be told they may disregard it. And it would be most exceptional ever to find it necessary to offer emergency contraception, to fully breastfeeding POP-users with amenorrhoea.

5.25 HOW LONG DOES IT TAKE TO ESTABLISH EFFICACY WHEN STARTING THE POP?

The contraceptive effect on the mucus develops very rapidly (Fig. 5.2). We do not know the minimum time needed to establish the anti-ovulation or anti-implantation effects. However, with a first-day start and hence taking at least seven pills before the earliest it would occur, any POP-induced interference with fertile ovulation ought theoretically to be as great as it will be in later cycles. So no extra precautions are now advised with a first-day start and this seems adequate.

5.26 WHAT THEREFORE ARE THE RECOMMENDED STARTING ROUTINES WITH THE POP?

See Table 5.4, and important footnotes.

TABLE 5.4 STARTING ROUTINES WITH THE POP

	Start when?	Extra precautions?
Menstruating	1st or 2nd day of period	No
Postpartum		
(a) No lactation*	Day 21 (see text & Q 8.22)†	No
(b) Lactation*	Day 21, or later (see Q 5.57)	No
Induced abortion/miscarriage	Same day or next day	No
Post COC	Instant switch	No
Post DMPA	Instant switch before or at 12 weeks since last injection	No

*Bleeding irregularities minimized by starting at or after the 4th week.
†See Q 8.22 re starting artificial hormones later on during postpartum amenorrhoea:
Provided there is certainty that there is no chance of an early pregnancy, can start POP (or COC) any time plus 7 days' extra precautions.

5.27 WHAT ADVICE SHOULD BE GIVEN TO A WOMAN WHO VOMITS A TABLET AND FAILS TO REPLACE IT SUCCESSFULLY WITHIN 2 HOURS?

Except during full lactation, she should take extra precautions as well as taking her tablets for the duration of the vomiting and for 7 days thereafter.

5.28 SHOULD ANY ACTION BE TAKEN IF A POP-USER REQUIRES ANTIBIOTIC TREATMENT?

Yes if the antibiotic is an enzyme-inducer! This means only rifamycins, (e.g. rifampicin) and griseofulvin. *Otherwise no action is required* since, as explained at Q 5.10, ordinary broad-spectrum antibiotics can have no effect on the blood level of the active exogenous progestagen.

5.29 SHOULD THE POP BE AVOIDED BY WOMEN USING ENZYME-INDUCING DRUGS?

Enzyme-inducers do lower progestagen as well as oestrogen blood levels, and the failure rate of the POP would therefore be expected to increase. Extra precautions should be advised during and for at least 7 days after any short-term treatment – and much longer after rifampicin, see Q 4.37. (The drugs concerned here are in Table 4.3, Q 4.34.)

Long term, a better hormonal option might be an injectable along with a shortened gap between injections (see Q 5.91). If the POP is preferred, Professors Back and Orme of Liverpool suggest that the dose be increased to two POP tablets per day – or even three tablets in the presence of factors like young age or obesity. Even then the woman should be warned that the efficacy of such a regimen is not well established. And as usual, since this is not supported by the Data Sheets, the 'named patient' criteria should be observed (page 507).

5.30 CAN THE SMALL DOSE OF PROGESTAGEN IN THE POP INFLUENCE OTHER DRUGS?

Since the effect of the COC on other drugs is for most practical purposes negligible (see Q 4.45), the effect of the lower dose in the POP can certainly be disregarded.

ADVANTAGES AND BENEFICIAL SIDE-EFFECTS

5.31 WHAT ARE THE ADVANTAGES OF THE POP?

Acceptable efficacy, in the range of 0.3–4/100 woman-years. Higher efficacy applies in the older women, for whom combined oral contraceptives (COCs) might be contraindicated.

No epidemiological proof, so far, of increased risk of either circulatory or malignant disease. Again this is not certain because of inadequate study; plus any (good or bad) effects may very well vary between women because of the variable impact of the POP on the hypothalamo–pituitary–ovarian axis.

Avoidance of all side-effects in which artificial oestrogens are implicated.

Minimization of any side-effects in which progestagens are implicated. *Minimal alteration in all metabolic variables* which have been measured (see Qs 5.40–47).

Good general tolerance – especially suitable for women who complain of side-effects with other hormonal methods, or in whom the latter are contraindicated.

Most minor symptoms of the COC are not a problem, such as weight gain, nausea, headaches and loss of libido.

8 *Return of women's fertility* on discontinuation more rapid than after the COC.

9 The tiny dose means *minimal effect on lactation*, and levels of the artificial steroids within breast milk seem to be negligible.

10 *No harmful effect from overdose*, even when taken by a child.

5.32 DO THE BENEFICIAL EFFECTS LISTED AT Q 4.50 ALSO APPLY TO THE POP?

1 Some do – most of the *contraceptive benefits*, for example.

2 Some women report improvement in *symptoms of the menstrual cycle*, notably premenstrual symptoms and dysmenorrhoea. Others report the reverse (see Qs 5.33 and 5.69).

3 Protection against *pelvic infection* is extremely probable through the mucus 'barrier' effect, though not yet proven for the POP (see Qs 4.58 and 5.93).

4 For the remaining items listed in Q 4.55 there is so far no evidence to suggest that the beneficial effect applies to the POP. And functional ovarian cysts are more, not less, frequent (see below).

MAIN PROBLEMS AND DISADVANTAGES

5.33 WHAT ARE THE MAIN PROBLEMS OF THE POP?

1 The need for *obsessional regularity* in pill taking (see Q 5.19). This is less critical during full lactation.

2 *Alteration of the menstrual pattern* is the main problem, except in breastfeeders. The reasons are explained at Q 5.5. According to that Swedish study one can predict to some extent the type of change that the POP will produce. Women whose own normal cycles had long follicular short luteal phases were more likely to be in Group 4 on the POP (tending to have episodes of amenorrhoea). Those with regular or short cycles – who had relatively short follicular but normal length luteal phases – were more likely to enter Group 1 and have the more regular bleeding.

In general, the duration and volume of flow may change, and there may be intermenstrual episodes. Alternatively the woman may develop amenorrhoea.

All in all cycle irregularity is the commonest reason for abandoning the method. Yet a woman can be told that irregularity means the method is probably more effective in her particular case (see Q 5.6). Another disadvantage therefore is that:

Precisely in those women with the most acceptable, regular cycles, the risk of pregnancy is greatest.

A small number of women develop symptomatic *functional ovarian cysts* (see Q 5.35), causing pain which may sometimes be severe enough to imitate an ectopic pregnancy.

Pregnancies in POP-users are more likely to be ectopic than are pregnancies occurring in the general population. As for the IUD (see Qs 6.29 and 6.32), it is not thought that the POP actually increases the risk of ectopics in a population of POP-users; indeed the reverse is true.

5.34 WHAT IS THE RISK OF ECTOPIC PREGNANCY? WHY DO ECTOPICS OCCUR IN POP-USERS?

When compared with sexually active non-pregnant controls studies have shown a *reduced* risk of ectopic pregnancy in POP-users. This is to be expected because the method often interferes with ovulation, and with fertilization. Moreover the effect of the POP on cervical mucus should reduce the risk of tubal damage in the first place, from pelvic infection.

However in some studies the likelihood of any breakthrough pregnancy which actually happens being ectopic is increased. Possible explanations include the following:

A selection effect, exactly as described for the IUD (see Q 6.30), if there is pre-existing tubal damage and fertilization occurs. The numerator of ectopics is reduced, but if the denominator of POP 'breakthrough' pregnancies is reduced even more, the *relative* frequency of ectopics among the conceptions will increase.

Progestagens may modify tubal function. Overall contractility and the rate of ovum transport are decreased, the latter probably from a reduction in the number of ciliated cells.

Of the two, the first explanation is thought by far the more important. See Qs 6.30–6.32. Ectopics can only happen if normal ovulation occurs, followed by fertilization; i.e. the risk relates only to a subgroup of Group 1 in Q 5.5.

5.35 HOW FREQUENT ARE FUNCTIONAL OVARIAN CYSTS AMONG POP-USERS?

In a Margaret Pyke Centre (MPC) study, functional ovarian cysts (FOCs) as diagnosed by ultrasound occurred in as many as half the POP-users (12/21), compared to four out of the 21 controls. Most of these were asymptomatic but seven women – all of them POP-users – complained of some pain; one required admission for rest and analgesia.

It is also clinical experience that some POP-users are diagnosed as cases of ectopic pregnancy (menstrual irregularity plus one-sided pain and a tender mass) but laparoscopy shows only a functional cyst, or evidence that one has recently ruptured.

5.36 WHAT IS THE CAUSE OF FOCs?

The precise causation of FOCs remains undefined. They are clearly due to an abnormality of ovulation (sometimes luteinization of an unruptured follicle) which is succeeded by accumulation of fluid. On the basis of the groups defined at Q 5.5 one would expect the frequency to be no different from a control population in Group 1, and actually reduced in the group with quiescent ovaries, Group 4. The increased frequency would be expected (though this is just my hypothesis) to manifest itself in Groups 2 and 3, especially 3 (see Q 5.54 for the clinical implications).

5.37 DOES THE POP AFFECT NEOPLASIA?

Little is known, for the reasons discussed at Qs 4.71 and 5.3. The UK National Case Control Study (1989) found a possible protective association with breast cancer, whereas the CGHFBC suggested an increased risk similar to that which they described for the COC (Q 4.81). So 'the jury is still out': if there is any real influence of the POP on carcinogenesis it will be subject to two important considerations:

1 Any effects may be (slightly) beneficial on some cancers, adverse on others (as for the COC, see Q 4.72), and usually related in each case to duration of use.
2 Intuitively, the effects are likely to depend in part on the amount of interaction with the woman's menstrual cycle, i.e. her 'Group' in Q 5.5.

For the present one can truthfully state to any woman: 'there is no evidence to suggest that any POP increases the risk of cancer'.

5.38 WHAT EFFECT DOES THE POP HAVE ON TROPHOBLASTIC DISEASE?

See Q 4.75 for a discussion of the reasons why in this country it is advised that the COC, and also for the time being the POP, should normally not be used until hCG levels are undetectable.

5.39 WHAT IS THE INFLUENCE OF THE POP ON BENIGN TUMOURS, SUCH AS BENIGN BREAST DISEASE AND FIBROIDS?

There is no evidence that any of the tumours mentioned at Q 4.91 are affected by use of the POP – but no evidence of no effect, either.

5.40 WHAT ARE THE EFFECTS OF THE POP ON METABOLISM?

Although this has been slightly better studied than the epidemiology, there are few good studies of modern POPs. Moreover, the studies can be faulted on at least one of the following counts:

1 Inadequate attention to confounding – meaning that the changes seen might be due to characteristics of the woman for whom a POP was chosen, rather than the POP itself.
2 Lack of attention to the different metabolic responses to be expected, according to whether the users respond to the POP as in the Groups 1, 2, 3 or 4 of Q 5.5. Figure 5.1 shows that the resultant metabolic effects might well vary: from (in Group 1) those of the normal menstrual cycle with normal ovarian oestrogen plus a small effect from the POP, to the situation (Group 4) where the progestagen is opposed by relatively little endogenous oestrogen production.

Despite these limitations, the overall findings of the metabolic studies are very reassuring, as discussed in the next questions.

5.41 WHAT ARE THE EFFECTS OF THE POP ON COAGULATION AND FIBRINOLYSIS?

1 Studies have shown that the POP, unlike COCs, has no important measurable adverse effect on blood clotting, platelet aggregation or fibrinolytic activity.
2 One interesting study looked at prostacyclin and thromboxane levels. Among COC-users prostacyclin levels were decreased (favouring platelet aggregation). There was no change in the POP group however, and in the latter, particularly among women using levonorgestrel alone, the thromboxane concentrations were depressed. Since thromboxane enhances platelet aggregation, this could even indicate a decreased risk of thrombosis in POP-users.

5.42 PRESUMABLY, THE POP MAY THEREFORE BE USED BY WOMEN WITH A DEFINITE PAST HISTORY OF THROMBOEMBOLISM, EVEN IF COC RELATED?

Yes, definitely (see Q 5.50). But most Data Sheets for POPs still do not say this!

The norethisterone products are particularly interesting. Past thrombosis is stated to be a 'contraindication' to the POP Noriday containing 350 μg of this progestagen and the Data Sheet recommends it is discontinued at least 4 weeks before elective operations. However, if you turn over just a few pages in the ABPI Data Sheet Compendium (1999) it is described that 'Utovlan' contains norethisterone 5 mg, which is regularly used for gynaecological indications such as menorrhagia, in doses up to 15 mg daily. Yet *past* thromboembolism is (rightly, in fact) not included as a contraindication and there is no mention at all about stopping the drug before major surgery! How come, when the same manufacturer's norethisterone is being given in 45 times the dose in Utovlan as in the Noriday POP, about which the Data Sheet creates anxiety about a past thrombosis history?! I rest my case.

5.43 WHAT ARE THE EFFECTS ON BLOOD LIPIDS, ESPECIALLY HIGH-DENSITY LIPOPROTEIN-CHOLESTEROL (HDL-C)?

The POPs currently available seem to have little effect on all the main aspects of lipid metabolism; but in one or two studies the important subfraction HDL_2-C was slightly depressed with POPs containing either levonorgestrel or norethisterone. This might be expected to happen less in those POP-users who have more endogenous oestrogen from their own ovaries – Groups 1–3 of Q 5.5.

5.44 WHAT ARE THE EFFECTS ON CARBOHYDRATE METABOLISM?

Once again a consensus view is that the effects are minimal. However, some studies have shown a slight deterioration in glucose tolerance and a tendency to hyperinsulinism, particularly in users of the levonorgestrel POPs. Some studies cannot exclude the possibility that adverse metabolic findings are the result of selection of the POP by users who have arterial disease risk factors, so that use of the POP is coincidental not causal.

5.45 MAY THE POP BE USED BY FRANK DIABETICS?

Certainly – after the diaphragm or sheath the POP can be the method of choice. Workers in Edinburgh have found that with 350 μg norethisterone POPs no increase in insulin dosage appeared necessary, and there was no change in the incidence and severity of retinopathy. They consider the POP to be an ideal choice from the metabolic point of view. In addition only one pregnancy occurred among 50 women during the period of observation (1050 woman-months) and the woman concerned omitted a number of pills.

Generally diabetics have exceptionally good compliance since they take their pill with each evening dose of insulin.

5.46 WOULD YOU USE CURRENT POPs IN A DIABETIC WITH EVIDENCE OF TISSUE DAMAGE, ESPECIALLY ARTERIOPATHY?

The uncertainty about metabolic effects makes this WHO 3, in my view (certainly not absolutely contraindicated), but other options like an IUD or IUS might be preferable.

5.47 HAVE ANY OTHER METABOLIC EFFECTS BEEN DESCRIBED?

1 When progestagens are administered alone they have little if any effect on hepatic secretion of plasma proteins – cf. the COC, Q 4.93.
2 Thyroid and pituitary-adrenal function also appear to be unaffected.
3 Progestagens beneficially affect the biochemistry and physiology of cervical mucus (see Q 5.16), thereby probably protecting the user against pelvic infection.
4 They also appear to improve aspects of erythrocyte metabolism in sickle cell anaemia (see Q 5.95).

5.48 SO, DOES THE POP AFFECT THE RISK OF CIRCULATORY DISEASE?

We lack adequate data. In the Oxford/FPA study there were just two cases of venous thromboembolism and two of stroke in 3303 woman-years of study. Considering the women were in the older age group and in general more likely to have other risk factors for circulatory disease, this seems a highly acceptable incidence.

Although we can be sure that the absence of artificial oestrogen does not increase the risk of thrombosis, we cannot be so sure about the effect on arterial wall disease.

5.49 DOES THE POP AFFECT BLOOD PRESSURE?

Reassuringly, apparently not. Studies have shown *neither* the slight rise in systolic and diastolic pressure which occurs in almost all individuals given oestrogen-containing preparations, *nor* any increase in the incidence of clinical hypertension. *COC-induced hypertension reverts to normal on the POP.* The same appears to apply to DMPA and other oestrogen-free methods in this chapter. *Progestagens appear adversely to affect blood pressure only if oestrogens are also administered.*

In a POP-user another cause (notably essential hypertension) should be sought if hypertension is diagnosed.

SELECTION OF USERS AND OF FORMULATIONS

5.50 FOR WHOM IS THE POP METHOD PARTICULARLY INDICATED?

As a working rule: *Contraindications to or side-effects with the COC, and a hormonal method is preferred? Try the POP.* Or, more specifically:

1 *Women above 35 who smoke cigarettes.* On present information it is acceptable to continue use of the POP even in a smoker on her say-so until beyond the average age of the menopause (i.e. about 50 years). See Qs 5.63–5.65 about establishing menopausal infertility)

2 *Oestrogen-linked contraindications or side-effects on the COC.* Some of those listed on the left of Table 4.17 (Q 4.246) may improve. The POP should not be chosen preferentially for conditions such as endometriosis, since it does not reliably suppress endogenous oestrogen. But the main point is that this category of indications for the COC also includes:

3 *History of or any predisposition to thromboembolism, including known prothrombotic coagulation factor changes*: since adverse effects on clotting mechanisms have not been demonstrated (see Qs 5.41 and 5.42). It follows, accordingly:

4 *Chronic systemic diseases* in which oestrogen is the hormone which might exacerbate the condition (e.g. *systemic lupus erythematosis (SLE)*) or where there is an extra thrombosis risk (e.g. severe cases of *Crohn's* or *ulcerative colitis* (Q 4.141)) and, again SLE (Q 4.142). *Sickle cell disease* is another example. But, see Q 5.95, for this DMPA may be an even better option.

5 Patients with *diabetes* or *obesity*. Diabetics do particularly well on the POP, especially with regard to compliance (see Q 5.45). There are *efficacy considerations for the obese* (see Qs 5.13–5.15).
6 Patients with *hypertension*, either related to the COC or other varieties if well-controlled by treatment.
7 Patients with *migraine* (including, with appropriate caution and advice, young women with migraines which are severe or with focal aura). See Qs 4.147–4.163.
8 During *lactation* (see Qs 5.55 and 5.56). This is a well-established indication, in which the method has the highest efficacy.
9 At the *woman's choice*: such as a reliable pill-taker who prefers a hormonal method, yet wishes to use the least possible amount of exogenous hormone.

5.51 WHAT ARE THE CONTRAINDICATIONS TO THE POP?

As we have seen, a long list of conditions contraindicating use of POPs may be found in the manufacturers' data sheets, but most are there for medicolegal reasons, with no epidemiological basis.

In general and with the exceptions suggested below, the absolute contraindications to the COC (WHO 4) are only relative contraindications (of varying importance, most commonly WHO 2) for the POP.

As before, any list of contraindications must be to some extent a matter of personal judgement (Q 4.132) and, with the POP, involve some informed guesswork – given the dearth of good data. ...

5.52 WHAT THEN ARE THE ABSOLUTE CONTRAINDICATIONS TO THE POP, IN YOUR VIEW?

So far as possible these are listed in the same order as for the COC (see Q 4.131), and here as in the next Questions the WHO categorization is used (WHO 4 throughout, here, unless otherwise stated).

1 *Past very severe arterial wall disease, or current exceptionally high risk of the same* (WHO 4, occasionally 3). Pending further information I would not normally prescribe the POP long term to a woman known to have current ischaemic heart disease including angina or to have already suffered a thrombotic stroke; nor to women with marked and multiple risk factors (e.g. a 45-year-old heavy smoking hypertensive diabetic!).

Severe hereditary lipid abnormalities with a poor prognosis come into this category because of 'exceptionally high risk'. However the POP may be prescribed with extra counselling and supervision in the presence of milder abnormalities with a good prognosis (WHO 3, see Q 5.53).

2 Any *serious side-effect occurring on the COC and not clearly due only to oestrogen* – or associated with past progestagen-only use. Liver adenoma or cancer, and severe past sex steroid-associated cholestatic jaundice would come here, since it is not clear with which of the two hormones in the COC they are primarily linked. Also in this category:

3 *Recent trophoblastic disease* (see Q 4.75) but only while the hCG is elevated.

4 *Acute porphyria*, past history of an actual attack (Q 4.218). See below if latent, with no history of past attack.
So it is a very short list, though as for all medical methods, we must add:

5 *Allergy* to a constituent.

6 *Undiagnosed abnormal genital tract bleeding* since the POP will confuse diagnosis.

7 Actual or possible *pregnancy*.

8 The woman's *own continuing uncertainty* about POP safety, even after full counselling.

5.53 WHAT ARE ONLY RELATIVE CONTRAINDICATIONS TO THE POP, IN YOUR VIEW (I.E. IT MAY CERTAINLY BE USED, BUT WITH CAUTION AND SOMETIMES SPECIAL MONITORING)?

Here there is much obvious overlap with Q 5.50. The WHO 2 'Broadly usable' category (which mainly applies, below) makes the POP an excellent second choice when the first choice was a *pill*, but the COC is now 'out' for some reason.

1 *Risk factors for arterial disease* (WHO 2, or 3 if severe or multiple). This category includes:
   (a) established *hypertension* once it has been diagnosed and controlled;
   (b) the presence of *more than one risk factor* can be tolerated more readily than with the COC. Prothrombotic coagulation factor abnormalities are rightly included above as 'indications', since they should not be worsened at all by the POP;
   (c) likewise, there is not the oestrogen-related concern about thrombotic stroke in migraine, including *migraine with focal aura* – though the headaches may be still be affected by the POP hormone.

(d) *Lipid abnormalities* might be slightly worsened by the POP, especially in Group 4 (see Q 5.5) amenorrhoeic women: however I still consider that if they have a good prognosis they are WHO 3. Hence elevation of cholesterol to above 8 mmol/l, which is usually a WHO 4 absolute contraindication to the COC, would only relatively contraindicate the POP (WHO 2).

2 *Past subarachnoid haemorrhage*: if there has been good recovery and definitive treatment such that the neurologists are confident recurrence is unlikely, this is WHO 2. But COC may also be usable (Q4.140).

3 *Sex-steroid-dependent cancer (WHO 3)*. In general, discuss this with the oncologist looking after your patient, particularly for breast cancer. There is no evidence that the POP affects the prognosis after breast cancer is diagnosed. Caution should still be exercised and the final decision should be the woman's own after counselling.

4 *Current liver disorders* (e.g. jaundice, cirrhosis) with persistent biochemical changes (WHO 2 unless severe changes). *FNH* is WHO 3 (Q 4.131).

5 *Acute porphyria*, latent without a past attack – but WHO 3, needs caution and full counselling of the woman regarding risk of a future attack (see Q 4.218).

6 *Relevant interacting drugs*. The dose can be increased in selected cases (see Q 5.29). Caution is also necessary in *severe* malabsorption states.

7 *Chronic systemic diseases* (see also Q 5.50). The same fundamental approach as at Q 4.135 for the COC applies here. The POP has the slight disadvantage of lesser efficacy, especially if pregnancy is made more dangerous by the particular disease. But this is balanced by the likelihood that if hormones were one day shown to worsen the prognosis, the tiny dose in the POP ought to have less effect than the COC.

Relative contraindications specific to the POP among pills:

8 Previous *ectopic pregnancy* (see Q 5.34), especially in a nulliparous woman. She is at risk of recurrence, plus a future second ectopic could endanger her future fertility as well as her life. Her remaining tube (or tubes) deserves maximum protection – which an anovulant method like the COC or DMPA or Implanon (Q 5.157) could provide.

On the other hand for an informed woman, especially if she is parous, this history is not quite an absolute contraindication, more like WHO 3.

9 *Functional ovarian cysts* (FOCs). These are definitely associated with the POP (see Qs 5.35 and 5.54). A past history of hospitalization for severe pain resulting in this diagnosis would be WHO 3. However, some

women may prefer to continue using the method, since most episodes of FOC formation will be practically asymptomatic.

10 *Unacceptability of irregular menstrual bleeding.*

11 Where *complete protection against pregnancy is vital*, especially if the woman is likely to be at all erratic as a pill-taker. In my view the method is therefore often (certainly not always) contraindicated for *teenagers* in general: chiefly because of its innately higher failure rate at this age (see Q 5.12) which may be increased by compliance problems.

5.54 WHAT ARE THE CLINICAL IMPLICATIONS OF AN INCREASED RATE OF FOCs?

1 Ultrasound studies suggest that most FOCs are asymptomatic – see Q 5.35.

2 It is likely that sex hormone production by functional cysts may explain some of the menstrual irregularity. For example, in half of the Group 3 women in the Swedish study (see Q 5.5) a high oestradiol followed by an abrupt fall was associated with a withdrawal bleed 72 hours later. This could well have been due to disappearance of a cyst (ultrasound scanning was not available).

3 The main risks of FOCs are those of unnecessary surgery, especially laparoscopy, and rarely also necessary surgery for acute events such as ovarian torsion. This is why the past history of *symptomatic* FOCs, either before use of the POP or while taking it, should now be considered WHO 3.

In my experience, however, some women so much prefer this method to the alternatives that they are prepared to take the risk of recurrences. They should be advised to take prompt medical advice as indicated. Given the problem of distinguishing this syndrome from ectopic pregnancy, pelvic ultrasound and ultrasensitive pregnancy tests should be utilized to avoid unnecessary laparoscopies or other surgery.

USE OF THE POP IN LACTATION

See Q 5.24 for the enhanced efficacy implications of the POP during breastfeeding. Worldwide, this is in fact the commonest context in which POPs are used.

5.55 WHAT ARE THE EFFECTS OF THE POP ON LACTATION?

The COC can reduce the volume and alter the constitution of milk. Some of the artificial steroids are transferred to the infant. By contrast the POP appears a suitable choice for lactating women. Indeed progestagens when administered alone, by any of the means discussed in this chapter, appear to reduce neither the volume of milk nor the duration of lactation, and some reports suggest that both may be increased. Careful studies on both norethisterone-and levonorgestrel-containing POPs show that the amount transferred to the milk is minute and most unlikely to present any hazard. Studies of the blood of suckling infants have been unable to demonstrate any progestagen, since the concentration is below the limits of the sensitivity of present assays.

Last, but not least, the contraceptive combination of lactation plus the POP is nearly 100% effective.

5.56 WHAT ARE THE IMPLICATIONS FOR PRESCRIBING THE POP DURING LACTATION?

1 First and foremost, the above findings need discussion. The prospective user may be interested to learn that, according to Scandinavian studies of 30-μg levonorgestrel POPs, after 2 years of lactation with regular POP-taking the infant will have received at most the equivalent of one tablet! If this is not sufficiently reassuring, of course, another method should be adopted.

2 Another advantage is that the main symptom with the POP – irregular bleeding – is unlikely during lactational amenorrhoea, except when it is first commenced postpartum (see Q 5.57).

5.57 WHEN SHOULD THE POP BE COMMENCED AFTER DELIVERY?

1 Since, unlike the COC, the POP does not affect lactation nor the risk of venous thrombosis, it is medically safe to start it in the immediate postpartum period. WHO calls such early use WHO 3, due to some concern that the neonate may be at some risk if exposure is in the first 6 weeks after delivery.

2 Studies have shown a greater likelihood of spotting and bleeding problems with starting early in the puerperium. So unless there are special reasons to start earlier, initiating the POP around day 21 is

recommended by the FPA (Table 5.4, page 280), as with the COC. Of course even a 6 week time of starting would be fully effective combined with full breastfeeding (Q 1.36).

5.58 HOW SHOULD WEANING BE MANAGED IN POP USERS?

Some women simply continue using the POP long term. However I well remember a clinic in which two consecutive women described how they had unwantedly conceived another pregnancy, through not being warned that the margin for error of their POP method would plummet once they weaned their child!

Therefore if greater efficacy is desired, the woman who is beginning to wean her infant should be prescribed in advance a suitable combined pill. She should be instructed to start taking it when breastfeeding frequency halves, or once solid food is being given or at the first bleed: whichever comes first. Relevant is the fact that the first fertile ovulation is more likely to happen without a first warning bleed, if it is more than 6 months since delivery.

The increased dose of hormones in the breast milk is not believed to have any relevance to the health of the baby, but the COC may very well hasten the end of lactation.

5.59 WITH OR WITHOUT LACTATION, WHICH POP SHOULD BE CHOSEN?

After consideration of the contraindications (see Qs 5.52 and 5.53), there are few guidelines.

- Neogest is not a very logical choice since it gives an added unnecessary dose of non-contraceptive dextro-norgestrel.
- During lactation, Microval and Norgeston are possibly preferable to the other POPs since such a negligible amount reaches the breast milk (see Q 5.56) – due to marked binding to SHBG in the blood.
- No study has shown statistically different rates of effectiveness between the levonorgestrel POPs (Microval, Norgeston, Neogest) and the norethisterone group (Micronor, Noriday and Femulen).
- A 'best buy' can also not be stated for menstrual disturbance or any other minor side-effects.

The initial choice of POP for cycling women is therefore an arbitrary one.

INITIAL MANAGEMENT AND FOLLOW-UP ARRANGEMENTS

5.60 WHAT ARE THE MAIN ASPECTS TO CONVEY DURING COUNSELLING?

- The truth of the phrase 'forewarned is forearmed' is never so clear as in counselling about the unpredictable bleeding pattern of the POP (as indeed for all the oestrogen-free methods in this chapter).
- Its good efficacy, second only to the combined pill and injectables, especially in older women, should also be stressed – provided always that the rules for successful pill taking are followed (see Qs 5.19–5.29).
- As for other methods, a supplementary leaflet (e.g. that produced by the FPA) should always be supplied.

5.61 HOW SHOULD POP USE BE MONITORED?

POP monitoring should be much as for the COC (see Qs 4.180 and 4.181), but almost all users can be put into the 'safer' category 2.

- A baseline blood pressure and weight are valuable.
- Routine cervical smear examinations are good screening practice, though (as before) not believed to have any special relevance to the contraceptive method.
- The woman should be seen 3 months after starting the POP and normally 6 monthly thereafter – but the interval may be extended, and all checks performed by the family-planning trained nurse, with recourse to a doctor only if problems arise, such as pelvic pain.
- Otherwise routine examinations should be kept to a minimum. Blood pressure may be recorded annually, once 6-monthly checks for 12 months have been entirely normal. Weight only needs to be measured in relation to decisions about whether to take two pills to maintain efficacy (Q 5.13).

5.62 FOR HOW LONG MAY POP USE BE CONTINUED?

At present the answer is 'indefinitely' as long as contraception is required, in the absence of contraindications, multiple-risk factors, or the occurrence of important complications.

5.63 HOW CAN THE MENOPAUSE BE DIAGNOSED IN OLDER POP-USERS?

If a POP-user develops prolonged amenorrhoea, yet was previously observing bleeding episodes, it can be difficult to distinguish between amenorrhoea secondary to the POP and the arrival of the menopause.

1 Symptoms, especially hot flushes, can be a useful guide.
2 There is also evidence that a high level of follicle stimulating hormone (FSH) may have some relevance at the menopause despite continued POP-taking. Low levels, on the other hand, suggest that the woman is in Group 4 of Q 5.5, still potentially fertile, and should certainly continue to use this or some alternative contraceptive method.

5.64 HOW DO YOU ACT IF THE FSH IS HIGH IN AN OLDER POP-USER? IS THERE A PRACTICAL PROTOCOL?

If the FSH is high (at menopause levels for the laboratory), my practice above age 50 is to suggest that the woman discontinues the POP and transfers to a simple barrier method. The FSH is then repeated at 4–6 weeks, on two occasions if there is any doubt.

If the woman is still amenorrhoeic, has vasomotor symptoms, and menopausal FSH results are again obtained, she may be advised that her chances of conception are low enough to discontinue alternative contraception – whether or not she now transfers to taking hormone replacement therapy (HRT).

No guarantee of total infertility can be given, however, and she is warned to return for advice should she develop any subsequent (non-HRT-related) bleeding. And women who want more complete reassurance should continue a simple method of birth control until 1 year after the last spontaneous bleed.

5.65 WHAT IF FSH MEASUREMENTS ARE LOW?

If she is amenorrhoeic, one's only concern relates to possible hypo-oestrogenism – see Qs 5.66 and 5.102. Since she needs contraception, the benefits of switching to using Delfen foam may be discussed (Q 3.64). Otherwise the POP may simply be continued into the 50s with periodic FSH checks.

5.66 SHOULD I BE CONCERNED ABOUT HYPO-OESTROGENISM IN ANY POP-USER WHO DEVELOPS PROLONGED AMENORRHOEA, UNRELATED TO THE MENOPAUSE (I.E. LOW FSH RESULT)?

This is a difficult one: as in the similar situation applying to DMPA, there are insufficient data. There has to be the *possibility* that some women in Group 4 at Q 5.5, with quiescent ovaries, may have very low plasma oestradiols (though most have more than adequate follicular activity despite no bleeds). That subgroup might then in the long term be like women with premature menopause. We know the latter are definitely at risk of early myocardial infarction and of osteoporosis, but no-one knows whether hypo-oestrogenism in a POP-user would have the same risks. If so, both those conditions would be further exacerbated by heavy cigarette smoking, which has known adverse effects on plasma oestrogens and (separately) on the risk of arterial disease. But the tiny progestagen dose makes this problem much less likely than with DMPA.

Arbitrarily, pending more data, I am currently suggesting that the same protocol is followed, after at least 5 years, as for long term DMPA-users: **please see the full account at Qs 5.102–5.106**. (*If* onset of the menopause in an older POP-taker is suspected, an FSH measurement would be done first, as in Qs 5.63 and 5.64 above). In the rare POP case who had very low oestradiol levels after counselling, taking natural oestrogen on an 'add-back' basis by any chosen route might then be advised.

5.67 IF ADD-BACK OESTROGEN IS TAKEN BY A POP-USER, WON'T THIS MAKE HER MORE LIKELY TO CONCEIVE?

Not in the circumstances just described, when she starts off in Group 4 of Q 5.5 which means she is not ovulating. She is not relying on the mucus effect for contraceptive efficacy, anyway, so it cannot enhance her fertility if the mucus is improved by the added oestrogen.

MANAGEMENT OF SIDE-EFFECTS OR COMPLICATIONS

5.68 WHAT SHOULD BE THE SECOND CHOICE OF POP IF BLEEDING PROBLEMS DEVELOP AND CANNOT BE TOLERATED?

First: examine the patient – for a coincidental gynaecological cause. (See Table 4.15 and Q 4.163!)

2   An understanding of the spectrum of individual reactions to the POP is of
    some help (see Qs 5.5 and 5.6). It would appear that the bleeding
    problems are concentrated in Groups 2 and 3. Group 1 cycles are generally
    the most acceptable. With good counselling, women in Group 4 can also
    accept their long episodes of amenorrhoea (but see Q 5.66). Careful
    assessment of the bleeding pattern therefore aids decision-making.

3   If it appears that a reduction in dose might transfer a woman from
    Group 2/3 to Group 1, one could for example switch from Femulen to
    Micronor/Noriday.

4   The reverse could be tried if reaching Group 4 seemed likely to be
    achieved thereby, i.e. a trial of Femulen, the strongest POP available.
    But this could be counterproductive, making the bleeding irregularity
    worse, if amenorrhoea did not result.

5   Switching between the levonorgestrel and norethisterone group POPs
    may be useful, but has to be empirical since their precise equivalence
    has not been worked out.

5.69 WHAT MINOR SIDE-EFFECTS HAVE BEEN DESCRIBED IN POP-TAKERS?

The short answer is that POP-users report almost any of the minor
side-effects reported by COC-takers, but in general less frequently. In the
Oxford/FPA study, headaches, psychological disturbance and hypertension
were particularly associated with COCs as a cause of discontinuation of
the method. However, menstrual disturbance and, interestingly, breast
discomfort, were reported more commonly among POP-users. Mildly
androgenic effects such as acne also occur.

5.70 WHICH SECOND CHOICE OF POP SHOULD FOLLOW IF NON-BLEEDING MINOR SIDE-EFFECTS DEVELOP?

The decision to change to a different POP has again to be empirical. For
example, if headaches occur on a levonorgestrel POP, it may be worth
transferring to one of the norethisterone group.

With support and reassurance, however, the subjective symptoms often
disappear after a few months of continuing to take the same POP.

When available, the new desogestrel POP (Cerazette, see Table 5.1) will
be a useful option for women with either bleeding or non-bleeding minor
side effects.

5.71 WHAT ACTION SHOULD BE TAKEN IF A POP-USER COMPLAINS OF LOW ABDOMINAL PAIN?

As usual, causes unrelated to contraception should be excluded. But two particular possibilities must be borne in mind, especially as both also cause menstrual irregularity and perhaps a unilateral mass:

- Ectopic pregnancy.
- Pain due to the formation/torsion or rupture of a functional ovarian cyst. Referral for ultrasound and (rarely) laparoscopy may be required. See Q 5.54.

5.72 WHICH SYMPTOMS SHOULD LEAD A POP-USER TO TAKE URGENT MEDICAL ADVICE? SHOULD SHE TRANSFER TO ANOTHER METHOD AT ONCE?

Abdominal pain is probably the only acute symptom requiring urgent advice. But neither for this, nor for any of the symptoms in the COC list at Q 4.191 (which are mostly irrelevant as they relate to oestrogen), should the woman discontinue the POP instantly without first arranging another method. Continuing to take the POP for a few more days can do no significant harm – whereas an unplanned pregnancy might.

5.73 WHAT SHOULD BE DONE IF A POP-USER IS IMMOBILIZED AFTER AN ACCIDENT OR REQUIRES EMERGENCY (OR ELECTIVE) MAJOR SURGERY?

There is no reason for a woman using any oestrogen-free preparation to discontinue the method in either of these clinical contexts.

5.74 WHAT ARE THE RISKS IF A WOMAN SHOULD BECOME PREGNANT WHILE TAKING THE POP?

1. If she *has* conceived, although the POP does not cause ectopics, a higher *proportion* of conceptions than usual prove to be extrauterine: so it would be clinically important to exclude the condition (see Q 5.34).
2. The available findings concerning teratogenesis are extremely reassuring. No cases of congenital abnormality have been reported, though there have been no good large studies. In the Oxford/FPA study

there were 30 accidental pregnancies in continuing POP-users. Of these seven were terminated, 15 ended in live births without malformations, one was ectopic and seven ended in spontaneous miscarriage.

See also Q 4.222. Given its small dose of only one hormone, the usual 'armchair thinking' about the POP would lead one to expect an even lower rate of fetal abnormalities in breakthrough POP pregnancies than with the COC. The rate for the latter (which is more firmly documented) is itself already remarkably low.

There is certainly no need to advise switching from the POP to another method for any arbitrary time before a planned conception (very debatably necessary even for the COC, see Q 4.224).

5.75 ARE THERE ANY RISKS OR BENEFITS FOR EX-TAKERS OF THE POP?

There are no data to support or refute any such ex-use effects. If they exist at all they are likely to be clinically insignificant.

QUESTIONS ASKED BY USERS ABOUT THE POP

The general public does not ask many questions about the POP, since few know of its existence as a separate method. Much confusion between these 'mini-pills' and low-dose combined pills has to be cleared up. The following short list may be instructive.

5.76 DOES THE POP EVER CAUSE AN ABORTION?

No. Although not its usual method of action, one possible way the POP operates on some occasions is by stopping implantation: the process by which a dividing fertilized egg becomes embedded in the lining of the womb. Stopping this is not now felt by most people to be causing an abortion, for the reasons explained at Qs 7.2 and 7.3. But the POP rarely if ever works this way, anyway and NEVER when combined with full breastfeeding (Q 5.24).

Reading the question a different way, deliberately taking a large number of POPs (or combined pills for that matter) is not a recognized abortifacient method: it is most unlikely to stop a fully established implanted pregnancy. (Even though they do work as emergency contraceptives, see Chapter 7.)

5.77 IF THE POP IS NOT SO EFFECTIVE AS THE COMBINED PILL, WHY ARE SOME WOMEN RECOMMENDED TO USE IT?

Taken regularly, this method is only a little less effective than the combined pill, especially in women above the age of 35. Indeed above the age of 40 it is as effective as the COC would be for a 25 year old. Otherwise the POP is chosen chiefly because of some medical reasons for not using the COC, which is the more normal first choice.

5.78 MY PERIOD IS OVERDUE ON THE POP – WHAT DOES THIS MEAN?

First, we must exclude the possibility that the method has let you down. Once that has been done, the most likely explanation is that the pill is preventing egg release. So paradoxically you will be more effectively protected from pregnancy than a girlfriend who is seeing regular periods on this pill (see Q 5.7).

5.79 I KNOW THAT COC USERS DO NOT SEE PROPER PERIODS – IS THAT ALSO TRUE OF THE BLEEDS I GET ON THE POP?

On the POP, some episodes of bleeding are caused like normal periods. In these the special structure in your ovary known as a corpus luteum stops producing the two hormones which stimulate growth of the uterine lining, and this leads to it coming away, and hence a period. However, many POP-users have other bleeding or spotting episodes as well. These are either shorter or longer than a normal period and can be lighter or heavier. They are caused by irregular shedding of the womb lining, in turn caused by combined effects from the artificial hormone of the POP and the oestrogen and progesterone produced by your ovary (see Qs 5.4–5.6 and Fig. 5.1).

5.80 I AM BREASTFEEDING MY BABY AND HAVE BEEN GIVEN THE POP – WON'T THIS HARM MY BABY?

Although a very tiny amount of the hormone does get into the breast milk, it has not been possible to show any changes in milk quantity or in quality.

There cannot be absolute proof that the POP hormone in the milk would be completely harmless: so if you are unhappy it would be important to discuss another method with your family doctor or a local clinic.

However, the amount taken by the baby is very small; for example with Microval or Norgeston your baby will take only the equivalent of one tablet if you continue to breastfeed for 2 years! In short, it is extremely unlikely that your baby will be affected at all (see Qs 5.55 and 5.56).

INJECTABLE CONTRACEPTIVES – DMPA AND NET EN

BACKGROUND AND MECHANISMS

5.81 WHAT ARE INJECTABLES?

The two available in the UK are progestagenic steroids given on a regular basis by deep intramuscular injection for contraception. Experience with them dates back to the early 1960s. DMPA (see below) has been used by over 20 million women worldwide.

5.82 WHAT INJECTABLES ARE AVAILABLE IN THE UK?

1 Depot medroxyprogesterone acetate (DMPA). This is available in aqueous microcrystalline suspension and is normally given in a dose of 150 mg every 12 weeks. Other regimens have also been tried and proved effective.
2 Norethisterone oenanthate (NET EN, Noristerat, Norigest). This is available in a vehicle of benzyl benzoate and castor oil, the dose being 200 mg every 8 weeks. Other regimens are not now recommended.

NOTE: DMPA is an example of a pregnane progestagen, which is more closely related to natural progesterone than either oestrane progestagens such as norethisterone or gonanes such as levonorgestrel – all derived from 19-nortestosterone.

5.83 WHAT IS THE STATUS AND AVAILABILITY OF INJECTABLES WORLDWIDE AND IN THE UK?

DMPA has been repeatedly endorsed by the WHO and the International Planned Parenthood Federation (IPPF) and virtually every other relevant authority. It is currently available for long-term contraceptive use in more than 130 countries, including the UK, Sweden, Germany, Denmark, the

Netherlands and New Zealand. It has been repeatedly recommended for similar licensing by the obstetrical and gynaecological subcommittee of the USA Food and Drug Administration (FDA), and finally received approval at the end of 1992. It is currently used by around 12 million women worldwide.

In the UK the Minister of Health agreed in 1984 to the earlier recommendation by the Committee on the Safety of Medicines (CSM) that the method could be used long-term for contraception, by selected women after full counselling about its long term (and slow to reverse) nature. It now has the status of a first-line option in the UK. Yet it is still chosen currently by a very small minority, only about 2% of women using reversible contraception in the UK. This low usage is largely provider-led: the option is offered so infrequently: most of those who do use it are very satisfied customers!

NET EN is used, chiefly in Germany and a number of developing countries, less widely. It is also available in the UK, a product licence for antifertility use having been granted. Although it is only officially for short-term use at present, longer-term use is acceptable in selected patients after counselling.

5.84 WHAT IS THE MODE OF ACTION OF INJECTABLES?

The primary action of the progestagen dose given by both injectables is, like the COC, to prevent ovulation. As with other hormonal methods, this is supplemented chiefly by contraceptive actions at the endometrial and mucus level (see Q 5.4 and Table 5.2.)

5.85 DO INJECTABLES PROVIDE A STEADY DOSE?

No – see Figure 5.3. Although the levels fluctuate far less than any oral method (COC or POP), there is a much higher level initially, declining exponentially thereafter. The release of hormone at a relatively constant or so-called zero-order rate is one of the advantages sought in newer injectables, and also rings and implants (see below).

5.86 WHAT IS KNOWN ABOUT INDIVIDUAL VARIATION IN BLOOD LEVELS?

This exists, as for the oral methods. However, the inter-individual variation is rather less marked since variable absorption from the gut and variable

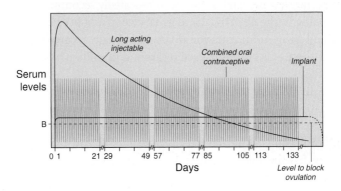

Figure 5.3 Blood levels of progestagen hormone in users of three delivery systems. Q 5.85. This is a schematic representation for DMPA. After an injection there is a relatively high level – B indicates the level to block ovulation – then a decline as time passes. Oral contraceptives (the POP would be similar, without a 7-day break) show wide fluctuations – a sawtooth pattern. Implants lead to remarkably constant blood levels. (Adapted from *Population Reports* K2 May 1983 Population information program. Johns Hopkins University, Baltimore, Figure 1)

'first-pass' metabolism (see Q 4.33) are not involved. Blood levels seem to decline more rapidly in thin women (see Q 5.89). *NET EN* has a shorter duration of action than DMPA.

5.87 WHAT EFFECTS DO INJECTABLES HAVE ON OVARIAN FUNCTION?

Since ovulation is generally inhibited, the 'spectrum effect' described at Q 5.5 for the POP is not observed with these agents. However follicular activity occurs, especially towards the end of the injection period and more in some women than others. Importantly, this follicular oestradiol keeps serum concentrations in the range normally found in the early to middle follicular phase (90–290 pmol/l). This prevents clinical hypo-oestrogenism (whether as symptoms or signs) in the majority of users. However there is some concern about a few who in long-term use are found to have abnormally low oestradiol levels (see Qs 5.99 and 5.102).

EFFECTIVENESS

5.88 WHAT IS THE OVERALL EFFECTIVENESS OF INJECTABLES?

Among available reversible contraceptives the use-effectiveness of these methods is in practice greater than the COC – since the factor of the user's memory is almost eliminated. The range of efficacy quoted for DMPA is 0–1/100 woman-years, and for NET EN 0.4–2/100 woman-years.

5.89 WHAT FACTORS INFLUENCE THE EFFECTIVENESS OF INJECTABLES?

As usual, the rate of failure is marginally higher in younger, more fertile women; and also paradoxically in women who are underweight, especially in studies from developing countries.

With either compound but especially NET EN it is essential not to massage the injection site (see Q 5.124) since this shortens the duration of action, increasing the failure rate in early studies. Local infection of the injection site may also be a factor (see Q 5.96 (11)). It is important to insert the complete dose without spillage and ensure it is truly intramuscular even in an obese woman.

5.90 WHAT ARE THE RECOMMENDED STARTING ROUTINES FOR INJECTABLES?

1   *In menstruating women* the first injection should normally be given before day 5 of the cycle (IPPF says day 7, and it can even be later if there has been 'believable abstinence or the equivalent' up to that date). With either drug the contraceptive effect is said to be immediate. Yet, because of the analogy with the COC (Table 4.4), and a couple of conceptions in my service (one was ectopic), I personally advise extra precautions for 7 days if the first dose is any later than day 2.

2   *If a woman is on the POP or COC*, and definitely not pregnant if amenorrhoeic on the former (see footnote to Table 4.4, Q 4.49), the injection can be given any time, and with no added precautions. The medical suitability of this 'overlap' of the two methods can be useful, for example in a combined pill-taker over the time of elective major surgery (Q 4.195).

3   *Postpartum* (whether or not the woman is breastfeeding). It is now clear that the first injection should *preferably* be postponed until 5–6 weeks

after the delivery. Earlier administration increases the likelihood of heavy and prolonged bleeding.

However this is not inevitable and DMPA can be given in the first week, exercising clinical judgement, if there is doubt whether the woman will return at the right time for her first dose. She must then be forewarned about the increased bleeding risk. Lactation is not inhibited.

4 *After miscarriage or termination of pregnancy* (first trimester). The injection is normally given within 7 days of the procedure and no extra precautions are required. See also Qs 4.75, 5.116 re trophoblastic disease.

5.91 DO INTERACTIONS WITH OTHER DRUGS POSE ANY PROBLEM WITH INJECTABLES?

1 There is certainly no problem with non-enzyme-inducing antibiotics, since the drug is not recycled from the gut.
2 Drugs inducing liver enzymes (see Q 4.36) pose a theoretical problem, particularly in the time just before the next injection is given (Fig. 5.3). As can be seen from the figure, increasing the dose may not usefully extend the duration above the level to block ovulation. It is therefore recommended:

that the interval between injections is shortened to 10 weeks for DMPA; or even to 8 weeks in the more high risk situations, e.g. when the ultra-potent enzyme-inducers rifampicin or rifabutin are used.

5.92 MIGHT INJECTABLES AFFECT THE ACTION OF OTHER DRUGS?

In clinical practice it seems that this possibility can be disregarded.

ADVANTAGES AND BENEFITS

5.93 WHAT ARE THE BENEFICIAL EFFECTS OF INJECTABLES?

These can be listed as follows:

CONTRACEPTIVE BENEFITS

1 *High effectiveness* – definitely greater than the COC (see Q 5.88). Freedom from 'fear of forgetting' – a problem with all pill methods.
2 *Highly convenient*, non-intercourse-related.
3 *Fully reversible* (though with some delay).

NON-CONTRACEPTIVE BENEFITS

Most of those at Q 4.55 are believed to apply.

4 In many women there is a reduction in the disorders of the menstrual cycle:
  (a) *less heavy bleeding*, often culminating in amenorrhoea (which can be a health benefit in reducing the risk of gynaecological disorders as listed at Q 4.56 – but with the caveats at Qs 5.102–5.107);
  (b) *less anaemia*, indeed the haemoglobin has been noted to rise regardless of the bleeding pattern, suggesting a direct haemopoietic effect as well as less quantity of loss;
  (c) *less dysmenorrhoea*;
  (d) *less symptoms of premenstrual tension* (not invariably – in some women similar symptoms (Q 5.96(10)) occur early in each injection interval);
  (e) *no ovulation pain*.

> **NOTE:** These improvements are variable, and dependent on the bleeding pattern experienced by individual women.

5 *Less pelvic inflammatory disease* (PID) – as for all progestagen-containing contraceptives (see Q 4.58). Confirmed by a WHO study (1985).
6 *Less extrauterine pregnancies* since ovulation is inhibited.
7 Possibly *less functional ovarian cysts* overall, for the same reason (see Q 4.59), but this has not been well studied.
8 *Reduction in the growth of fibroids.*
9 A possible reduction in the rate of *endometriosis*, which indeed can be treated by these agents.
10 Overdose extremely unlikely and would not be fatal.
11 *Beneficial social effects*, especially because the method is under a woman's control.
12 Protection against endometrial cancer (see Q 5.111).

It is not known how many of the other benefits described for the COC (Q 4.55) apply also to injectables, namely a reduction in risk of benign breast disease, thyroid disease, rheumatoid arthritis, toxic shock syndrome, *Trichomonas vaginitis* and above all ovarian cancer. On theoretical grounds most are likely benefits, only waiting to be firmly established.

BENEFITS NOT (NECESSARILY) SHARED WITH THE COC

13 Beneficial effects on frank *sickle cell disease* (see Q 5.95).

14 *Aggression, mood swings and epileptic attacks*: especially in patients with severe learning disabilities, DMPA is reported as very beneficial if the timing of these problems is regularly premenstrual or menstrual. 'Tricycling' of the COC may be a way of obtaining a similar benefit (see Q 4.31).

15 *Lactation* is not suppressed, may even be enhanced due to increased production of prolactin – but POP appears even better, see Q 5.120.

16 Complete freedom from side-effects due to oestrogen.

5.94 IN VIEW OF THE ABOVE ADVANTAGES, WHY HAS THERE BEEN SO MUCH ADVERSE PUBLICITY OVER THE YEARS ABOUT INJECTABLES?

Mainly because of:

1 Unfounded excessive anxiety about *cancer* (the balance of the evidence is actually favourable! Q 5.111);

2 The possibility of *abuse* (by providers, 'pushing' the method on women or, worse, giving it without their knowledge or consent). This is a potential problem with any injection but one that is not best solved by banning a good product.

3 If side-effects occur, the impossibility of removing the injection once it has been given.

Yet overall safety is clearly greater than the COC, which itself is amazingly safe. Wherever injectables have been made available as a realistic choice, continuation rates are better than for most other methods.

5.95 WHAT IS THE EFFECT OF DMPA ON HOMOZYGOUS SICKLE CELL DISEASE?

A careful trial in the West Indies demonstrated a highly significant improvement in the haematological picture, and a reduction in the number of painful crises, in patients treated with 3-monthly injections of DMPA. It is suggested that this may be the method of choice both in SS and SC disease.

There are theoretical reasons for believing that all progestagen-containing contraceptives would be similarly beneficial, including the POP (see Q 5.47), NET EN, implants (see Q 5.152) and even perhaps the COC – though with the last the artificial oestrogen content has its own potential disadvantages (see Q 4.139).

MAIN PROBLEMS AND DISADVANTAGES

1 First and foremost, the fact that *the injection cannot be removed once given*. This means that the method is irreversible for at least 2–3 months (depending on the injectable used), and early side-effects would therefore have to be tolerated for a long time.

2 *Disturbance of menstruation* when it occurs can be so marked and variable over time, that it has been called 'menstrual chaos'. With reassuring counselling *amenorrhoea* is usually very acceptable (see Q 5.123); however:

3 Possible, as yet unconfirmed, *risks of long-term hypo-oestrogenism* (see Q 5.102).

4 *Delay in the return, but no loss, of fertility* (see Q 5.119).

5 *Weight gain.* Most women gain weight, up to 2 kg (4.5 lb) in the first year, and a few do so very rapidly after the very first dose. This possibility must be discussed with users in advance. The increase is thought to be due to increased appetite plus possibly an anabolic effect. It is not associated with fluid retention and diuretics are useless.

6 Possible *adverse effects on the fetus* (see Q 5.135).

7 *Galactorrhoea* may occur, with a raised prolactin (usually within the normal range).

8 *Mildly androgenic effects* such as acne are surprisingly uncommon.

9 *Enuresis* may recur in women who were enuretic at adolescence. This is believed to be caused by a relaxing effect of the progestagens on smooth muscle.

10 *Subjective effects.* These are many and varied, as with all hormonal methods. Some may be truly attributable to the method and in some cases they may be placebo reactions. The following have been reported;
   (a) loss of libido, vaginal dryness (relatively rare, but biologically plausible, see Qs 5.102 and 5.106);
   (b) lassitude;
   (c) depression (see Q 5.130) and other mood changes;
   (d) bloatedness;
   (e) dizziness;
   (f) breast symptoms (increase in size and tenderness);
   (g) leg cramps;
   (h) headaches.

ii *Local complications*:

(a) haematoma of the injection site (particularly in patients using anticoagulants, which are therefore a WHO 3 contraindication to the method);

(b) infection of the injection site. I am aware of a legal action alleging that an abscess caused failure of the method. In this rare event that particular injection should be deemed to be ineffective.

5.97 WHAT ARE THE EFFECTS OF INJECTABLES ON METABOLISM?

Although many studies have been reported (particularly on DMPA) they tend to be poorly controlled especially for cigarette smoking, and may not be standardised for the time since the last injection was given, individual variation, the presence or absence of ovarian activity, and so on.

Endogenous oestrogen has a vital part to play in most women, more than with the COC, particularly in the last half of the time of effectiveness of each injection. However, neither ovulation nor functional cyst formation are common, and overall there is less individual variation between women in the amount of ovarian activity than with the POP (see Q 5.5).

5.98 WHAT ARE THE EFFECTS ON BLOOD COAGULATION AND FIBRINOLYSIS?

To summarize much research, there is no proven effect of any significance on either of these. In the WHO Collaborative Study (1998) there was a small and non-significant increase in the odds ratio for venous thromboembolism. This may well have been related to selective use of the methods by women at greater risk, and diagnostic bias.

For the present it remains good practice to use either DMPA or NET EN where there is a past history of venous thromboembolism (WHO 2).

5.99 WHAT ARE THE EFFECTS ON BLOOD LIPIDS, ESPECIALLY HDL-C?

Available data about blood lipids are scanty and difficult to interpret. Most researchers have reassuringly found no effect or even a decrease in triglycerides or total cholesterol with both injectables. A few DMPA studies show a less encouraging increase in LDL and decrease (of around 10–15%) in HDL-C levels with DMPA. In a prospective study of NET EN, HDL-C declined more markedly, by about 25% after the first injection, but did not change further with up to 4 years of use.

These results may at least partly be related to the lower endogenous oestradiol production in users of injectables. Their relation to amenorrhoea and the overall clinical significance for arterial disease are not clear – see discussion below at Q 5.102 and, with regard to contraindications, Qs 5.116 and 5.118.

5.100 WHAT ARE THE EFFECTS ON CARBOHYDRATE METABOLISM?

Some reports find an increase in insulin levels with both these injectables, but most report no change. The development of overt diabetes in women using DMPA for contraception has not been reported, and WHO does not consider this a contraindication to the method.

5.101 ARE THERE ANY OTHER METABOLIC EFFECTS?

- In general only minimal effects have been shown.
- Since all progestogens appear capable of causing attacks of *acute porphyria*, and injectables cannot be rapidly reversed, they are absolutely contraindicated even in *latent* acute porphyria (WHO 4, see Q 4.218 and 5.116).
- Injectables do not appear adversely to affect liver function. Injectables can be used safely by women with a history of jaundice or current liver disease, including hepatitis B infection. But they should be used very cautiously if liver function tests are grossly abnormal (WHO 3) – the POP would normally be preferred.

5.102 WHAT IS THE PRESENT INFORMATION ON HYPO-OESTROGENISM AND PROGESTAGEN-ONLY INJECTABLES?

For DMPA the evidence is still too scanty to give any confident answer, and data are all-but absent for NET EN. There is some cause for concern, in my view, as follows:

1 It has been known since the 1970s that oestradiol levels in long-term DMPA users are low, as in the follicular phase of the cycle, and in some individuals very low (well under 100 pmol/l, compared with 150–200 pmol/l as the target bone-sparing threshold level in low-dose oestrogen replacement after the menopause).

Recent work shows that levels can be very low whether women are seeing bleeds (bleeds from the endometrium in DMPA users not being 'periods' anyway), or have complete amenorrhoea. (Contrariwise, other long-term users with complete amenorrhoea do have enough ovarian follicular activity for perfectly adequate oestradiol levels to be measurable (see Q 5.106(4).)

2   It is also well established that premature menopause (idiopathic or after bilateral oophorectomy) increases the risk of acute myocardial infarction (AMI) and osteoporosis thereafter, unless the missing oestrogen is replaced.

So the big question is: *does hypo-oestrogenism in DMPA users signify similar long-term risks to having a premature menopause?*

5.103 WHAT DO WE KNOW THEN ABOUT OSTEOPOROSIS RISK IN LONG-TERM DMPA USERS?

Cundy *et al.* from New Zealand published their results in the *British Medical Journal* in 1991. In brief, that was a cross-sectional study of 30 current users of DMPA with a minimum 5 years' previous use and all with continuous amenorrhoea, compared with 30 premenopausal volunteers and 30 postmenopausal controls. The bone density values in the DMPA users were lower by about 7% compared with the premenopausal women. This is too small a reduction for any fracture risk and moreover the values were higher than in the postmenopausal women, whose mean duration of relative oestrogen deficiency was similar (about 10 years).

There are many problems with this study. The laboratory and technical work may be good but they were let down by the basic design (there could be no knowledge of the bone status of the DMPA-users *prior to* starting the method), and the attempted matching process could not correct for gross disparity between the studied groups. Four times as many DMPA users were smokers (40%) as the premenopausal controls, though the DMPA-related difference persisted when the (only) 21 women who were concordant for smoking habits were compared.

Moreover, a later report from the same workers documented recovery of bone density, with the restoration of more normal oestradiol levels, when DMPA users were monitored before and after stopping DMPA. Subsequent studies in the world literature are mostly (not all) reassuring about osteoporosis; but the jury is still out as to whether there is a minor adverse effect on bones in long-term users – especially in smokers, the underweight and in adolescents who are building their peak bone mass.

5.104 ARE THE BONES THE MAIN CONCERN? WHAT DO WE KNOW ABOUT THE RISK OF HEART ATTACKS AND OTHER ARTERIAL DISEASES IN LONG-TERM DMPA USERS?

WHO and IPPF are a little uneasy on behalf of teenagers under 16 whose bone mineral density is still being established post-menarche, and in 1997 put usage under that age generally in WHO category 2 ('Broadly usable', benefits outweigh possible risks) and not as previously in WHO 1 ('Always usable').

My chief concern is not with the bones at all, except as a *marker* that the oestrogen levels of long-term users may have somatic effects. My concern is far more about whether the analogy with premature menopause means that long-term DMPA users will resemble women with (premature) menopause for subsequent risk of *arterial disease*, especially in smokers. Some of the metabolic (lipid) changes (described many years ago) in long-term users are not entirely reassuring (Q 5.99).

The WHO Collaborative study (*Contraception* 1998;57:315–24) is encouraging about all arterial disease including AMI in *current* injectable users. However they admit that their study has a 'major limitation', 'the potential for false negative findings ... resulting from the small numbers of cases and control subjects'.

I would add that a significant difference in AMI risk may only be detectable in *ex-users*, and many years later, since women (fortunately) have so low a risk of AMI in the childbearing years.

5.105 WE ALL WANT TO PRACTISE EVIDENCE-BASED MEDICINE, SO WHAT DOES THIS ADD UP TO?

Given the biochemical 'surrogate markers' of possible risk, and the whole corpus of data that it is good for women's arteries to have sufficient oestrogen circulating, we all face a dilemma. I summarize it in the following completely true statements:

1 *There is no evidence that long-term hypo-oestrogenism in DMPA-users actually increases the risk of a later heart attack or other arterial event.*
2 *There is insufficient evidence that long-term hypo-oestrogenism in DMPA-users does not increase the risk of a later heart attack or other arterial event.*

Both statements cannot be refuted. It becomes a matter of clinical Judgement, with a capital 'J'!

I prefer to act on the precautionary principle. One day the evidence will be incontrovertible. I will find it easier to look my patients in the eye *if* it then emerges that I have over the years unnecessarily changed some women to using another method (even if this has led to some unwanted pregnancies), or given them 'add-back' oestrogen – than *if* it turns out they have been exposed for years to a real and possibly long-term increased risk of AMI.

There is no simple answer. Below you will find the protocol I currently recommend at the Margaret Pyke Centre. But I have to report that many other UK authorities (and staff-members in my own service!) consider this, as they are perfectly entitled to do, an over-reaction. They would not proactively raise the issue of arterial disease with any long-term user. They would rarely if ever arrange an oestradiol measurement, and only consider change of method or add-back oestrogen on the basis of relevant 'menopausal'-type symptoms. In this they are being reassured by statement I above – and they are well supported by all recent publications of WHO and IPPF which simply do not discuss the arterial issue!

5.106 BUT HOW DO YOU PERSONALLY FEEL LONG-TERM USERS OF INJECTABLES SHOULD BE MANAGED?

1 Arbitrarily after 5 years' use the issue should be *reviewed* with the woman herself, and at any time earlier if she has actual symptoms suggestive of hypo-oestrogenism (notably dryness of the vagina, loss of libido, hot flushes).

2 *Consultation*

(a) If she has relevant symptoms, or if she is a smoker she may choose to change her method anyway. If she wishes to continue, she is offered the choice of blood tests. She may well decide, given all the genuine scientific uncertainty about what a low oestradiol means for health, and all the other risks she takes in life anyway (specially relevant thinking for a smoker!) that she will never want the test done: because almost whatever it showed she would choose to continue with DMPA. If so, this fact should be recorded, and the question readdressed (by discussion) perhaps at 5-yearly review visits. Otherwise, go to 3 below.

(b) If she is keen to continue the method, symptom-free and a non-smoker, after this discussion oestradiol measurements may still be reasonably *deferred* (and again, never done at all if she either decides to limit her own use of the method to 5 years, or if she insists she does not want to know her oestrogen status). But we do not defer the oestradiol levels (see below) for smokers and those with relevant symptoms. They are done by around 3 years not 5.

Note: Oestrogen levels are more likely to be good anyway in a moderately *overweight* individual, due to peripheral conversion of androgenic precursors to oestrogens.

3 *Testing*

Once the decision is made to test for hypo-oestrogenism, in a woman wanting to continue, what test and when? There is no point in doing FSH levels since these will always be low, due to pituitary suppression. There is also not much point in doing expensive bone scans or lipid assays *unless there is another specific indication* (e.g. relevant family history).

So we do a plasma oestradiol, on or shortly before the day of her next injection, *not in the weeks just after an injection*, to get some measure of the levels *well after* the peak levels of the DMPA have subsided (see Figure 5.3, Q 5.86).

4 *Results*

(a) Sometimes the first result is good, well above 100 pmol/l, implying, according to present knowledge, ovarian follicular activity sufficient both for arterial and bone health. If so, and the woman is happy with the injectable, it may continue to be used (long term), plus the usual follow-up.

(b) If the first oestradiol is less than 100 pmol/l or borderline it is repeated (see above regarding timing). The laboratory will stress that results are not accurate at this low end of the sensitivity range, they are only 'plus or minus 20–25 pmol/l' anyway. This does not matter, since we are only looking for results significantly below 100.

5.107 WHAT CHOICES DO YOU THEN DISCUSS WITH THE DMPA USER IF TWO OESTRADIOLS LATE IN THE INJECTION INTERVAL ARE UNDER 100 pmol/l?

Obviously, another contraceptive method may be chosen. If she shifts to the combined pill (and sometimes in a very forgetful young pill-taker she might even do this *and* continue on DMPA! since the two go together well, see Qs 4.195, 5.90 and 5.128) she will get oestrogen from that product. In almost all other cases, including if she shifts to using an

IUD or male or female sterilization, she will now obtain sufficient oestrogen from her own ovaries.

2 'Add-back' natural oestrogen by any chosen route, usually cyclically but it could be tried continuously if preferred. Older amenorrhoeic DMPA-users would almost always benefit from this form of HRT, and all in all I think it is wise to discontinue progestagen-only injectables by 45 anyway (Q 5.126). Do not retest oestradiol levels in any 'add-back' cases.

3 What if she insists on just carrying on with the DMPA? To me this suggests *poor counselling* earlier, since it would have been better not to do the tests at all if they are not going to be acted on (Q 5.106 (2b)). However her autonomy is paramount, and especially in a woman under 30 she could continue with her (documented) choice, using DMPA alone under supervision.

Option 2 is of course using the DMPA to prevent hyperstimulation by the add-back oestrogen of the endometrium, and although 'Provera' tablets are used this way it is an unlicensed use. So it is safest to follow the 'Named Patient' routine (page 507) – including documenting the good explanation of the plan to the woman herself, stressing effective future follow-up.

5.108 WHAT PROTOCOL WOULD YOU FOLLOW FOR NET EN USERS? OR IF A POP-USER HAS LONG-TERM AMENORRHOEA?

There are no good data to help us, again. With DMPA it is primarily long-term use that is relevant since, as we have seen, the occurrence of some bleeding is no guide to oestrogen levels. But with the POP and NET EN bleeding seems to be a better marker of oestrogen status, and I would only follow the above protocol after continuous *amenorrhoea for 5 years* (3 years in smokers, or earlier if relevant low-oestrogen symptoms).

Note FSH levels ARE of some use in (older) POP users – if high the protocol of Qs 5.63 and 5.64 should be followed, without the need for an oestradiol measurement. The latter would only be required perhaps in a younger woman, with 5 years amenorrhoea as above.

NOTE: All these proposals (Qs 5.102–5.108) are tentative, for the time being, and until we have better data.

5.109 WHAT EFFECTS DO INJECTABLES HAVE ON BLOOD PRESSURE?

Here is some good news: studies show no consistent and certainly no significant change in either systolic or diastolic blood pressure in women using either injectable.

Interestingly, neither WHO nor IPPF in their latest guidelines recommend regular blood pressure measurements, aside from the first visit to assess pre-existing hypertension. In this country it is usual to check BP at least every 6 months. Yet would not annual checks be more than adequate after the first year, and surely doing it at every 12-week visit for an injection is over the top?!

5.110 DO INJECTABLES AFFECT NEOPLASIA IN ANIMALS?

Given enormous doses of DMPA, Beagle bitches (which are by nature prone to breast lumps) can develop malignant tumours of the breast. Two out of 12 rhesus monkeys given 50 times the human contraceptive dose in a 10-year trial developed endometrial carcinoma. No cases were observed in monkeys treated with the human dose or 10 times the human dose.

The animal models (Beagle bitches or rhesus monkeys) are believed by most authorities to be manifesting species-specific reactions which are not applicable to the human, or the doses used have been irrelevantly high.

5.111 WHAT ARE THE LATEST DATA ABOUT DMPA AND CANCER IN THE HUMAN?

Recent (1991) publications by WHO from good hospital-based case-control studies in developing countries provide the best data to date. The findings can be summarized as follows:

1 *Endometrial cancer* – a protective effect, in fact a fivefold reduction in risk. There was also an ex-use protective effect detectable for at least 8 years after cessation of DMPA use. It seems the reduction in risk is as great for DMPA as for the COC.

2 *Epithelial ovarian cancer* – protective effect as with the COC was (surprisingly) not demonstrated: but certainly no increase in risk either. It may be that protection would only be shown in a population of DMPA users at high risk of ovarian cancer (not so far studied).

3 *Primary liver cancer* – no increased risk, and this was in countries (Thailand and Kenya) where hepatitis B is endemic.

4 *Cervical cancer* – no increased risk. This is the finding of a larger and better WHO study than the earlier one reported in 1984, which showed a small association with DMPA use. It confirms the suspicion at the time that the association was due to confounding by factors such as sexual activity and smoking.
5 *Breast cancer* – see Q 5.112, below.

Overall these results are very favourable to this much maligned method!

5.112 DOES DMPA INCREASE THE RISK OF BREAST CANCER?

In the large WHO hospital-based case-control study from five centres, reported in *The Lancet* in October 1991, there was no link with breast cancer in the total population (869 cases, 11 890 controls), nor any increased risk with increased duration of use.

The only statistically increased risk was for use in the first 4 years after initial exposure, mainly in women under 35. There was no increase in risk among women who started DMPA more than 5 years previously.

DMPA may perhaps be bringing forward the appearance of cancers which would have become manifest later. On the other hand it is very plausible that the association in the WHO study is entirely caused by *detection bias*; recent users (who would necessarily be young) or their physicians being more likely to discover breast lumps in the first 4 years of DMPA use.

The CGHFBC study differs slightly, giving similar results to those for the COC (Q 4.80): i.e. a possible but non-significant increased risk in current users, diminishing to nil after 10 years in ex-users. More data are needed.

5.113 MAY DMPA BE USED IN CASES OF TROPHOBLASTIC DISEASE?

In the UK it is recommended that DMPA, like all contraceptive steroids, should be avoided until hCG is undetectable (see Q 4.75). Thereafter there is no objection to this method, which can be a very suitable means of preventing pregnancy for the 2 years of designated follow-up.

5.114 IS THERE ANY EVIDENCE THAT INJECTABLES AFFECT THE DEVELOPMENT OR GROWTH OF BENIGN TUMOURS?

The growth of uterine fibroids is usually inhibited, presumably because of hypo-oestrogenism. Most other benign tumours appear to be unaffected, though benign liver tumours have been reported.

SELECTION OF USERS AND OF FORMULATIONS

5.115 FOR WHOM ARE INJECTABLES PARTICULARLY INDICATED?

1 First and foremost, if a *systemic, non-intercourse-related method* is chosen by the woman and other options (particularly those containing oestrogen) are contraindicated, or disliked.

This includes the categories:

(a) post venous thromboembolism or known prothrombotic abnormality of coagulation (WHO 2). A good example of the latter is severe *SLE* (see Q 4.142);

(b) to cover *relevant elective surgery* (Q 4.195);

(c) *forgetful pill-takers.*

2 Women in whom *long-term progestagens are indicated anyway*, e.g. some with perimenopausal problems, fibroids and endometriosis.

3 As an *alternative to the IUD* where the risk of PID is held to be high (e.g. the young woman whose partner may have multiple partners).

4 *Sickle cell disease* (see Q 5.95).

5 *Past history of a tubal ectopic pregnancy*: because like the COC it is an anovulant and will prevent pregnancy in any location (Q 5.111).

6 *Epilepsy*: the frequency of seizures can sometimes be reduced.

7 At the woman's *choice.*

5.116 WHAT ARE THE ABSOLUTE CONTRAINDICATIONS TO INJECTABLES?

These are identical to the first six relating to the POP (see Q 5.52), with the need for a little more caution (as also in Q 5.118 with respect to relative contraindications) because:

- The dose is larger, and lipid changes greater.
- There is the aforementioned reversibility problem after any given injection is given.
- Amenorrhoea is more frequent (see Q 5.102)

Past *severe arterial disease*, or current exceptionally high risk of the same. Pending further information I would not prescribe an injectable long term to a woman known to have current ischaemic heart disease including angina or to have already suffered a thrombotic stroke; nor to women with marked and multiple risk factors (e.g. a 45-year-old heavy smoking hypertensive diabetic!) – or if so one would certainly only use the method as a short-term expedient (see Qs 5.99, 5.102). *Severe hereditary lipid abnormalities* with a poor prognosis come into this category because of 'exceptionally high risk'. However, the injectable might be prescribed with extra counselling and supervision in the presence of milder abnormalities with a good prognosis.

2 Any *serious side-effect occurring on the COC and not clearly due only to oestrogen* – or associated with past progestagen-only use.

- *Liver adenoma* and severe past *steroid-associated cholestatic jaundice*, also current *severe liver impairment*.

Also in this category:

- *Recent trophoblastic disease* (see Q 4.75), until hCG is undetectable.
- *Acute porphyria*, WHO 4 even if only the latent condition, without a past attack history, see Q 4.218.

As for all medical methods, we must also add:

3 *allergy* to a constituent; (particularly the methyl parabens excipient);
4 *undiagnosed abnormal genital tract bleeding* since the injectable will confuse diagnosis;
5 actual or possible *pregnancy*;
6 the woman's own *continuing uncertainty* about the safety of DMPA or NET EN, even after full counselling.

5.117 WHY IS PAST ECTOPIC PREGNANCY AN INDICATION RATHER THAN A CONTRAINDICATION TO INJECTABLES, WHEREAS THE POP WOULD NOT BE RECOMMENDED?

Because, like the COC, injectables almost always block ovulation and hence virtually eliminate the risk of an ectopic. The woman with damaged tubes of course remains still at risk of getting her ectopic later, when the anovulant treatment cases.

5.118 WHAT ARE THE RELATIVE CONTRAINDICATIONS TO INJECTABLES?

See Q 4.132 – here is my list:

1 *Risk factors for arterial disease*. This category includes established hypertension once it has been diagnosed and controlled and also migraine with focal aura (see Q 4.147). The presence of more than one

risk factor can be tolerated more readily than with the COC – but there are limits. Prothrombotic coagulation factor abnormalities are actually included above as 'indications', since they should not be worsened at all by an injectable. Likewise, there is not the oestrogen-related concern about thrombotic stroke in migraine, including migraine with focal aura – though it may be affected.

Lipid abnormalities might perhaps be worsened by the injectables, especially in amenorrhoeic women. The POP, having less metabolic effects, would normally be a better choice (see Qs 5.53 and 5.66).

Sex steroid-dependent cancer (WHO 3). The POP is lower dose, more readily reversible (see Q 5.53). But seek the advice of the oncologist looking after your patient. There is no evidence that injectables worsen the prognosis after *breast cancer* – usually started when in remission: but there is no proof of the opposite either.

Active liver disease, with moderately abnormal liver function tests – caution required (WHO 3). *FNH* is also WHO 3 for DMPA (Qs 4.91, 4.131).

Other chronic systemic disease. The same comments as at Q 4.135 for the COC apply. The great effectiveness as a contraceptive often helps to outweigh the continuing uncertainty as to what effect (either way) an injectable might have on the disease. With that proviso and given the reversibility problem, DMPA may be a good choice (WHO 3) for the conditions listed as absolute (see Q 4.131) or relative (see Q 4.133) contraindications to the COC – including severe SLE or diabetes with tissue damage.

Unacceptability of menstrual irregularities, especially cultural/religious taboos (e.g. Islam and Orthodox Judaism) associated with bleeding – *or* amenorrhoea.

Obesity – though further weight gain is *not* inevitable and see Q 5.106 (2b)

Past *severe endogenous depression* (above-average support needed).

Any woman who is *planning a pregnancy in the near future*. This contraindication would become 'absolute' if she wished to conceive within 6–9 months of the proposed injection.

In the *years leading up to the menopause*. There are five concerns, none of which are insuperable:

(a) the effect on HDL-C (see Q 5.99), particularly if the woman were a smoker;

(b) the possibility of hypo-oestrogenism and its uncertain implications (see Q 5.102).

These objections (a) and (b) might, in selected cases, be overcome by 'add-back' oestrogen replacement (see Q 5.106)

(c) irregular bleeding may necessitate endometrial sampling;
(d) the menopause may be masked (see Q 5.127);
(e) the method is perhaps too strong, a 'contraceptive overkill' (see Qs 8.32 and 8.49).

In practice, it may be appropriate to switch to the POP at around age 45.

5.119 WHAT EFFECTS DO INJECTABLES HAVE ON FUTURE FERTILITY?

Return of fertility is slow, especially with DMPA, but complete. In the largest study (Figure 5.4) of parous women in Thailand, the mean time to conception was 9 months after the last injection. Now the last injection has a significant antifertility effect for about 15 weeks (the 12-week injection frequency being set to prevent, not the average, but the most DMPA-resistant woman from conceiving). So the true delay after stopping the method is a median of only 5.5 months, comparing very favourably with discontinuation of the COC (mean delay 3 months – see Fig 5.4). Underweight women regained their fertility faster.

The same study showed that 91% of DMPA-users had conceived by 2 years from discontinuation, as just defined, compared with 95% of

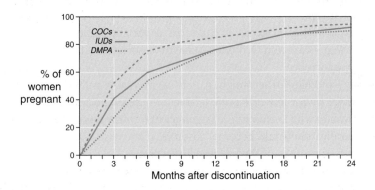

Figure 5.4 Cumulative conception rates for women discontinuing DMPA, COCs, and copper IUDs to become pregnant. *Note*: Researchers assumed that users 'discontinued' DMPA 15 weeks after their last injection. Source: Pardthaisong, *Journal of Biosocial Science* 1984; 16: 23–34

former COC users – not a statistically significant difference, and confirming the lack of any permanent fertility loss.

Secondary amenorrhoea does persist in a minority and should be investigated and treated if it lasts for more than 9 months after the last injection (Qs 4.61–4.66). This is extremely treatable by standard ovulation induction methods.

5.120 WHAT ARE THE EFFECTS OF INJECTABLES ON LACTATION?

1 Both injectables appear to increase the volume of breast milk.
2 Most studies suggest no important change in its composition.
3 The amount of hormone transmitted to the infant in breast milk is very small, less than 0.5% of the maternal dose. The amount of exposure to hormone is even less with NET EN.

Although no long-term effects on infant growth and development have been reported, the amount of exposure to an artificial hormone is obviously greater than with the POP. In view of this minimal uncertainty, in my view it would be preferable *in this country* for most lactating women to use the POP, transferring to the injectable as one option when the child is weaned. (The combination of POP plus full lactation is already almost 100% effective contraception.)

If DMPA or NET EN are used in lactation they should ideally be given 5–6 weeks after delivery, this delay being helpful to minimize bleeding problems. But it is sometimes right to give an injectable much earlier than this.

5.121 WHICH INJECTABLE SHOULD BE CHOSEN?

1 The natural first choice is DMPA, since its effects are better known, and it is marginally more effective. The injection is less uncomfortable and only needs to be given four times a year.
2 Possible reasons for selecting NET EN include:
   (a) more bleeds, reduced likelihood of complete amenorrhoea;
   (b) shorter time until spontaneous reversal of the effect if unacceptable side-effects were to develop after the first injection;
   (c) more rapid return of fertility after the last injection;
   (d) less risk of marked weight gain;
   (e) if DMPA proves unsatisfactory, as an empirical second choice.

INITIAL MANAGEMENT AND FOLLOW-UP ARRANGEMENTS

5.122 WHAT SHOULD BE DONE AT THE FIRST VISIT PRIOR TO GIVING AN INJECTABLE?

1 A good *medical history* should be taken with special reference to the absolute and relative contraindications (see Qs 5.116 and 5.118).
2 Record the *weight*. This is more important than with other hormonal methods.
3 Record the *blood pressure*. The evidence suggests it is not specially relevant to the method (Q 5.109), but it is desirable as a baseline.
4 Discuss breast self-examination/awareness with a good leaflet – not leading to a nerve-racking ritual. *Offer to examine the breasts* if she has any concern, and with a lower threshold in women above age 40 (as a baseline).
5 Carry out a pelvic examination and cervical smear only if due, as good preventive medicine. It may be clinically indicated after childbirth to exclude the possibility of retained products; and sometimes to exclude a clinical pre-existing pregnancy.

5.123 WHAT IS THE MINIMUM INFORMATION WHICH SHOULD BE CONVEYED AT COUNSELLING?

Failure to counsel adequately has been the main cause of adverse publicity in this country. The following should be discussed.

1 *Amenorrhoea.* As Dr Wilson of Glasgow has declared, reassurance that a 'monthly clean-out' of the 'bad blood' is not necessary for good health may make all the difference between happy acceptance and chronic anxiety and dissatisfaction.
2 The opposite possibility of *frequent irregular bleeding*. Reassure the woman that medical advice is available if this should occur (Q 5.128).
3 *Weight gain.* Not inevitable, as it is mainly caused by increased appetite.
4 *Delay in fertility return.* Women should be told on average it may take 9 months from the time of the last injection to conceive.
5 Theoretical *long-term risks*. The cancer balance seems on present evidence to be rather favourable to the method (see Q 5.111). The issues of arterial disease and osteoporosis, especially if there were to be prolonged amenorrhoea, are still not fully resolved (see Qs 5.102 and 5.106).

How much is told must depend on the doctor's judgement of the patient's understanding and background, but an opportunity for questions must be given and they must be frankly answered.

The information leaflet agreed between the manufacturing company and the UK Minister of Health should be given to each woman. She should be given time to read it before making up her mind, and any further questions then answered. The FPA also supplies a useful leaflet.

5.124 HOW ARE THE INJECTABLES GIVEN?

By deep intramuscular injection, in this country usually from the pre-loaded syringe into the upper outer quadrant of the buttock or outer thigh.

The DMPA ampoule should be very thoroughly shaken to remove any sediment. NET EN should preferably be warmed to body temperature. The site of either injection should not be massaged.

See also Q 5.89. If any of the dose is spilled, the amount lost should be carefully (over-) estimated and replaced by another injection.

5.125 WHAT ARE THE REQUIREMENTS FOR SUCCESSFUL MONITORING AND FOLLOW-UP?

1 Careful planning of the date for the next dose when each is given. Try to avoid the complexities of Qs 5.133 and 5.134 by explaining that if a planned date proves inconvenient, it is far better to ask for the next dose a week or two early than to be late. ...

2 Equally important is ready access between injections to medical advice by telephone or in person, to deal with any anxieties arising.

3 Blood pressure is checked annually (see Q 5.109) and weight at each visit in the first year; but thereafter, if stable, mainly at the patient's request.

4 Cervical screening is performed according to local policies.

5.126 FOR HOW LONG, AND TO WHAT AGE, MAY USE OF INJECTABLES BE CONTINUED?

There are no known reasons for arbitrarily restricting the duration of use in younger women with adequate endogenous ovarian activity. The implications and management of prolonged amenorrhoea are discussed at Qs 5.102–5.106. At around age 45 a review is appropriate (earlier for those with multiple arterial CVS risk factors): transferring to another method or add-back of natural oestrogen should in my view be considered then.

With difficulty – the scheme for the POP at Q 5.64 is not appropriate for injectables. The method has to be discontinued and alternative contraception practised e.g. the POP in fact, then following Q 5.63–5.64 protocol.

Injectables are by way of being a 'contraceptive overkill' around the climacteric (see Q 8.50). Transfer to another method before age 45 is therefore normally preferable as just suggested (Q 5.126), with the added advantage of simplifying diagnosis of the menopause.

MANAGEMENT OF SIDE-EFFECTS AND PRACTICAL PROBLEMS

1 The patient should be examined to *exclude an unrelated cause*: notably retained products of conception, polyps, *Chlamydia*, or carcinoma. An ultrasound scan may be required. If the uterus is firm and non-tender, with a normal closed cervical os, it is unlikely that the bleeding has any cause other than as a side-effect of the injectable.

2 *Drugs*: ensure she has not recently been commenced on an enzyme inducer (Q 5.91)

3 *Possible treatments*:
   (a) *Best*: give oestrogen (if not contraindicated). Simply giving one or more packets of any convenient 30 μg COC stops the bleeding in most cases, if not contraindicated. The extra progestagen matters not at all, so this is often convenient. Otherwise use conjugated oestrogens (Premarin 1.25 mg daily for 21 days), repeated as necessary if unacceptable irregularity follows the withdrawal bleed.
   (b) *Other options* (rarely successful):
   - Give the next dose early; but no earlier than 4 weeks since the last
   - Haemostatics such as tranexamic acid and ethamsylate have been tried. They rarely work well, and their risks would therefore usually outweigh the benefits for this indication.

Iron treatment is very rarely indicated to correct anaemia (Q 5.93(4)). The actual amount lost over many days is usually not great.

It may be possible to help a woman through initial difficulties, *particularly by the use of one or sometimes more courses of oestrogen*. But irregular bleeding remains the commonest reason for discontinuing the method. The problem is most pronounced postpartum, often helped by delaying the first dose to 5–6 weeks.

5.129 HOW SHOULD AMENORRHOEA BE MANAGED?

1 Pregnancy should be eliminated as the (very rare) cause.
2 Secondly, the woman should be counselled as at Q 5.123(1). I find it helpful to say 'there's no blood coming away because there *is no blood to come away*'. The establishment of prolonged amenorrhoea can often be the best solution for women with bleeding problems.
3 One cycle of the COC or a natural oestrogen to cause a withdrawal 'period' can sometimes be helpful as an adjunct to reassurance.

See also Qs 5.102 and 5.106 above, regarding the issue of hypo-oestrogenism, especially relevant to smokers.

5.130 WHAT ABOUT OTHER MINOR SIDE-EFFECTS?

Management can only be empirical, for example, switching to the other injectable or another method. Weight gain is the commonest complaint: dieting is possible but difficult. Diuretics are useless. Pyridoxine treatment may be tried if depression is reported (see Q 4.199), but there have been no good studies.

5.131 WHAT SYMPTOMS SHOULD LEAD AN INJECTABLE-USER TO TAKE URGENT MEDICAL ADVICE?

Specifically related to the method, there are none – apart from the very rare occurrence of massive uterine 'flooding' (see Q 5.128).

5.132 ARE PROLONGED IMMOBILIZATION OR MAJOR SURGERY CONTRAINDICATIONS TO INJECTABLES?

There is no need to discontinue either DMPA or NET EN before any kind of surgery. Indeed an injectable may be a very satisfactory option instead of the combined pill for women at high risk of pregnancy while on the waiting list for major surgery. See Q 4.195 for the practical management.

5.133 HOW SHOULD ONE HANDLE THE PROBLEM OF OVERDUE INJECTIONS? HOW CAN ONE MAINTAIN CONTRACEPTION WITHOUT AVOIDABLY RISKING FETAL EXPOSURE TO THE DRUG?

This is very difficult. Even if the woman is not amenorrhoeic, any bleeds she has give no information about when she may ovulate.

The manufacturer of DMPA is much more cautious in the UK (see *Note* below); but *according to WHO there is a full 2 weeks of leeway for late injections with BOTH injectables*. The likelihood of conception when 1 week overdue (during the 13th week with DMPA and the 9th week with NET EN) is acceptably low, so I recommend the following protocol for this common problem (subtract 4 weeks or 28 days from all numbers if the injectable is NET EN not DMPA).

OVERDUE INJECTIONS

Assuming regular intercourse has been continuing:

1 *Up to 13 weeks (91 days)*: give the due dose, advising also added precautions for 7 days. Beyond that the chances of a blastocyst being in the genital tract increase. Assuming intercourse has been continuing:

2 *If the due dose is late by a further 3 days (94 days)*: hormonal postcoital contraception (either combined or progestagen-only) can be given plus an immediate DMPA injection – plus 7 days added precautions.

3 *Up to 96 days*: if the earliest ovulation is assumed to be at 13 weeks and hence the intervention is still before implantation 5 days later: a copper IUD can be inserted in good faith, plus an immediate injection plus later removal of the IUD – *or* neither of the latter, if the woman chooses to switch to the IUD as her future method.

  Up to 96 days it would also be legitimate to offer one of the hormone postcoital methods, which are not in fact contraindicated beyond 72 hours... it is only that how much their efficacy will be reduced when required to work as an anti-implantation method 5 days after ovulation is unquantified (Q 7.8). The ethical/legal situation is, surely, the same, 5 days after the earliest postulated ovulation, as with the copper IUD option.

In all these cases added precautions for a further 7 days are advisable, plus 100% follow-up with exclusion of pregnancy 3–4 weeks later. Counselling must include discussion of the (very low) potential of harm to any fetus. It should be recorded that no promise has been made that she will not conceive, nor that any fetus would be born normal.

Note: Given that the manufacturer states (in sharp contrast to the WHO!) that the safety margin of DMPA is only up to 89 days after the last dose, some authorities cautiously recommend reducing the total durations at nos. 1, 2 and 3 above by 2 days in each case.

5.134 WHAT IF THE INJECTION IS MORE THAN 5 DAYS BEYOND THE 1 WEEK ASSUMED SAFETY MARGIN FOR THE FIRST POSSIBLE OVULATION?

This means beyond 96 days with DMPA. In a currently sexually active user one would have to follow the policy described at Q 8.22.

In brief, insist that she agrees to avoid all risk of conception – by abstinence, combinations of methods, whatever – for a total of 10 days since the last intercourse. She then returns with an early morning urine.

If this gives a negative result by one of the ultrasensitive pregnancy tests now available for primary care use (with a minimum sensitivity of at least 25 mIU/l – e.g. 'Clear-view'), this can be interpreted as no fertilization up to 10 days previously, since when she had additionally agreed to be 'safe'.

After discussion, recorded as in the italicized penultimate paragraph of Q 5.133, the next due injection may be given. For extra security the couple should use the condom for a further 7 days and, again, there *must* be a follow-up visit to exclude pregnancy after 3–4 weeks.

The above protocol (Qs 5.133–5.134) is surely preferable to the medical paranoia which has led to refusal to give the late DMPA dose at all in these circumstances.

5.135 WHAT ARE THE RISKS IF A FETUS IS EXPOSED TO INJECTABLES?

1 There is no evidence of an increase in ectopic or miscarriage rates.
2 There is some concern that offspring of women exposed to DMPA during pregnancy, especially in the 4 weeks after an injection, are at increased risk of low birth weight and subsequent infant mortality. But it has been suggested this could be due to *confounding*, e.g. by social class.
3 Masculinization of the female fetus, particularly transient enlargement of the clitoris, and a possible increase in the incidence of hypospadias in males exposed to medroxyprogesterone acetate and similar hormones, have been reported. But no serious fetal malformation risks have been established with the very low doses used for contraception in DMPA and

NET EN. Meaningful conclusions about what must be very low potential teratogenic risks are unlikely ever to be reached, because proceeding to term after exposure to injectables is such a rare event.

Every effort must of course continue to be made to prevent fetal exposure (see Qs 5.133 and 5.134).

5.136 ARE THERE ANY KNOWN RISKS OR BENEFITS FOR EX-USERS OF INJECTABLES?

There are no established teratogenic effects on pregnancies among recent ex-users of injectables.

The only known problem is prolonged amenorrhoea and delayed return of fertility (see Q 5.119). There is a definite ex-use protective effect against carcinoma of the endometrium.

QUESTIONS ASKED BY USERS

GENERAL

Most questions asked are about DMPA, or Depo-Provera as it is best known by the general public.

5.137 WHAT ARE IN PRACTICE THE MOST EFFECTIVE PURELY HORMONAL CONTRACEPTIVES CURRENTLY AVAILABLE?

Implants and injectables. The COC fails far more often – through human error.

5.138 DO INJECTABLES CAUSE CANCER IN WOMEN?

This currently seems very unlikely and one cancer (of the lining of the womb) is less frequent (see Qs. 5.110–5.113).

5.139 BUT IS IT SAFE? HOW DOES THE SAFETY (FREEDOM FROM HEALTH RISK) OF DEPO-PROVERA COMPARE WITH 'THE PILL'?

Overall, since it contains no oestrogen, its safety is believed to be greater than that of the combined pill. No deaths have ever been clearly blamed upon it (see Q 5.94).

5.140 WHY ARE SOME PEOPLE SO OPPOSED TO DEPO-PROVERA?

Mainly because of its *potential* for abuse, and the fact that if side-effects occur – and there are fewer overall than with the pill – the drug's action cannot be reversed once given. You have to wait for the last injection to wear off (see Q 5.96).

5.141 IS IT A 'LAST RESORT' METHOD?

In the UK its licence used to require it to be used only after discussion of all the alternatives and after special counselling with the special leaflet. But it is now approved as a 'first-line' option.

5.142 CAN I BE TOO YOUNG TO BE GIVEN DEPO-PROVERA?

Some doctors are reluctant to give it to very young teenagers, who are just beginning their normal menstrual cycle. There is no proof that it will cause fertility or osteoporosis problems even then, and injectables would normally be preferable to insertion of an IUD, if that was the alternative choice (see Qs 5.104 and 5.115).

5.143 CAN I BE TOO OLD TO BE GIVEN DEPO-PROVERA?

Above the age of 45 injectables are stronger contraceptives than are really required, and there is an increasing risk of disease of the arteries. Many other good choices are now available, so other methods are usually preferable, especially in smokers not seeing 'periods' (see Qs 5.99 and 5.127).

5.144 CAN THE INJECTION BE GIVEN BY MY FAMILY DOCTOR AS WELL AS THROUGH A CLINIC?

Yes – though some GPs still feel a bit uncertain about using the method. (Perhaps they should read this book!)

5.145 WHERE (ON THE BODY) IS THE INJECTION GIVEN?

Usually into the upper outer region of the buttocks, on either side; but it can sometimes be given into the shoulder or thigh muscles.

QUESTIONS ASKED BY CURRENT USERS

5.146 WHY CAN THE INJECTION NOT BE GIVEN RIGHT AFTER MY BABY?

If given too soon it tends to cause more bleeding problems in the weeks after childbirth. These are less if it is given at about 5–6 weeks; but since it does not have any thrombosis risks it can sometimes be given much earlier, if you are prepared to accept some irregular bleeding.

5.147 HOW LONG DOES THE INJECTION LAST?

Officially for 12 weeks, and each injection should be on time. This is for maximum safety against pregnancy. However, some women (and we do not know who they are in advance) go on being affected for much longer (see Q 5.148).

5.148 HOW FAR AHEAD SHOULD I DISCONTINUE INJECTIONS IF PLANNING ANOTHER BABY?

You should plan for about one year after the last injection, since it is quite usual (and nothing to worry about) for conception to be delayed that long.

5.149 EXCESS BLEEDING – WILL IT HARM ME IN ANY WAY IF I CAN LIVE WITH IT?

The short answer is 'no'. You ought to be examined to eliminate any cause not related to the Depo-Provera. A blood test may sometimes be done to check that you are not anaemic. Some treatments may be tried to stop the bleeding (see Q 5.128). Otherwise if you can live with an unpredictable bleeding pattern it will do you no harm. If you choose to have intercourse during bleeding that too is medically harmless.

COMBINED INJECTABLES

5.150 WHAT ARE THE MONTHLY COMBINED INJECTABLES?

One problem with DMPA and NET EN is the initially too high levels which subsequently fall off rather unpredictably (Fig. 5.3). An approach actually making use of this decline in levels began in South America and became very popular: once a month combined injectable contraceptives (CICs) containing either NET-EN 50 mg plus oestradiol valerate 5 mg (Mesigyna) or DMPA 25 mg plus oestradiol cypionate 5 mg (Cyclofem/Cycloprovera). This approach seems to give much more predictable bleeding patterns, the first bleed occurring about 2 weeks after the first injection, and then monthly, lasting for about 5 days, and without loss of efficacy.

Around 1 million women are already using CICs and Cyclofem is the CIC expected first on the UK market. Experiments with self-injection using a special disposable system have been successful: it remains to be seen if this would be British women's preferred method of administration.

SUBDERMAL IMPLANTS

I think not! It is sadly true of Norplant that the media, combined with legal action, destroyed public and professional confidence in what, since 1994, had been a very satisfactory option for many women. But the implant *route* is not defunct.

Implants contain a progestagen in a slow-release carrier, made either of dimethylsiloxane (as in Norplant with six implants and the very similar two-rod Norplant II, now called Jadelle™) or EVA, ethylene vinyl acetate (Implanon™). After an initial phase of several weeks giving higher blood levels they deliver almost constant low daily levels of the hormone (Figure 5.3).

Implanon™ is now (1999) the only marketed implant in the UK. Its main features are summarized in Table 5.2 at Q 5.4. It works primarily by ovulation inhibition, supplemented by the usual mucus and endometrial effects.

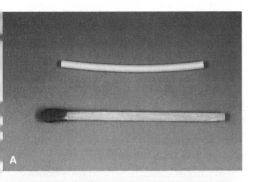

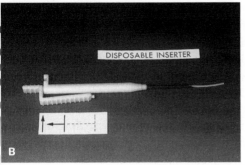

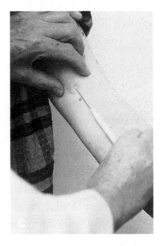

Figure 5.5 Implanon.

5.152 WHAT IS IMPLANON™? HOW EFFECTIVE IS IT?

It is a single 40 mm rod, just 2 mm in diameter, inserted far more simply than Norplant straight from a dedicated sterile preloaded applicator with a cleverly shaped wide-bore needle (Figure 5.5), by a simple injection/withdrawal technique. The implant contains 68 mg of etonogestrel – the new name for 3-keto-desogestrel. This is dispersed in an EVA matrix and covered by a 0.06 mm rate-limiting EVA membrane.

- Its duration of use is for 3 years, with the unique distinction of a zero failure rate in the trials to date (1999) – though the 95% confidence interval ranges up to 7 in 10 000.
- Since in the international studies serum levels do tend to be lower in heavier women, contraceptive efficacy might be lower in the obese, especially in the third year (consider reimplanting sooner).
- If enzyme inducer treatment is necessary, additional contraceptive precautions are recommended.

5.153 HOW IS IT INSERTED, AND WHEN?

Though not difficult, specific training is essential. The upper arm is the best site (Figure 5.5), under LA: implants at other sites may migrate.

TIMING OF IMPLANON™ INSERTION

- Day 1 to 5 of the woman's natural cycle. If later than day 2, at MPC we would recommend additional contraception for 7 days.
- Following first-trimester abortion: immediate insertion is best.
- Following delivery or second-trimester abortion: Implanon™ insertion on day 21 is recommended, and if later, with additional contraception for 7 days. If still amenorrhoeic pregnancy risk should be excluded – see Q 8.22.
- If breast feeding, the manufacturer urges caution. Uncertainty about possible effects of the tiny amount of etonogestrel reaching the breast milk must be discussed (as for the POP, Q 5.55–Q 5.56).
- Changing from combined pill or any (other) progestagen-only method: Implanon™ may be injected on any convenient day. Condoms should then be used or the preceding method continued for 7 days.

5.154 WHAT ARE THE ADVANTAGES AND BENEFITS OF IMPLANON™?

- Above all efficacy and convenience, if the bleeding pattern suits it is a 'forgettable' contraceptive.

- Long action with one treatment (3 years), plus very high continuation rates.
- Absence of the initial peak dose given orally to the liver.
- Blood levels are steady rather than fluctuating (as the POP) or initially too high (as injectables). This minimizes metabolic changes: HDL/LDL lipid ratios remained essentially unchanged and there were no important changes in clotting factors – as for Norplant.
- Oestrogen-free, therefore usable if past VTE (this is WHO 2, in my opinion). An excellent choice for many diabetics (Q 4.143).
- Median systolic and diastolic blood pressures were unchanged in trials for up to 4 years.
- Being an anovulant, special indications include past ectopic pregnancy (Q 5.115 (5)), intractable Mittelschmerz.
- The implant is rapidly reversible. After removal serum etonogestrel levels were undetectable within one week. Within 3 weeks 44 out of 47 women were ovulating normally.

5.155 WHAT ARE ITS PROBLEMS AND DISADVANTAGES?

- **Altered bleeding pattern**. In the premarketing randomized comparative trial of Implanon™ with Norplant, the bleeding patterns – analyzed in 90 day reference periods – were very similar, with one main difference. As expected for an anovulant method, amenorrhoea was significantly more common (20.8% versus 4.4%). The infrequent bleeding and spotting rate was 26.1%. Normal cycling was reported by 35%. But the combined rates for the more annoying 'frequent bleeding and spotting' and 'prolonged bleeding and spotting' totalled 18% (actually more than the 12% for Norplant).
  Treatment: the best short-term treatment is cyclical COC therapy, logically with 'Marvelon', after which the bleeding may become acceptable.
- **'Minor' side-effects** reported in frequency order were: acne, headache, abdominal pain, breast pain, 'dizziness', mood changes (depression, emotional lability), libido decrease, hair loss. The frequencies were amazingly similar to Norplant, and placebo studies suggest they would often not be drug related.
  Body weight: in a comparative study the mean weight increase over 2 years was 2.6 % with Implanon™ and 2.9% with Norplant, but in users of an IUD the weight increase was 2.4%! Though this implies a normal increase over time, by 24 months 35% had put on more than 3 kg.

As with DMPA forewarning is essential: some individuals do put on an unacceptable amount of weight.

- **Possible hypo-oestrogenism?** Since Implanon™ suppresses ovulation and does not supply any oestrogen, the same long-term concerns as with DMPA arise (Q 5.102). We need more data, but the initial findings on oestrogen levels and bone density are reassuring.
- **Local adverse effects.** Discomfort at insertion and removal can be minimized by good training. Infection of the site, migration, difficult removal and scarring are very infrequent.

5.156 WHO MIGHT CHOOSE THIS METHOD?

Indications: these really follow from Q 5.154, especially for women wanting effectiveness without the finality of sterilization.

ABSOLUTE CONTRAINDICATIONS (WHO 4) – A VERY SHORT LIST!

- *Progestagen-dependent tumours* (including active trophoblastic disease, liver adenoma).
- *Severe hepatic disease* with markedly abnormal liver function.
- Known or suspected *pregnancy*.
- Undiagnosed *vaginal bleeding*.
- *Hypersensitivity* to any component.
- Acute *porphyria* (see Q 4.218).

The manufacturer adds 'active venous thromboembolic disorder', but in my view this history (past or present) would be WHO 2. There is no evidence that Implanon™ would increase the risk.

RELATIVE CONTRAINDICATIONS

In my view these are as for DMPA which are listed at Q5.118 – EXCEPT for number eight in the list, since Implanon™ is immediately reversible. They are nearly all WHO 2. *Breastfeeding:* maybe WHO 2, see Q 5.153.

5.157 WHAT ABOUT FOLLOW-UP? AND REMOVAL OF IMPLANON™?

No treatment-specific follow-up is necessary, including no BP checks. There should be an 'open house' policy to discuss possible side effects, without any provider pressure to persevere if the woman really wants the implant out.

Removal is usually easy, with training. In the comparative study the mean insertion time was 1.1 minutes (range 0.03–5 minutes) and the mean removal time 2.6 minutes (range 0.2–20 minutes). This was approximately four times faster for both procedures than for Norplant.

Implanon™ is radio-translucent. If an implant cannot be palpated it should be removed under ultrasound control.

5.158 WHAT FURTHER IMPLANTS CAN BE EXPECTED?

Implants which slowly biodegrade would never need removing: but they should remain removable if desired.

A much improved oestradiol implant, releasing steady levels for 1-3 years (rather than as currently, with declining levels over 6 months) is in the pipeline. We can anticipate combined implants of progestagen with this oestrogen, also that other contraceptive compounds will be delivered by this route, such as gonadotrophin-releasing hormone antagonists.

VAGINAL RINGS

5.159 WHAT ARE VAGINAL RINGS?

Like implants, current versions use a Silastic carrier, which is in the shape of a ring between 5 and 6 cm in diameter and 4–10 mm thick. There are two main designs. In core-rings all the hormone is in a central core. In the shell design the inner core is hormone free, but encircled by a narrow hormone-filled band. Both types are then covered by Silastic tubing, giving controlled (zero-order) release to the vaginal mucosa.

Research into vaginal contraceptive rings generally received a set-back during a study of a levonorgestrel-releasing ring at the MPC during 1991–92. Asymptomatic erythematous patches were discovered, apparently associated with the areas of contact of the rings with the vaginal fornices. It is still not clear whether these were caused by physical pressure or a chemical effect. The long-term effects on the vagina and cervix of all future rings will certainly need careful monitoring.

5.160 WHAT IS CLINICALLY THE MOST PROMISING TYPE OF RING?

The combined type. The combined pill is after all a very successful model from which to start. Workers in Brazil and Israel in the early 1980s showed that a standard pill (LNG 250 μg plus EE 50 μg), as formulated for oral use, was effective when taken vaginally. Symptoms such as nausea were less frequent, though it is possible that this was partly due to achieving lower blood levels of oestrogen.

Vaginal pills have never become popular, probably because daily compliance is still necessary. But a combined ring which releases 3-keto-desogestrel and EE has been studied at the MPC and elsewhere and shows promise. It gives excellent cycle control with very few contraceptive failures. It can be retained for 3 weeks and removed for a withdrawal bleed during the fourth, thus closely imitating the combined pill. Alternatively it can be used continuously perhaps for 3 calendar months at a time (analogous to tricycling, see Q 4.31).

5.161 WHAT IS THE NATURAL PROGESTERONE RING?

This is a WHO ring designed especially for *lactating women*. It releases over 3 months 5–10 mg/day of progesterone, thereby minimizing concerns about the composition of breast milk. With this method I would foresee (as with the POP) the need for great care to transfer to a more effective method during weaning: if unwanted conceptions are to be avoided when the progesterone is no longer supplemented by the contraceptive effect of full lactation.

OTHER DEVELOPMENTS

5.162 WILL THE TRANSDERMAL ROUTE BE USED FOR CONTRACEPTION?

Already we have transdermal oestrogen and combined oestrogen and progestogen patches for HRT. At MPC we have recently been involved in a multicentre trial of the first commercial combined patch for contraception, which has given promising results – the standard regimen is for each patch to be used for a week at a time over 3 weeks followed by a 'patch-free interval'. Forgetting to change patches for up to three days makes little difference to the efficacy of this percutaneous 'combined pill', which should be a compliance advantage. This new choice for women is also keenly awaited! It is expected to be marketed as 'EVRA™'.

5.163 WHAT ARE OTHER THEORETICAL ROUTES?

For completeness, one should mention the rectal, transnasal and sublingual routes, all of which are in current use for other drugs. There are no known plans at present for routine contraception by those methods.

6 Intrauterine devices

BACKGROUND AND MECHANISMS

6.1 HOW WOULD YOU DEFINE AN INTRAUTERINE DEVICE?

This is any solid object which is wholly retained within the uterine cavity for the purpose of preventing pregnancy. Such devices are usually inserted via the cervical canal and may have marker thread(s) attached which are visible at the external os. There are three main types with frames: inert, copper-bearing and hormone-releasing (often called 'systems'). There are now also two frameless (implantable) varieties: copper-bearing (GyneFIX™ being the sole representative thus far) and hormone-releasing.

6.2 SHOULD THEY BE ABBREVIATED IUD OR IUCD?

Underlying this question is the possibility of confusion of 'intrauterine device' with 'intrauterine death' of a fetus. Hence many gynaecologists prefer IUCD, for IntraUterine Contraceptive Device. But this leads to problems in translation and moreover IUD is now well established in the world literature. An amusing compromise adopted by an expert committee of the World Health Organization (WHO) in the 1970s was the following: to use IUD (without full stops) for intrauterine device, and I.U.D. for intrauterine death! This agreed notation will be used here.

6.3 WHAT IS THE HISTORY OF IUDs?

An oft-quoted but poorly substantiated story describes the first IUD as a stone or stones placed in the uterus of camels in North Africa, to prevent pregnancies during long caravan journeys. One version of the story, however, suggests that the stones were actually put in the vagina, making the method more akin to a chastity belt than an IUD! Over 2500 years ago Hippocrates is credited with using a hollow lead tube to insert pessaries or other objects into human uteri. (The translations differ as to whether this was for contraception or other purposes.) Casanova recommended a gold ball; and as recently as 1950 one woman apparently used her wedding ring as a do-it-yourself IUD!

Cervicouterine stem pessaries were used from the late 19th century. They were made from material as exotic as ivory, glass, ebony and diamond-studded platinum, and were used for many purposes – including contraception. Some were shaped like collar-studs or had V-shaped flexible wings inserted into the lower uterine cavity. When the devices fractured, as they sometimes did, leaving just the intrauterine part in position, it was learnt that the latter (rather than the surface cap covering the external os) was the contraceptive. The first completely intrauterine device was a ring made of silkworm gut, described by Dr Richter of Braslaw. Later, silver wire was wound around the silkworm gut by Grafenberg and it is of interest that later versions were made of German silver, an alloy which contains *copper*. Now made of coiled stainless steel, the design is still one of the most widely used in the world (because it is so popular in China).

Many of the early devices were used as abortifacients as well as contraceptives, and the resultant haemorrhage and pelvic infection led to widespread condemnation by the medical profession. This retarded acceptance of the method, which was only really achieved in 1962 at the first International Conference on IUDs in New York City. The Lippes Loop was presented to this conference by its inventor, and became the standard inert device (see Fig. 6.1) against which many newer devices were compared: many now being bioactive, bearing copper or releasing hormones. The 'lay' terms 'loop'/'coil' are out-of-date and best not used.

6.4 HOW PREVALENT IS USE OF THE IUD?

It is estimated that about 110 million IUDs are in use worldwide, about 50 million of them in one country – China. In Britain, according to a recent survey (1995), IUDs were fitted in a mere 4% of women in the childbearing years. This is far fewer than might be predicted from the method's advantages (Q 6.19) and, in fact, current usage is on the increase.

6.5 WHAT ARE THE EFFECTS OF IUD INSERTION ON THE GENITAL TRACT?

Many cellular and biochemical changes have been described, but it is now clear that any IUD in situ long term acts chiefly by interfering with gametes and fertilization (Q 5.7).

All types of IUD lead to a marked increase in the number of leukocytes, both in the endometrium and in the uterine and tubal fluid. All the different types of white cell involved in a typical foreign body reaction are represented.
Inert and copper devices lead to elevated levels of many prostaglandins.

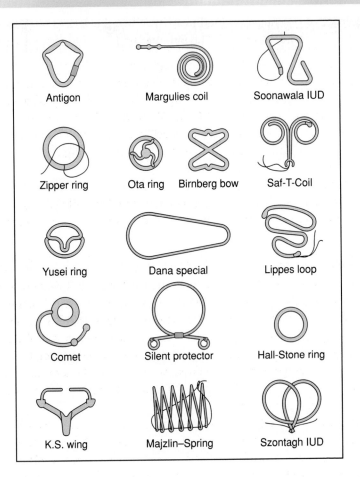

Figure 6.1 Past inert IUDs – see Figures 6.10, 6.12 and 6.13 for bioactive IUDs. Q 6.3.

3 Copper enhances the foreign body reaction and leads to a range of biochemical changes in the endometrium, affecting enzyme systems and hormone receptors.

4 Copper ions are also toxic to sperm and blastocyst.

5 Progestagen-releasing IUDs alter endometrial histology with a decidual reaction and glandular atrophy, and block oestrogen and progesterone receptors. They also markedly reduce the sperm penetrability of mucus to sperm.

6.6 ARE THERE ANY KNOWN SYSTEMIC EFFECTS OF IUDs (OUTSIDE THE GENITAL TRACT)?

An increase in some circulating immunoglobulins has been reported, but neither this nor the minute amount of copper entering the systemic circulation in copper IUD users is thought to be of clinical significance except in Wilson's disease, see Q 6.85). Absorption of hormones or any other chemicals which are carried by bioactive devices must always be presumed; but systemic effects of the progestagen-releasing IUDs are small (and depend on the release rate).

Inert and copper IUDs have no effect on the pituitary or ovary. However uterine shedding starts 2–3 days before circulating levels of oestrogen and progesterone have reached the levels usual at the start of the menses in non-IUD-users.

6.7 SO WHAT IS THE MAIN MODE OF ACTION OF IUDs?

The main effect is now believed to be by the blocking of fertilization. The inflammatory cells of the fluid in the whole genital tract (including the tubes) appear with all IUDs to impede sperm transport and fertilization. Actual phagocytosis of the sperm has been reported. Copper is probably also directly toxic to the sperm and ova. In various studies of long-term IUD users viable sperm have very rarely been found in the uterine cavity, the tubes or in aspirates of the pouch of Douglas, in clear contrast with the findings in sexually active controls.

However, an implantation-blocking effect is a back-up contraceptive mechanism. The remarkable effectiveness of *copper* IUDs when inserted postcoitally, up to 5 days after ovulation, indicates that they can still be exceptionally effective when the action cannot be by blocking fertilization. To work by this mechanism IUDs seem only to require to be present in the uterus for the last 9 days of each cycle. This implies the need for caution whenever IUDs are removed (see Qs 6.13 and 6.14).

The progesterone or progestagen-releasing IUDs (see Qs 6.143–6.149) markedly impair the sperm penetrability of cervical-uterine fluid, as well as sometimes stopping fertile ovulation. But they also have an anti-implantation effect, one that builds up too slowly for the LNG-IUS to be a reliable postcoital contraceptive (Q 6.146, 7.5, 7.33).

From this point until Q 6.139, unless otherwise stated, I shall deal only with modern copper IUDs. The important and often different features applying to the LNG-IUS are dealt with later.

6.8 SO HOW DO IUDs MAINLY ACT WHEN THEY ARE IN SITU LONG TERM?

They mainly act pre-fertilization. The postfertilization effects are potential but rarely utilized with all in situ IUDs. But it cannot be guaranteed to a prospective long-term user that her IUD or IUS will never in an occasional cycle block the implantation of a blastocyst. If she has ethical problems about that possibility she should perhaps only use anovulant, barrier or natural methods (or sterilization). See also Q 7.2.

6.9 WHY ARE INERT DEVICES NOW NO LONGER USED IN THE UK?

Their market was taken by the copper IUDs. As the surface area of inert devices is reduced, so the bleeding and pain side-effects are minimized but the failure rate increases. By virtue of its additional contraceptive actions (see Q 6.5), copper enables smaller devices to be used without loss of efficacy. The major advantage of inert devices (long-term use through to the menopause) is disappearing with the steady increase in permissible duration of use of copper IUDs.

EFFECTIVENESS

6.10 WHAT IS THE OVERALL FAILURE RATE?

For all current devices this is low, in the range of 0.2–2.0/100 woman-years including pregnancies which are due to unrecognized expulsions (estimated at about one-third of the total) – in the first year.

Three IUD designs stand out as the most effective currently available. These are the *Copper T 380, GyneFIX™* and the *levonorgestrel-releasing (LNG)-IUS* discussed later (see Q 6.142). Based on no less than 16 000 woman-years of use in multicentre WHO and Population Council studies, the first of these is now the 'gold standard' among copper devices. *At 10 years of use the cumulative failure rate was 1.4/100 women*, putting it in the same league as female sterilization! The LNG-IUS is even more effective, but the former market-leader the Nova T has a much higher failure rate, see Figure 6.2 and Qs 6.94 and 6.97.

6.11 WHAT FACTORS INFLUENCE FAILURE RATES (AND OTHER PROBLEMS) OF IUDs?

1 In fact, by far the most important is competence of the doctor or other professional inserting the device into the correct high fundal position.

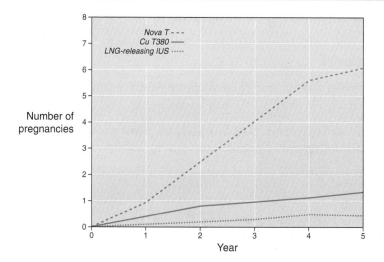

Figure 6.2 Five-year cumulative gross pregnancy rates per 100 women: for 937 women using Nova T; 1821 women using a 20 µg/24 h levonorgestrel-releasing device; and 1121 women using the Copper-T 380 (recruited in a separate Population Council RCT). From Andersson *et al.* 1994. *Contraception* 49: 56–72 and Sivin *et al.* 1990. *Contraception* 42: 361–78.

Comparative studies invariably show that the difference between doctors, for all the problems (summarized at Q 6.22) is greater than the difference between devices.

2 The second most important factor in comparative studies is the age and hence relative fertility of the population. Above 35, the first-year failure rate (of 0.1–0.5/100 woman-years with any device) is so good that IUDs become the method of choice for many older women (see Qs 6.20 and 6.23).

3 Duration of use (see Q 6.132).

6.12 ARE THE VARIOUS ASPECTS OF DEVICE DESIGN ALMOST IRRELEVANT THEN?

No. Attention to the shape and size of a device and of its introducer, and the insertion technique, can all influence efficacy. The ideal design would maximize delivery of any bioactive agent such as copper to the most important (high fundal) zone, and minimize:

1 the likelihood of malposition (especially too low in the cavity);
2 the likelihood of expulsion;

3 the liability to and seriousness of uterine perforation (see Qs 6.42 and 6.44).

Also, if possible:

4 the severity and duration of bleeding and pain (see Q 6.76).
5 any liability to exacerbate pelvic infection (see Q 6.61).

The implantable GyneFIX™ (Q 6.139) approach looks promising, particularly in regard to expulsion, malposition, and device-related pain.

6.13 HOW CAN INSUFFICIENT CAUTION WHEN REMOVING AN IUD CAUSE IATROGENIC PREGNANCY?

The answer follows from Q 6.7 above. If *one* of the major actions of IUDs is to block implantation, removal at any time before the last 9 days of the cycle can enable the blastocyst to arrive at a non-IUD-bearing uterus. Pregnancy could therefore result even if a women were being sterilized at the time of removal, and this has in fact been reported. A more serious risk would be a clip-induced ectopic, due to trapping the blastocyst in the tube. These events are quite rare because of the strong pre-fertilization effects of in situ IUDs (see Q 6.5), but they are entirely preventable (see below and Q 8.16).

6.14 HOW CAN SUCH PREGNANCIES BE AVOIDED?

Either by removal during a period, or more usually by following a '7-day rule', that is advice in advance to abstain or use a barrier method for 7 days before any IUD is removed. Seven days is believed to allow sufficient time, namely that between ejaculation and the latest likely implantation, for the IUD to have its antinidatory effects in that cycle. The 7-day rule is particularly important prior to sterilization, for fear of that iatrogenic tubal ectopic. It is also wise before any attempted replacement of an IUD.

Occasionally an IUD has to be removed midcycle although it has been recently relied upon (e.g. see Q 6.66). Postcoital hormone treatment should be considered in such cases (see Ch. 7).

6.15 HOW CAN EXCESSIVE CAUTION ABOUT THE TIME OF INSERTION OF IUDS CAUSE IATROGENIC PREGNANCIES?

By slavish adherence to the *myth* that it is best to insert only during or just after the menses! If women are told to wait until after their next period, not a few return pregnant. Several US-based studies have shown that IUDs can be inserted with relative safety *on the day they are requested*, if the woman's history indicates she will not have an implanted pregnancy.

Especially relevant was a US study which showed a statistically significant doubling of the rate of *expulsion* if copper-T IUDs were inserted on days 1–5 of the cycle as compared with days 11–17. Since the patients were unaware of the expulsion (usually partial) in nearly 40% of the cases, extra pregnancies could actually be caused by only inserting IUDs during the menses.

Finally, of course, deliberate postcoital IUD insertion up to day 19 of a 28-day cycle (adjusted for cycle length) is very effective (see Q 6.7).

6.16 WHAT IS THE LIKELY EXPLANATION FOR A HIGH EXPULSION RATE WHEN IUDS ARE INSERTED VERY EARLY IN THE CYCLE?

The main increase in expulsion rate occurs when IUDs are inserted during the menstrual flow, and is probably linked with extra myometrial activity at that time due to prostaglandins. The intraluminal pressure can rise above 100 mmHg and the fundal cavity is also narrower at this time than it is midcycle.

6.17 SO WHEN ARE IUDs BEST INSERTED?

The answer is – not during heavy days of the menses but at any time from their ending phase through until about midcycle. At the Margaret Pyke Centre (MPC) we target days 4–14 of a normal cycle. Beyond that if intercourse has been continuing, postcoital insertion in good faith is still permissible up to 5 days after the calculated ovulation day (see Q 7.15), but with caution and counselling, good records and follow-up.

6.18 SHOULD ADJUNCTIVE CONTRACEPTIVE MEASURES BE RECOMMENDED TO IUD-USERS FOLLOWING INSERTION?

Many women select this method precisely because they desire a non-intercourse-related method. However, there are three arguments for a very positive attitude to this approach, ideally using a male or female condom, or if not a spermicide:

- There is particular logic in condom use for any intercourse in the first 3–4 days following insertion or reinsertion of any IUD or IUS: insertion being the time when there is interference with the protective barrier to upper genital infection provided by the cervix (Q 6.55). Moreover, sperm seem able to act as bio-vectors of STIs.

2 To provide some protection longer term against both sexually transmitted and non-specific pelvic infection (see Qs 6.48 and 6.49), since there is good evidence that 'spermicides are also germicides'. Nonoxynol-9, in most spermicides, is insufficient protection against HIV though, hence condoms are preferable.

3 To provide some protection in the event of unrecognized expulsion, which is common especially in early months, and may be unnoticed in the menstrual flow.

ADVANTAGES AND BENEFITS

6.19 WHAT ARE THE ADVANTAGES OF IUDS?

These can be listed:

1 Effective:
   (a) highly, comparable to female sterilization;
   (b) postcoitally (not the LNG-IUS);
   (c) postabortally.
2 Safe:
   (a) mortality 1:500 000;
   (b) no known, unwanted *systemic* effects (not LNG–IUS);
3 Independent of intercourse.
4 Does not require any day-to-day actions, such as taking a pill.
5 Motivation is chiefly required around the time of insertion and never subsequently if side-effects are acceptable – it then being truly a 'default' method, for over 10 years duration of use in the case of Cu T 380.
6 Relatively cheap and easy to distribute.
7 Does not influence milk volume or composition.
8 With sympathetic providers the method is under a woman's control and (a point of occasional relevance) if the threads are removed, can be undetectable by her partner.
9 Continuation rates high.
10 Nearly always reversible (see Q 6.137).

What a remarkable list of advantages! It makes one wonder why we do not at least offer this choice far more, as a routine to all parous young women in stable relationships?

6.20 FOR WHOM ARE IUDs INDICATED?

The answer is: *upon request* for contraception, unless the absolute contraindications apply (see Qs 6.84 and 6.85) or if the relative contraindications are unacceptable to the woman herself after discussion in the light of alternatives. More specifically, in view of the threats to fertility (see Q 6.23(d)), and the fact that these are not only more serious when there is no family but also more probable in the young, IUDs are still not first-choice methods for most women until they have had children.

After childbearing, IUDs are an excellent 'holding manoeuvre' until the time that the couple are certain that their family is complete (and the man perhaps volunteers for his vasectomy!). Alternatively the method may be so acceptable that it remains in use until final removal 1 year following the menopause.

6.21 IS IT POSSIBLE THAT NEWER IUDs MAY BROADEN THE INDICATIONS?

Certainly. The LNG-IUS (see Qs 6.143 and 6.144) in particular 'rewrites the textbooks' in relation to use by women with heavy menses. Because it has some apparent protective action against PID it may also be more suitable for those at some risk than framed copper IUDs.

MAIN PROBLEMS AND DISADVANTAGES

6.22 IN SUMMARY, WHAT ARE THE MAIN PROBLEMS AND DISADVANTAGES OF INTRAUTERINE CONTRACEPTION USING COPPER?

These can be listed briefly as follows:

1. *Intrauterine pregnancy* – increased risk of miscarriage, hence of infection.
2. *Extrauterine pregnancy* (but no increase in overall population risk, see Q 6.30).
3. *Expulsion* with risks of pregnancy (see item 1).
4. *Perforation* with risks of pregnancy, also risk of IUD penetration of bowel/bladder and adhesion formation – and the risks of surgery;

5 *Malposition* of the device which may cause items 1, 7 and 8 in this list, as well as 'lost threads'.

6 *Pelvic infection/salpingitis* – though IUDs are definitely not the initiating cause, see Q 6.48.

7 *Pain.*

8 *Abnormal bleeding* – this may be increased in amount, duration, and/or frequency.

> **NOTE:** All available data are reassuring concerning *carcinogenesis*, whether of endometrium or cervix. Rare problems are considered at Qs 6.72, 6.87, 6.117 and 6.125.

6.23 CAN THE PROBLEMS IN Q 6.22 BE INTERCONNECTED? PLEASE GIVE EXAMPLES.

1 *Insertion* – is capable (either directly or indirectly) of causing any one of the eight problems.

2 *Pain* – may be a symptom of 1–6. Hence these should first be excluded before terming it a side-effect (i.e. something that the woman may or may not be able to 'live with'). Beware the stoical woman or the one who tries too hard to avoid troubling the doctor!

3 *Bleeding* – might mean numbers 1, 2, 3, 5 (definitely) and 6 (sometimes – could be *Chlamydia*. So this too is not necessarily just a side-effect.

4 *Fertility* – (indirectly or directly) can be impaired by any of 1–6 (see Qs 6.25, 6.33, and 6.48). Hence the general view that nulliparae should think twice before using this method.

5 *'Lost threads'* – may signify any of 1, 3, 4 and 5 (see Q 6.34).

6 *Malposition* of the device may cause numbers 1, 3, 7 and 8 in this list, as well as 'lost threads'.

7 *Age* – increases the risk of 2 (ectopics) and of 8 (heavy bleeding), anyway whether or not an IUD be present. But it definitely *reduces* the risk of 1, 3 and 6 (see Qs 6.11, 6.37 and 6.52).

8 *Duration of use* – may increase the risk of 2 (mainly, it is thought, through increasing age). But it *reduces* almost all the other problems! i.e. 1, 3, 6, 7 and 8 (see Q 6.132–3).

INTRAUTERINE PREGNANCY (IUD IN SITU)

There is absolutely no evidence for an increased risk of any of the commoner fetal abnormalities, whether the device be present at the time of conception or during organogenesis – at least for the inert and copper-containing types. Proof of this is (as usual) impossible, especially as 2% of all babies have an abnormality, and most particularly for the rarer disorders.

There are as yet no adequate data concerning any possible effects of a high local dose of progestagen on a continuing pregnancy (Q 6.145).

6.25 SHOULD THE DEVICE BE REMOVED, AND IF SO, SURELY THIS WILL INCREASE THE RISK OF MISCARRIAGE?

Counter-intuitively, the 'obvious' course of action – which is to leave the device alone, so as to avoid disturbing the pregnancy – has been shown to lead to a high rate of miscarriage (above 50%). Moreover, more often than expected this occurs in the second trimester with dangerous complications, particularly haemorrhage and sepsis. Septic second-trimester abortions were 26 times more frequent in one study. There is also evidence that the risks of antepartum haemorrhage, of preterm delivery and of stillbirth are increased if the IUD remains present.

Such problems are not restricted to the Dalkon Shield, although first reported for that device. Tatum (inventor of the first T-device) produced good evidence that removal of a copper device in the early part of pregnancy reduced the spontaneous abortion rate from 54% to 20%. So the slogan is:

If an IUD fails and a woman wishes to proceed to full-term delivery, do not leave the device in situ.

6.26 HOW SHOULD REMOVAL OF THE DEVICE BE MANAGED?

1. First, the woman should be counselled and warned that she is at increased risk of miscarriage whatever is done, but that the risk can usually be reduced considerably by gentle removal of the device.
2. Arrange an ultrasound scan. Rarely, the device may be identified above the pregnancy sac and it may be judged that removal would cause excessive trauma/rupture of the membranes. But far more commonly

the device is below the sac (displacement having been the cause of failure of the method, in fact).

3 Removal should then be performed, at the earliest possible stage in pregnancy, whenever the threads of the device are still accessible. In rare cases of heavy bleeding or leakage of liquor thereafter, the woman may need immediate admission. Usually she may continue as an outpatient, with appropriate advice about the subsequent occurrence of any pain, or more bleeding than the slight show to be expected at IUD removal.

If the threads are (already) missing, consider the possibility of perforation, not only of expulsion; and in all cases categorize/supervise the pregnancy as 'high risk' (see Q 6.25).

See also Q 6.28 re-ensuring that the location of the IUD is established after delivery.

6.27 WHAT IF THE OUTCOME AFTER COUNSELLING IS TO BE A LEGAL ABORTION?

Clearly the removal of the device is then best performed at the time of termination. In my view there should be routine *Chlamydia* testing and antibiotic cover for all such procedures. The latter is essential:

1 if the woman is first seen with an IUD-associated incomplete abortion (take swabs first), or
2 if medical induction of the termination be planned, with mifepristone and/or prostaglandins (PGs). This is because of anecdotes of severe infections, implying that the presence of the foreign body increases the sepsis risk. The IUD should be removed at the time of the first administration of the treatment, whether mifepristone or PG pessary, and not left to come away with the products of conception.

6.28 WHAT IF THE ORIGINAL IUD IS NEVER FOUND FOLLOWING SPONTANEOUS OR INDUCED ABORTION? OR AT FULL TERM?

It is unbelievable how often the original presence of an IUD gets forgotten, especially after delivery. There should be a thorough search for it in the placenta and membranes, and its presence or otherwise recorded. Otherwise women may finish up at a later stage with two intrauterine IUDs, or one in their uterus and one still at large, free in the abdomen. ... Many legal cases have resulted, and they are indefensible.

One can readily exclude either an embedded or perforated device with plain abdominal X-rays supplemented by ultrasound scanning (see Q 6.36).

EXTRAUTERINE PREGNANCY

6.29 WHAT IS THE RISK OF EXTRAUTERINE PREGNANCY WHEN AN IUD-USER BECOMES PREGNANT, AND IS THE RATE REALLY INCREASED?

No! to the second question. First and foremost, since the last edition of this book it is now clearly established that: *copper IUDs do not increase the overall risk of ectopics in a population, as compared with suitable non-IUD-using controls.*

The rate of ectopics is fundamentally dependent on the rate of pelvic infection (see Q 6.49) in that community. Because in situ copper IUDs drastically reduce fertilization rates (see Q 6.7), even women with damaged tubes, who will be at definite risk of an ectopic when they come to try for a pregnancy, may well escape this while using an IUD.

The risk among current users of the Progestasert (progesterone-containing) IUD appears to have been truly higher; but the more potent LNG IUS seems to block fertilization so well that in the Population Council study (1990, Figure 6.2) no ectopics at all occurred during a massive 3371 woman-years of use! However they do very rarely occur even with the IUS.

6.30 BUT SURELY ECTOPICS ARE COMMONER AMONG IUD CONCEPTIONS?

Precisely so, but this does not invalidate the above answer. As a working rule, the ratio increases roughly tenfold. Thus approximately 1 in 10–20 IUD-associated pregnancies will be extrauterine if the background rate is 1 in 100–200 pregnancies among non-IUD users. My assessment of the literature is as follows:

IUDs do not prevent extrauterine pregnancy (through the anti-fertilization effect) quite as well as they prevent intrauterine pregnancy (with the added anti-implantation effect). Hence there will be such a great reduction in the *denominator* of uterine pregnancies as to lead to an increased *rate*, even though the *numerator* of ectopic pregnancies is also reduced (but not by so much). It may help to use real numbers (Table 6.1)

TABLE 6.1 ECTOPIC PREGNANCY RISK WITH IUDs

	Annual conceptions (no.)	Ectopics (no.)	Ratio
Ordinarily, in a society, let the ectopic rate be 1 in 100 pregnancies.			
Assuming no infertility, if 1000 women use no contraception:	1000	10	1:100
If the same 1000 women use a copper IUD with a 1st-year failure rate of 1/100 woman-years:	10	1	1:10
Reduction:	990	9	

Thus although 1 in 10 among the IUD conceptions is ectopic, this is actually a valuable *reduction* of 9 in the expected number in the population. The numerator of the first ratio is truly lower, so it is myth that IUDs cause ectopics; but the denominator of total conceptions is so massively reduced (by 990) as to allow there to be *relatively* more ectopics among the few conceptions.

The ectopic problem is caused by pre-existing tubal damage and should not be blamed on the IUD. Very probably, even the one woman who has an ectopic while using the IUD was due to get one (along with the other nine women) in the future, anyway, when trying to conceive.

A similar explanation holds for the apparently increased *rate* of ectopics among conceptions with the POP, which nevertheless also protects against ectopics as compared with non-contracepting controls.

6.31 IS THERE AN INCREASED RISK OF ECTOPICS WITH DURATION OF USE?

Some studies show this, others, especially of the new *banded* IUDs, do not. It is presently thought that the apparent association is mainly because longer-term users are also older – and the proportion of pregnancies which are ectopic rises with age in the general population.

6.32 WHAT ARE THE IMPLICATIONS FOR MANAGEMENT?

The main point is that, even if only by the above *selection* mechanism (more ectopics being allowed to happen *relative* to the intrauterine pregnancies), once an IUD-user is pregnant she could well have an ectopic. So the clinical slogan is:

Every IUD-user with menstrual irregularity and pelvic discomfort has an ectopic pregnancy till proved otherwise.

In practice every IUD-user in whom pregnancy is suspected, with or without a positive pregnancy test, should have a pelvic examination to detect adnexal tenderness; and each IUD-user should be warned prospectively, backed by a leaflet, that any marked pelvic pain should always receive prompt medical attention, particularly if her period is late.

Beware also of the IUD-user who has just been sterilized. She could have a clip-induced ectopic if she was not advised appropriately (Qs 6.13 and 6.14) not to rely on the IUD for 7 days pre-surgery.

6.33 IS PAST TUBAL PREGNANCY A CONTRAINDICATION TO IUD USE?

In my view this is a relative contraindication (WHO 3) in parous women and 'almost absolutely' contraindicates the copper IUD method for nulliparae (WHO 4, but could be 3 if the 'right' device is chosen – see end of this answer). Although *the method does not increase the overall risk of ectopics in a population*, it does as we have seen sometimes selectively fail to prevent them. The woman concerned should surely use a method which will provide maximal protection to her one remaining tube. Another poor choice would therefore be the progestagen-only pill (see Q 5.34).

Good choices would be the combined pill, an injectable, or Implanon™ (Q 5.157) all being anovulants and therefore equally good at stopping ectopics and intrauterine conceptions.

If a copper device is nevertheless chosen, the Cu T 380 or the GyneFIX™ should be used, since ectopics like all conceptions are much less frequent than they are with the Nova T. The LNG-IUS would be another option with this history, since an ectopic was more than 10 times less likely in the randomized European trial than among Nova T users.

'LOST THREADS'

6.34 WHAT IS THE DIFFERENTIAL DIAGNOSIS OF 'LOST THREADS' WITH IUDs?

The first possibility is that the threads are in fact present but not being palpated by the user. This may be due to her inexperience, or the threads may have retreated to just within the external os. If the threads are truly absent then the differential diagnosis is as shown in Table 6.2.

6.35 WHAT ARE THE 'DO'S AND DON'TS' OF THE MANAGEMENT OF 'LOST THREADS'?

The first message from Table 6.2 is another IUD 'slogan', namely that:

IUD-users with lost threads either are already pregnant, or at increased risk of becoming pregnant.

This is hardly surprising: the device is just as bad at preventing pregnancy, just as *absent* from the uterine cavity, after perforation (under the liver ...) as after expulsion (in the toilet ...). And if the IUD was only malpositioned this might still leave part of the cavity unprotected and increase the conception risk.

1 All such women therefore need to be advised to use an alternative contraceptive method until the protective presence of an IUD has been established.
2 Consider also the possible need for postcoital contraception, especially if recent expulsion is diagnosed (see Q 7.23).
3 In general, X-rays and any form of intrauterine manipulation should be arranged in the follicular phase of the menstrual cycle, for fear of disturbing a pregnancy.
4 Above all, women with this problem need full explanations and supportive counselling throughout the management, which is described below (see Q 6.36).

6.36 WHAT IS THE RECOMMENDED PROTOCOL FOR THE MANAGEMENT OF 'LOST THREADS'?

I recommend the following very practical scheme (Fig. 6.3). Diagnosis and treatment are simultaneous in most cases, with minimum use of hospital facilities:

TABLE 6.2 DIFFERENTIAL DIAGNOSIS OF 'LOST THREADS' WITH IUDs

Main diagnoses A: Not pregnant	Clinical clues	B: Pregnant	Clinical clues
(1) **Device in uterus** Threads cut too short, or caught up around device during original insertion or avulsed at a previous removal attempt; or device itself malpositioned	(a) Periods likely to be those characteristic of IUD in situ (b) Uterus normal size	(4) **Device in situ + pregnancy**	(a) Amenorrhoea (b) Pregnancy test likely to be positive, with clinically enlarged uterus (sufficient to pull up thread)
(2) **Unrecognized expulsion**	(a) Recent periods as woman's normal pattern (b) Uterus normal size	(5) **Unrecognized expulsion + pregnancy**	(a) Amenorrhoea, following one or more apparently normal periods (i.e. unmodified by IUD) (b) Signs of pregnancy variably present (may be too early on first presentation) or pregnancy test positive
(3) **Perforation of uterus**	As (2) plus (rarely) mass or actual IUD palpated on bimanual examination	(6) **Perforation of uterus + pregnancy**	As (5) plus (rarely) mass or actual IUD identified on bimanual examination

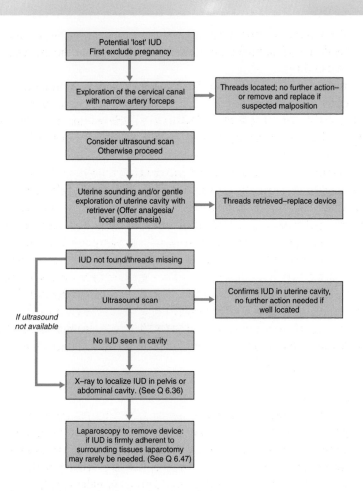

Figure 6.3 Management of 'lost' IUD threads. Q 6.36

1 *Exclude implanted pregnancy.* Take a careful menstrual history, do a bimanual examination and if indicated perform the most sensitive pregnancy test available. If the woman is pregnant, the management is primarily that of the pregnancy itself. *Note: However,* if an IUD is not recovered in the products of conception, or at full term in the placenta, an X-ray should be taken before assuming expulsion (as opposed to perforation or malposition).

In the absence of pregnancy, proceed as follows: *during the follicular phase of the cycle*, but preferably *not* during heavy days of the menstrual flow (see Q 6.16):

2 First insert *long-handled Spencer-Wells forceps* or equivalent into the endocervical canal. In a recent (1992) MPC study of 400 women with 'lost threads', almost 50% of the IUDs were retrieved this way! Meaning that they had a wasted trip, since this could so easily have been done by the referring doctor.

If the threads are readily located and the IUD judged (perhaps after sounding) to be correctly located, no further action need be taken; but disappearance of the threads may be a sign of malposition. So it is often advisable (after discussion with the woman) to remove and replace the device. *An ultrasound scan* may be helpful here (see point 6 below).

3 Try the use of *thread-retrievers*. The most established of these in the UK is the Emmett retriever, which is available presterilized and disposable. It has a handle to which is attached a thin plastic strip with multiple notches designed to trap the threads, when the edge is used like a curette against each surface of the fundus. There is also the Retrievette. The 'MI-Mark Helix' was found to be significantly less effective than either of these in the MPC study.

What about analgesia?

(a) Ideally (and this is MPC policy) a prostaglandin inhibitor such as mefenamic acid should be routinely given about 30–60 minutes before any intrauterine manipulations – as for all IUD insertions.

(b) A few women, especially nulliparae, require a paracervical block with local anaesthetic (see Q 6.110). Sterile anaesthetic jelly (Instillagel) via a special quill is also recommended by some.

(c) If cervix is stenosed, pretreatment with ethinyloestradiol (EE; 30 μg daily for 5 days) may be given to soften and dilate the canal. Misoprostol 200 μg *vaginally* as a single dose the night before is a very satisfactory alternative (but see page 507).

4 Various *resterilizable IUD retrieving forceps* (made by Rocket or Zeppelin), with short jaws opening wholly in the uterine cavity, may next be tried with success. Other options are suction using a Karman curette, and hysteroscopy; all require good analgesia, but a general anaesthetic should usually be avoidable.

6.36 continued

5 Next try *small, blunt IUD-removal hooks (Grafenberg pattern)*. In skilled hands these metal devices can be used to hook down either a thread or part of the device itself. Excessive traction is dangerous (see Q 6.47).

6 Arrange *appropriate imaging*. If the facilities are available, an ultrasound (US) scan may be arranged at this point. This should be done earlier in order not to cause unnecessary discomfort, if the device was not readily located by sound or retriever at Stage 3 above. Confirmation of correct intrauterine location within a non-pregnant uterus can be helpful for a woman who wishes to continue using the same device; but if there is any suspicion that it is malpositioned (e.g. too low or rotated), appropriate steps should be taken for its removal as above.

  Local anaesthesia is nearly always sufficient. General anaesthesia should very rarely be required for any device which is in utero.

  If the scan shows unequivocally that the uterus is empty, an X-ray is then required to differentiate between expulsion and perforation (see Qs 6.37–6.47).

7 *What if ultrasound facilities are not available?* It may then be useful to arrange an *X-ray with a uterine marker*. The most practical marker is another IUD, preferably of a different pattern from that originally fitted. There are three possible X-ray findings:

(a) Only the newly inserted device visible. This implies unrecognized expulsion of the first device.

(b) Two IUDs shown on the abdominal radiograph in close proximity. If a lateral view also shows that the IUDs are contiguous this means that the first device is actually in utero. This should be a rare finding if the X-ray is arranged only after stages 1–4 above. However, it is well worth removing the second IUD, as this may bring down part of the original device.

(c) The IUDs may be clearly separated on the X-ray. This establishes the diagnosis of complete perforation (translocation) (see Qs 6.42–6.47).

EXPULSION

6.37 WHAT IS THE FREQUENCY OF PARTIAL OR COMPLETE EXPULSION?

In most large studies of *framed* IUDs this ranges widely, from about 3 to 15/100 women at 1 year. The rates are influenced by:

1 characteristics of the woman (age, parity and uterine shape) – also the timing of insertion in relation to the menses (see Qs 6.15–6.17);
2 the size and nature of the device: the implantable GyneFIX™ has it is claimed the lowest rate (0.4% in the first year);
3 above all, the skill of the person performing the insertion.

6.38 WHEN DO EXPULSIONS MOST COMMONLY OCCUR?

During the menses, most particularly the first or second menstruation after insertion. About one-third of first year pregnancies among IUD-users occur after unnoticed expulsion. This should not happen if women are instructed to check for the presence of the threads (and the absence of any part of a partially expelled device), after each period and prior to relying on the device for that cycle. Among users for more than 3 years, the expulsion rate with most devices approaches nil. (See also Qs 6.35 and 7.23)

6.39 WHAT EFFECT DO AGE AND PARITY HAVE ON THE EXPULSION RATE?

Nulliparous women have higher expulsion rates for all devices than do parous women. After the first child there is a negligible effect of increasing parity on the expulsion rate. However, IUD expulsion rates seem to decline in a fairly linear fashion with increasing age. In studies either of parous or of nulliparous women, the rates of expulsion are about half above the age of 30 as compared with women under that age.

6.40 WHAT IS THE EFFECT OF THE SIZE AND SHAPE OF THE UTERUS?

If the cavity of the uterus is significantly distorted, either congenitally or by fibroids, there will be an increase in uterine activity (and cramps) after insertion and an increased likelihood of both malposition and expulsion. Ideally, therefore, such women should avoid framed IUDs, though the GyneFIX™ is often usable.

Careful sounding as described at Q 6.111 during the insertion may lead to a change of plan, but in practice quite gross distortions of the uterine cavity may be difficult to identify clinically. (see Fig. 6.7 and Q 6.92.) If in doubt, a good pre-insertion ultrasound scan of the contours of the uterine cavity is invaluable; and this should always be done if fibroids are identified.

6.41 WHAT IS THE EFFECT OF THE SIZE AND SHAPE OF THE DEVICE ITSELF?

Different expulsion rates between devices certainly exist. For example, the rate for the now obsolete Copper 7 (particularly for partial expulsions) was considerably higher than that for the T-shaped IUDs even after controlling for other variables. However, aside from insertion skill, expulsion rates are probably more correlated with the precise fit of the device within the uterus of different women. It is becoming clear that many framed IUDs are too wide for the uterine cavity at the fundus in vivo, particularly during menstruation; and also too long for many nulliparae.

The GyneFIX™ solves the problem of fitting different sizes and even shapes of uterus comfortably in a unique way (see Q 6.139) and so has a particularly low expulsion rate.

PERFORATION

6.42 WHAT PROBLEMS ARE ASSOCIATED WITH UTERINE PERFORATION?

1 Pregnancy. Most perforations first present as a pregnancy with 'lost threads'.
2 If the device is bioactive (copper or progestagen-containing) it leads to adhesion formation or may penetrate the wall of bowel or bladder. 'Closed' devices (e.g. rings) are particularly associated with bowel strangulation.

6.43 SHOULD PERFORATED DEVICES BE REMOVED? SHOULD IT BE CONSIDERED AN EMERGENCY?

In countries with developed medical services the benefits of removal always outweigh the risks. There are usually no specific symptoms so removal can be elective but prompt after diagnosis (see Q 6.36).

While waiting for hospital admission the patient should be warned to use alternative contraception, and that any abdominal pain, particularly if there is associated diarrhoea, must be reported promptly. Serious complications involving the bowel have been reported (including one death from peritonitis in a Copper 7-user).

6.44 WHAT IS THE FREQUENCY OF UTERINE PERFORATION FOLLOWING IUD INSERTION?

The true incidence is difficult to establish but is commonly quoted as around 1 per 1000 insertions. It is probably even lower for T-shaped IUDs that are positioned by a 'withdrawal' technique. Only one perforation in 1815 insertions of such devices was reported by Chi in 1987 (see also Q 8.23).

6.45 WHAT FACTORS AFFECT THE PERFORATION RATE?

The rate is affected by the usual three kinds of variable.

1 *Features of the woman.* The main factor here is recent pregnancy. Puerperal insertion is notorious in this respect, though any additional effect of *breastfeeding* is not so clear. See Q 8.23.
2 *Features of the device.* Linear devices such as the Lippes Loop, which were inserted by a 'push' technique (rather than the 'withdrawal' techniques now more commonly used) were more likely to perforate. An important safety factor is to avoid loading any IUD into its inserter too far ahead of the insertion, so that the plastic loses its 'memory' see Q 6.113).
3 *Features of the inserting clinician.* This is by far and away the most important factor. As Lippes himself observed: 'IUDs do not perforate. For this to happen we need a practitioner.' Almost all perforations are produced at insertion even though the diagnosis may be long delayed (and frequently emerges only when the empty uterus permits a pregnancy). Perforations are commoner:
   (a) when the operator is inexperienced;
   (b) when the position of the uterus is misdiagnosed (especially unrecognized retroversion) and probably:
   (c) when a holding forceps or tenaculum is not used to steady the cervix (see Q 6.111).

6.46 WHAT IS THE BEST WAY TO REMOVE PERFORATED DEVICES?

This can sometimes be done with minimal trauma by simple colpotomy (when the device is palpable in the pouch of Douglas); or more commonly at laparoscopy.

Even if there are adhesions, the device can usually be grasped at one end or the other and pulled through its own 'tunnel'. However, great care is necessary as devices can sometimes be adherent to the actual wall of bowel or bladder. Laparotomy may be required, but very rarely these days. If operative laparoscopic removal is not successful I would consider arranging more detailed imaging and referral to an expert in minimal access surgery, before necessarily proceeding to a laparotomy under the same anaesthetic.

6.47 ARE THERE ANY SPECIAL POINTS ABOUT EMBEDDING AND PARTIAL PERFORATION?

If part of a partially translocated device can be grasped within the uterus, it may be possible to remove it transcervically. However, this should be done with great gentleness. It is possible for the part of the device which is through the uterine wall to be adherent to bowel or bladder. Removal at hysteroscopy under ultrasound or laparoscopic control is much safer in such cases (see also Q 6.123 and Figure 6.11).

PELVIC INFECTION

6.48 DO IUDs CAUSE OR AGGRAVATE PELVIC INFLAMMATORY DISEASE (PID)?

There can be little doubt of this being an *associated* hazard. But to what extent if at all is the association causal? Studies have repeatedly shown an increased risk of such infections in IUD-users as compared with controls, though the controls are usually *protected* (see Q 6.49). When they occur, in some studies, attacks do appear to be of greater severity than in cases without the associated foreign body.

Now according to Westrom, one severe attack of laparoscopically diagnosed PID of any type carries a 1 in 8 risk of infertility due to tubal occlusion; two attacks, a 1 in 3 risk; and three attacks a 1 in 2 risk. So this infection risk has rightly become the greatest single anxiety about the IUD method, particularly for use by nulliparae.

NOTE: PID is primarily caused by people, not by devices; and the people are most often *MEN*, bringing the infection in to what the woman believed to be a monogamous relationship.

6.49 WHAT IS THE ACTUAL FREQUENCY OF PID AMONG IUD-USERS?

The absolute risk varies enormously according to the background rate of (sexually transmitted) PID in the population studied. The problem is that in most comparative studies the controls have been themselves *protected* against infection, either by using barrier methods or the combined pill. Progestagen-containing (i.e. mucus-altering) contraception, generally, about halves the risk of PID (see Q 4.40).

Westrom (1980) studied all women aged 20–29 in the town of Lund, Sweden and found the incidence of PID per 1000 woman-years to be 52 for IUD-users, as compared with 34 for sexually active users of no contraception, 14 for barrier method-users and nine for pill-users.

That study usefully shows that the lion's share of the sixfold difference at that time (early 1970s) when IUDs were compared with pills was caused by the protective effect of the latter: four-fold compared with users of nothing.

6.50 AS SHOWN BY THAT WESTROM STUDY, A DOUBLING OF THE RISK OF PID THROUGH USE OF THE IUD WOULD SURELY STILL BE IMPORTANT?

Definitely. But even that is an exaggeration. Factors like diagnostic bias are operative: PID is more likely to be thought about/diagnosed when pelvic symptoms occur in IUD-users. *Several studies have shown low or absent risk in women claiming only one sexual partner* – and that's even without good information about what their partner is up to! More convincingly, in the massive WHO study described below, *there was not one single case of PID reported among 4301 women fitted with IUDs in China in the 1980s, a country where true (two-sided) monogamy was then a reality!*

6.51 SO WHAT FACTORS HAVE BEEN SHOWN TO AFFECT THE RATE OF PID IN IUD-USERS?

In summary, and in order of clinical importance, the factors are:

1 woman's risk of acquiring PID from a partner;
2 the insertion process – combined with point 1 (see also Q 6.53–6.54 below);

3 features of the IUD:
  (a) foreign body effect;
  (b) the cervical tail(s).

The IUD itself has the least influence on risk.

6.52 WHAT FEATURES OF THE WOMAN CAN INFLUENCE THE PID RATE?

Age, acting as a marker for the risk of sexually transmitted infections. The risk is highest in young women under 20 and declines in a linear fashion as age increases (Fig. 6.4). In a study at the MPC in London, the incidence of infection was 10 times greater below the age of 20 than it was above 30 – although the 871 women were all nulliparous, had received the same type of IUD (Copper 7), at the same centre and all in the first 10 days of the cycle. Since:

1 there is no evidence that the uterus becomes more resistant to infection with age, and since:
2 the isolation of specific cervical pathogens and rates of PID in non-IUD-users show a decline with age and correlate with sexual lifestyle;

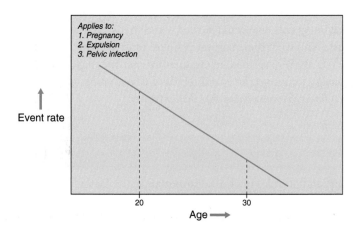

Figure 6.4 Effect of age on IUD performance. Qs 6.11, 6.39 and 6.52.

this again is indirect evidence that the vast majority of cases of PID in IUD-users are primarily sexually acquired.

It needs to be stressed again that, of course, the infection is often transmitted to the woman who is practising monogamy (*serial* monogamy, anyway) by her partner who is less so – or at the time of partner change. Very often if the right questions are asked, the attack of PID comes after a recent partner change. After the age of 30, it is an observed fact that partner change becomes less frequent.

6.53 SO HOW SHOULD WE QUESTION AND COUNSEL WOMEN WHO WISH TO USE THE IUD METHOD?

Questioning about frequency of partner change is of relevance but never sufficient: in an MPC study during the mid-80s the background rate of *Chlamydia* carriage was 2.4% in the general clinic population, but higher, 8.2%, in the pre-IUD group who had first been sensitively questioned about their likely exposure!

Thus in most metropolitan areas of the UK today I consider it suboptimal to fit copper or progestogen-releasing devices without microbiological screening: the money for pre-insertion *Chlamydia* testing must just be found. This argument is greatly strengthened by the WHO study depicted in Fig. 6.5 and the discussion below.

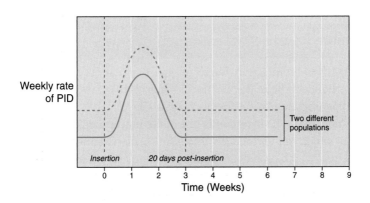

Figure 6.5 Graphic representation of PID rates post-IUD insertion. Farley *et al. Lancet* 1992; 339: 785–88.

6.54 WHAT LIGHT IS THROWN ON THIS PID PROBLEM BY THE THOROUGH REVIEW OF 12 INTERNATIONAL WHO STUDIES PUBLISHED IN 1992 (FARLEY *ET AL.*, *LANCET* 1992; 339: 785–88)?

One of ten types of IUD were inserted in 22 908 women (almost all parous) from 1975 to about 1990, and there were no less than 51 399 years of follow-up. The overall rate of PID was low, 1.6/1000 woman-years of use (contrast Lund in the 1970s, Q 6.49!). The most important findings were:

1 PID risk was more than six times higher specifically during the first 20 days after insertion than later; the risk was constant and relatively low thereafter for up to 8 years, with no evidence that it was then any higher than the local background rate (see Fig. 6.5).
2 PID rates varied by geographical area, highest in Africa and nil in China, and were inversely associated with age. This mirrors exactly the background risk of sexually transmitted diseases (STIs).
3 Whether considered individually or grouped by type, the PID rates for copper-bearing, hormonal and inert IUDs were statistically indistinguishable. For all these devices this makes a specific IUD factor in the attacks very improbable, especially as previous studies were readily able to show that one device, the Dalkon Shield, did specifically increase PID risk (see Q 6.62).
4 In China, 4301 IUDs were inserted, and not a single case of PID was reported either in the critical first 3 weeks or later!

6.55 IT LOOKS THEN AS THOUGH INSERTION TIME IS THE MAIN DANGER TIME FOR IUDs, BUT WHY?

- The post-insertion infection 'bulge' of Figure 6.5 cannot be because of bad insertion technique (i.e. the doctors introducing new organisms), only happening among the doctors outside China.
- We do know that IUD insertion is one of the procedures (like induced abortion) which can temporarily impair the protective mechanisms at a cervical level which protect the upper genital tract from infections.
- Although the doctors in all the centres were searching for monogamous women, they may well only have been successful in this search in China. In mainland China through the 1970s and 1980s (it would not be true now) monogamy was the norm, and it was also two-sided, with a consequential very low incidence of STIs of all kinds.

- Since there was no systematic pre-screening, in the other countries PID-causing organisms (especially *Chlamydia trachomatis*) are presumed to have been present in a proportion of the women. (In a later study from California, Walsh *et al.* 1998, where there was effective pre-screening, the post-insertion 'bulge' of PID was not detected even when antibiotics were not given).
- So in the WHO studies the process of insertion would therefore enable clinically silent infection to spread from the lower genital tract where it had previously resided into the upper genital tract including the fallopian tubes, becoming symptomatic. *Everywhere except in China.*

In summary:

1. The greatest risk of PID is in the first 20 days, believed to be caused by pre-existing carriage of sexually transmitted diseases (STDs).
2. Risk thereafter, like pre-insertion, relates to the background risk of STDs.
3. Insertion through 'Chinese cervices' does not cause an IUD-related post-insertion 'bulge' of PID, as in Figure 6.5.

6.56 WHAT ARE THE PRACTICAL IMPLICATIONS FOR ARRANGEMENTS AT IUD INSERTION, IN ANY SOCIETY WITH A MODERATE OR HIGH PREVALENCE OF STIs?

Defining 'moderate prevalence' arbitrarily as over 3% *Chlamydia* carriage, it is my view that, today:

1. all prospective IUD-users should be closely questioned about their own STI risk (see below) and then:
2. all cervices should be screened at least for *Chlamydia* prior to all IUD insertions or re-insertions.
3. Evidence of a purulent discharge from the cervix indicates more detailed investigation, ideally at a genito-urinary medicine clinic.
4. If *Chlamydia* is detected it should be treated vigorously (e.g. doxycycline 100 mg bd for 7 days, or azithromycin 1 g stat), other STIs looked for, first, contact tracing arranged and IUD insertion postponed – maybe indefinitely. There should certainly be a serious re-appraisal of the implications of (mainly her partner's) lifestyle for use of this method – most particularly, as usual, if she is nulliparous.
5. In the presence of a negative *Chlamydia* test and with no pelvic tenderness on examination, this cervix should still be inspected

carefully. A mucopurulent discharge may signify the need for GUM referral, to search for other pathogens.

6 In all cases this, now identified to be 'a Chinese cervix', should be very thoroughly physically and antiseptically cleansed, before the device is inserted following the manufacturer's instructions with minimum trauma.

7 Timing of insertion: it seems also advisable generally to *avoid insertion during the heavy days of menstrual bleeding*. There is not only a higher expulsion rate following insertion at that time (Qs 6.15–6.16), but also the suspicion of an increased infection risk.

6.57 WHAT IF THE (COPPER) IUD NEEDS TO BE INSERTED BEFORE THE RESULTS OF SCREENING ARE KNOWN, ESPECIALLY IN EMERGENCY CONTRACEPTION CASES?

Normally antibiotic treatment as at Q 6.56 (4) should be given, with 100% follow-up for contact tracing if the *Chlamydia* test does return positive.

6.58 WHAT ARE THE IMPLICATIONS OF FIGURE 6.5 FOR FOLLOW-UP?

At MPC, our initial reaction to the WHO publication was to arrange a (new) first post-insertion visit after 7 days (additional to the routine 6-week follow-up): designed to pick up any women with post-insertion infection (during the 'hump' of Fig. 6.4). We would still do that if we did not have the pre-screening option. However, subsequent to effective *Chlamydia* screening being available, we now find it is sufficient to give screen-negative women a hand-out, at the insertion visit, with a list of the symptoms suggestive of PID:

- low abdominal or pelvic pain, especially if the post-insertion symptoms had initially improved;
- dyspareunia;
- abnormal vaginal discharge;
- a temperature above 38.3°C especially preceded by rigors.

She is instructed to telephone our Advice Sister should she be in the slightest doubt. In General Practice, as a minimum a similar handout could be used, and it might be advisable for the woman to be asked routinely to 'touch base' by telephoning the practice nurse about a week post-insertion.

6.59 HOW DO YOU MANAGE THOSE WHO REPORT PROBLEMS?

If examination reveals cervical excitation tenderness and/or adnexal tenderness, then full PID treatment (see Q 6.65) is begun. The IUD (or IUS) may need removal, especially in nulliparae.

6.60 COULD ONE NOT SIMPLY ELIMINATE THE POST-INSERTION 'HUMP OF INFECTION' BY ROUTINELY PRESCRIBING THE APPROPRIATE ANTIBIOTICS?

Yes. Indeed, in an RCT by Penney *et al.* (1997) of post-abortion infections, which are similarly caused by cervical pathogens being enabled by the procedure to get to the upper genital tract, the group routinely receiving antimicrobial therapy did *better* than the group screened and selectively treated. This can be explained by false negatives for *Chlamydia*, or the presence of rarer pathogens which are nevertheless susceptible to the therapy.

But contact tracing is impossible without screening and the woman is at risk of reinfection later by her partner.

Hence if the resources could be found, there is a lot to be said in favour of *both* pre-screening *and* chemoprophylaxis for everyone. Considering that a Copper T 380 costs only around £10 for 10 years (and just one course of IVF for blocked tubes costs £1500) the extra expense of £50 or so for such a cost-effective method is fairly easy to justify!

6.61 WHAT FEATURES OF THE DEVICE ITSELF MIGHT INCREASE RISK OF PID, AND HOW MIGHT THEY BE CHANGED?

As we have seen, PID is primarily a 'self- or partner-inflicted wound'. Yet all IUDs are foreign bodies, and as such they have the potential to facilitate primary (sexually transmitted) infection, or to promote secondary invaders and the severity and chronicity of attacks. Indeed, aside from insertion (fully discussed above), the main IUD-factor in PID seems to be this potential to make it more clinically manifest (worse when it happens).

By definition, the foreign body effect of IUDs cannot be eliminated; however it may be reducible by device design, perhaps by:

1 avoiding embedding of part of the device in the myometrium;
2 elimination of the plastic carrier as in the GyneFIX™ (see Q 6.139);
3 release of progestagens into the cervical/uterine fluid, to hinder transfer of pathogens to the upper genital tract (as with the LNG-IUS, see Q 6.144)
4 experimentally, by similar release of antiseptic substances.

6.62 WHAT COULD BE THE EFFECT OF THE THREADS TRAVERSING THE CERVICAL CANAL?

The thread of the now defunct Dalkon Shield was multifilament in design and this was shown to act as a 'wick'. This was disastrous, and since a very few Dalkon Shields are still in situ they should always be removed on suspicion of their presence.

Even when using IUDs with monofilament threads, however, elegant pre-hysterectomy studies by Sparks and Elstein showed that symptomless bacterial infection of the lower part of the uterine fundus is almost invariable. However the uterus was always sterile if the threads were excised prior to insertion (even from Dalkon Shields).

6.63 SO SHOULD WE GO BACK TO USING THREADLESS IUDS?

On balance, I think not. An early study in 1967 by Professor Elstein showed more infections among users of Lippes loops (with threads) than in threadless Birnberg bows. A (randomized) comparison from Sweden reported in 1992 a lower risk of clinical upper and lower genital tract infections at follow-up if the threads of Multiload Cu-250 devices were deliberately pushed into the uterus at insertion, than in normal Nova T controls.

However other studies including a large international clinical trial of 1250 women randomly assigned old TCu-200 IUDs with or without threads reported no significant difference in incidence of PID, STIs or other infections.

More importantly, the WHO studies among others, have shown vanishingly low rates of important infections among threaded device users so long as they are at low risk of STIs, above all in China in the 1980s! (Q 6.50).

Pending more data any adverse influence of the threads must be very small in practice, and more than outweighed by their usefulness during IUD follow-up and to simplify device removal.

6.64 HOW WOULD YOU SUMMARIZE *PRACTICAL* IMPLICATIONS, ESPECIALLY OF THE WHO STUDIES (Q 6.53–6.60)?

1 Monogamous parous women with monogamous partners as in China in the 1980s may use IUDs without fear of PID.
2 Monogamous nulliparae may consider the option, but always as a second choice, since they do not have 'that cushion, of one or more babies already in the cot'.
3 All others need to be informed/reminded where the infection really comes from, since as the WHO authors put it: 'exposure to sexually transmitted disease rather than type of IUD is the major determinant of PID'.
4 Around the crucial time of *insertion*, the measures described in Qs 6.56–60 need to be implemented.
5 There should be very vigorous treatment and contact-tracing of PID when it happens.
6 Providers should minimize the number of (dangerous) reinsertions by choosing devices with the longest possible long-term efficacy (see Q 6.132).

6.65 HOW SHOULD SIGNIFICANT IUD-ASSOCIATED PELVIC INFECTION BE MANAGED?

Laparoscopy may be indicated in severe cases to establish the diagnosis.
Bearing in mind the high likelihood that this is a sexually transmitted infection (see Q 6.52), ideally full bacteriological screening at a genitourinary medicine clinic should be performed. If such detailed bacteriology is impossible, often because treatment is urgent, at least endocervical swabs should be taken first into the appropriate transport media. The usual first choice of antibiotic would be a tetracycline (preferably for at least 2 weeks, in order to treat the most common and possibly most harmful pathogen, namely *Chlamydia*), with 5 days of metronidazole to deal with the frequently associated anaerobes such as Bacteroides.

6.66 SHOULD THE IUD BE REMOVED?

There is controversy as to whether it should *always* be removed. My own threshold for doing this at the outset of treatment is very low in young nulliparous women – with consideration of the possible need for postcoital contraception according to the menstrual and coital histories (see Qs 6.13 and 6.14). The device should always be removed if there is no response to treatment within 48 hours, not omitting to arrange with the woman concerned a new method of birth control.

6.67 SHOULD THERE BE ANY OTHER ACTION, AFTER IUD-ASSOCIATED PID?

Regrettably healthcare providers in most cultures still pussyfoot around this matter, but sexual contacts of all such women should be traced and appropriately treated. There are a minimum of three individuals to be treated, the index case, her partner and his other partner.

Moreover, a very clear warning should be given about the disastrous effects of *recurrent* PID (reaching after three hospitalized attacks a tubal occlusion rate of one in two), along with advice about condom use to avoid that other risk she may also be running, of HIV infection. All this is not being judgemental, just good preventive medicine.

6.68 IS PELVIC INFECTION *ALWAYS* A CONTRAINDICATION TO AN IUD?

If currently acutely or chronically present, this is an absolute contraindication. All women reporting deep dyspareunia, or exhibiting tenderness of the pelvic organs whether on palpation or caused by cervical excitation, should not receive an IUD until infection has been excluded.

6.69 WHAT ABOUT A HISTORY OF PAST PELVIC INFECTION?

If this was not severe, more than 6 months ago and there has been no recurrence, and currently the woman is free of any symptoms or signs, then (after full discussion and counselling) IUD insertion is only relatively contraindicated. It would still be preferable that such a woman should have at least one living child.

Re-screening for STIs especially *Chlamydia* should be done, and there should be serious consideration of tetracycline 'cover' for the insertion. The woman may need to be advised to use condoms as well, subsequently. She should also be warned to return exceptionally promptly at the first sign of another PID attack.

Past infection always contraindicates the IUD in a case at risk of endocarditis (see Q 6.89).

6.70 WHAT IS *ACTINOMYCES ISRAELI*?

This bacterium is normally a harmless commensal in the mouth and gastrointestinal tract. In the lower female genital tract it is almost never detected by cytology or culture except when a foreign body is present, the commonest being an IUD or IUS.

There is also an association with *bacterial vaginosis* (BV) – which itself has been found commoner in IUD-users than controls (Q 6.174).

6.71 HOW OFTEN ARE *ACTINOMYCES*-LIKE ORGANISMS (ALOs) FOUND IN THE CERVICAL SMEARS OF IUD USERS?

The frequency with which routine smears show these organisms appears to relate in a linear fashion to the duration of use of the device: whether inert, copper or LNG-containing. After 1 year's use 1–2% of smears are positive, rising to 8–10% after 3 years and over 20% after 5 years.

It was at first though that copper prevented the carriage of these organisms. It is now believed that the main explanation for lower incidence is the shorter average duration of use of copper than inert devices (plus, in the past, frequent *changes* – see Q 6.74).

6.72 WHAT IS THE MOST SERIOUS POTENTIAL SIGNIFICANCE OF THE FINDING OF ALOs IN THE CERVICAL SMEAR?

Frank actinomycosis is an extremely serious and debilitating condition, featuring granulomatous pelvic abscesses. A fatal outcome has been reported once in an IUD-user, and other young women have been known to require pelvic clearance as a lifesaving measure. However, the incidence of this complication is extremely low, even allowing for under-diagnosis among women with severe IUD-related infections.

It seems clear in short that *actinomycosis represents a very small part of the spectrum of pelvic infection associated with IUDs*.

6.73 WHAT ACTION SHOULD BE TAKEN WHEN A CERVICAL SMEAR REPORT SHOWING ALOs IS RECEIVED?

The advice which follows is substantially that of the Faculty of Family Planning as issued in January 1998.

The patient should be recalled without delay and carefully questioned about the occurrence of pain, deep dyspareunia, intermenstrual bleeding or excessive discharge. If there is even mild adnexal or uterine tenderness on examination, or cervical excitation tenderness, in my view the knowledge that ALOs are present should markedly lower the threshold for IUD removal. Endocervical swabs should be taken and sent with the removed device (threads excised) for appropriate bacteriology, ideally after speaking personally with the microbiologist.

Arrange appropriate referral for women with marked symptoms, either to a department of genitourinary medicine or especially if there is an adnexal mass to a gynaecologist. If the laboratory recommends antibiotic therapy, penicillin is the usual choice but *in high dose for several weeks*, and the usual course of metronidazole 400 mg bd for 5 days as well if BV is also diagnosed.

The patient should be followed up to check for cure, and another method of birth control arranged.

6.74 WHAT ACTION SHOULD BE TAKEN IF ALOs ARE REPORTED AND THERE ARE *NO SYMPTOMS* OR SIGNS AT ALL (PELVIC INFECTION NOT SUSPECTED)?

If over 20% of long-term IUD-users carry ALOs, and so very few ever develop symptoms, more morbidity (through resulting pregnancies) could be caused by insisting on ceasing the method than by simply monitoring the situation.

An asymptomatic woman should be counselled about the potential (small) risk and taught the symptoms of pelvic actinomycosis. At MPC we have a helpful leaflet describing the two management options:

1   *Removal or change of the IUD or IUS.* A popular course of action, particularly for copper IUDs, since it usually leads to a more reassuring situation for the woman, is simply to remove the device and replace it *immediately* with a new one. In 1984 a study at the MPC showed that this schedule – device removal, *with or without* immediate reinsertion, and without any antibiotic treatment – was followed by disappearance of the ALOs from the subsequent cervical smears. Although later experience shows that such clearance is not invariable, we find that most women after counselling now elect to try device replacement. If successful (checked by a cervical smear first at 6 months and then at normal intervals as advized locally for routine cytology), this option reduces both *her* ongoing anxiety about harbouring a potential pathogen and *our* burden of responsibility for long-term follow-up.

2 *Leave the IUD or IUS in situ, with monitoring*: by regular follow-up arranged every 6 months. This is for a bimanual examination and enquiry (and reminder) about relevant symptoms. The woman is advised that if they ever should occur she should return even before her next routine visit. She should agree to be contacted at home or through her general practitioner if she fails to attend. Cervical smears are likely to remain showing the ALOs and are hence only repeated at the frequency of local screening guidelines.

In both cases if BV is diagnosed (characteristic odour and history with pH more than 4.5) it should be treated with metronidazole, as above (Q6.73).

PAIN AND BLEEDING

6.75 WHAT IS THE MOST FREQUENT COMPLAINT OF COPPER IUD-USERS?

In practice, the most frequent problem is increased bleeding, frequently accompanied by cramp-like menstrual pain and the two are often considered together. However, it is a good working slogan that:

Pain plus bleeding in an IUD-user has a serious cause until proved otherwise.

Thus to label these as a 'side-effect' should only be after exclusion of more important causes – listed at Q 6.22–6.23 above.

6.76 WHAT TYPES OF BLEEDING PATTERN ARE OBSERVED BY IUD-USERS?

The loss at the menses may be heavier and/or longer: the latter typically because of light premenstrual bleeding or spotting, before and after the flow proper. There may also be intermenstrual bleeding or spotting, too light to cause anaemia, but often very troublesome to the woman.

6.77 HOW OFTEN DO IUD-USERS DISCONTINUE THE METHOD BECAUSE OF PAIN OR BLEEDING?

About 5–20% of inert or copper IUD-users have the device removed because of bleeding and pain within the first 12 months. Of the remainder, approximately half will admit to annoying bleeding symptoms which they have learnt to live with, and some will subsequently discontinue the method for the same reason. (Measurement of the loss has shown that inert devices roughly double the measured volume of flow, whereas the smaller copper ones only increase the amount by about 50%, that is about 20–30 ml on average.) Nevertheless removal rates were not dramatically improved when copper devices arrived. This is doubtless because they (even GyneFIX™) have not eliminated the problems in some women of prolongation of duration of flow and intermenstrual spotting.

These last two bleeding problems are still features of at least the early months of use of progestagen-releasing devices like the LNG-IUS, even though they positively reduce the measured volume of loss and often eliminate pain. Perseverance is usually rewarded by frank amenorrhoea or infrequent light bleeds (see Q 6.145).

6.78 IS COPPER A HAEMOSTATIC AGENT?

Menstrual blood loss measurement studies of my own in the 1970s, comparing Lippes Loops with and without copper bands (but otherwise identical) showed clearly that the measured mean volumes were similar. Indeed the *duration* of loss in the copper-using group was slightly but significantly increased. Hence it is possible to be definite, that the reduced amount of bleeding with copper devices is a function merely of their smaller size and surface area (see Q 6.9).

6.79 WHAT IS THE CAUSE OF THE INCREASED BLEEDING AS AN IUD SYMPTOM, WITH OR WITHOUT PAIN?

1 Various types of *malposition* can cause both symptoms.
2 The fact that the cavity of the uterus is *distorted* congenitally or by *fibroids* may be missed, causing pain as the uterus attempts to expel the device. Coincidental *polyps* are also possible.
3 Especially in *nulliparae* whose cavities tend to be smaller, the fitting of a device which is *too long or too wide* (see Q 6.93) may similarly cause cramping pain. The stem of a device which is too long projects into the sensitive isthmic part of the uterus, and pain may also result from penetration of the myometrium by the side arms.
4 *Perforation of the cervix* by the stem of the device may result from partial expulsion and also cause pain (see Fig. 6.11 and Q 6.123).

In all these cases following bouts of cramping, some at least of the observed intermenstrual bleeding (IMB) may be caused by mechanical trauma to the endometrium.

According to some X-ray studies, small *devices which float too loosely* in a large cavity may also cause some IMB but without pain.

he LNG-IUS has the same mechanical limitations as the Nova T whose hape it shares, but GyneFIX™ (Q 6.139) generally eliminates or minimizes ll of these problems 1–5 above, through its unique implantable technology.

6.80 WHAT IS THE UTERINE MECHANISM FOR IUD-RELATED BLEEDING AND PAIN?

nsertion of IUDs leads to a high concentration of plasminogen activators vhich increase fibrinolytic activity and hence lead to more blood flow. inked in some way with these changes are alterations in the prostaglandin esponses of the endometrium during menstruation. Prostacyclin activity is ncreased and this causes vasodilatation and inhibition of platelet function. n increase in other prostaglandins probably explains the increased nenstrual cramps, but not why some are affected so much less than others.

6.81 ARE THERE ANY DRUGS THAT CAN REDUCE THE MENSTRUAL FLOW AND PAIN IN IUD-USERS?

here is no very effective therapy for the problem of prolonged spotting. lowever, for the heaviness of flow at the menses antifibrinolytic agents are ertainly effective. Tranexamic acid is available, but it is not certain whether ne benefits of treatment outweigh its well-documented risks (see Q 5.129), articularly as it is not an analgesic.

The pain-relieving prostaglandin synthetase inhibitors (PGSIs) are nerefore normally preferable, particularly mefenamic acid (1500 mg), uprofen (1200 mg) and naproxen (1500 mg). (Amounts in parentheses re totals for each day, to be taken in divided doses.) These drugs need nly be taken from the onset of menstruation, for so long as the patient eels the benefit from treatment. Response is very variable (Fig. 6.6), but ome women report that the flow diminishes rapidly within an hour of king a tablet.

6.82 DO MANY WOMEN PERSEVERE FOR LONG WITH AN IUD F THEY HAVE TO TAKE DRUGS REGULARLY TO COPE WITH BLEEDING AND/OR PAIN?

ot as a rule. Few women would be happy to continue for years taking owerful drugs with each menstruation and doctors too would be worried

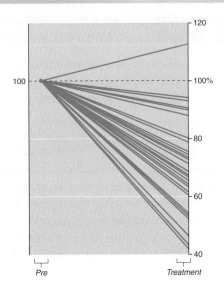

Figure 6.6 Percentage change in menstrual blood loss with mefenamic acid. Q 6.81. The figure shows the percentage reduction in menstrual blood loss with mefenamic acid 1500 g daily for a maximum of 7 days. The mean of two treatment periods is compared for each individual woman with the mean of two previous control periods expressed as 100%. (From Guillebaud J *et al*. Reduction by mefenamic acid of increased menstrual blood loss associated with intrauterine contraception. *British Journal of Obstetrics and Gynaecology* 1978; 85: 53–62, Figure 1)

by possible long-term risks. Antiprostaglandin drugs are certainly very useful to reduce the cramps at IUD insertion, and both pain and bleeding over the first few cycles. In practice, however, few women continue to take them (except intermittently for dysmenorrhoea) and the majority either live with their symptoms or eventually give up the IUD method.

A better alternative may often be to exchange the IUD for an IUS (Q 6.143).

SELECTION OF USERS AND OF DEVICES

CONTRAINDICATIONS

Please see general discussion re the WHO classification of contraindications at Q 4.130.

6.83 WHAT ARE THE ABSOLUTE CONTRAINDICATIONS TO IUD/IUS USE (WHO 4)?

These mostly relate to the adverse side-effects which we have now considered. They can be classified into temporary absolute contraindications, which imply some variable delay before possible later insertion, and permanent contraindications. In general absolute contraindications apply to both IUDs and IUSs, but relative contraindications do not always apply to the IUS (see below).

6.84 WHAT ARE THE (POSSIBLY) TEMPORARY ABSOLUTE CONTRAINDICATIONS TO IUDs AND IUSs?

1 Undiagnosed irregular *genital tract bleeding*. This is for fear of wrongly attributing post-insertion bleeding to the IUD, when in fact due to important uterine pathology, such as carcinoma of the endometrium.
2 Suspicion of *pregnancy*.
3 Post *septic abortion*, current *pelvic infection* or undiagnosed pelvic tenderness/deep dyspareunia or *purulent cervicitis* (see Q 6.88).
4 Therapy causing *significant immunosuppression* – i.e. more profound than use of low dose corticosteroids (see Q 6.88).
5 *Malignant trophoblastic disease, with uterine wall involvement.*

6.85 WHAT ARE THE PERMANENT ABSOLUTE CONTRAINDICATIONS TO IUDs AND IUSs?

1 Markedly *distorted uterine cavity*, or cavity sounding to less than 5.5 cm depth (see Fig. 6.7 and Q 6.92). (*Note: However this finding signifies only category WHO 2 (Broadly usable) for the GyneFIX™ frameless device (Q 6.139)*
2 Known *true allergy* to a constituent (see Q 6.87).
3 *Wilson's disease* (copper devices only).
4 Past attack of *bacterial endocarditis* or of severe pelvic infection in a woman with an anatomical lesion of the heart; or after any *prosthetic valve replacement* (Q 6.89).

6.86 WHAT ARE THE RELATIVE CONTRAINDICATIONS TO COPPER IUD USE?

These often *do not apply* to the LNG-IUS, see Box below.
   They vary in their importance: the WHO classification is useful, see Q 4.130): WHO 3 meaning use very cautiously, other options usually

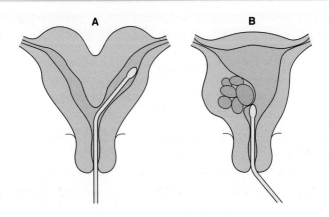

Figure 6.7 Uterine cavity distorted – congenitally or by fibroids. Q 6.85. *Note* in A that it is easy to obtain a normal sounding depth despite a septate uterus. Careful sounding will detect the abnormality, however, and will also identify a submucous fibroid as in B.

preferable, and WHO 2 meaning broadly usable, benefits outweigh risks. The factors listed are WHO 2 unless otherwise stated. Some are considered in more detail at subsequent questions.

1 *48 hours to 4 weeks postpartum* (excess risk of perforation; WHO 3).
2 Known *HIV infection or AIDS* (Q 6.88). Eventual interference with the immune system by the virus can be expected to increase the risk of severe infection (WHO 3).
3 Recent exposure to *high risk of a sexually transmitted disease* (e.g. after rape). Ideally the insertion should be delayed until after full investigation; but in emergency situations such as for postcoital contraception copper IUD may be permissible (WHO 3) with full antibiotic cover (after swabs for bacteriology taken). See Qs 7.24 and 7.28.
4 *Valvular heart disease* with risk but not as Q 6.85 (4) above; no past history of bacterial endocarditis (see Q 6.89; WHO 3).
5 Past history of tubal *ectopic pregnancy* (see Q 6.31) in *nulliparae*, WHO 3 if most effective copper IUDs or the LNG-IUS used (*not* the Nova T); but better to use an anovulant method. Also past history of tubal surgery, or other very high ectopic risk, in those still wanting a child. In parous women recurrence risk remains a need for caution and use of the most effective among intrauterine methods.

6 Any prosthesis which can be prejudiced by blood-borne infection, e.g. *hip replacement* (see Q 6.90) – IUDs certainly usable, just antibiotic cover for the insertion advised.

7 *Benign trophoblastic disease* while blood HCG still detectable (see Q 4.75).

8 Past *history of definite pelvic infection* (see Q 6.69).

9 Lifestyle *risking STIs*.

0 Suspected *subfertility*, WHO 2 for any cause, or WHO 3 if the questionable fertility relates to a tubal cause.

1 *Nulliparity and young age*, especially less than 20. The reason this is WHO 2 is both increased *risk* of infection and also the more serious *implications* thereof. Summation with other factors in this list may make the caution even stronger (WHO 3). Expulsion is also commoner, though not with GyneFIX™.

2 *Diabetes* – WHO 2 for infection risk, but IUD often acceptable, and LNG-IUS may be preferable. See Q 6.91.

3 *Fibroids or congenital abnormality* without too marked distortion of the uterine cavity (see Q 6.92). WHO 2 for framed IUDs or IUSs, WHO 1 for the GyneFIX™.

4 Severely *scarred uterus*, e.g. after myomectomy (WHO 3).

5 Severe *cervical stenosis* (WHO 3). Pretreatments may help. See 6.36 3(c).

6 *Heavy periods*, with or without *anaemia* before insertion for any reason, including anticoagulation. This is an *indication* for the LNG-IUS, of course, WHO 1.

7 Severe *primary dysmenorrhoea*. GyneFIX™ or LNG-IUS may be tried.

8 *Endometriosis.* (There is no proven link, but part of the mechanism of endometriosis may be retrograde menstruation. Hence prudence dictates it might be preferable not to increase this with a copper IUD. However a progestagen-releasing IUS is a good option, WHO 1.)

9 *Penicillamine* treatment, whether for Wilson's disease or rheumatoid arthritis. (There are one or two anecdotes of in situ pregnancy occurring in penicillamine-treated copper IUD-users – possibly due to interference with the contraceptive action of the copper. This is unproven; inert or progestagen-releasing IUDs would not be affected.)

0 After *endometrial ablation/resection* – see Qs 8.60 and 8.61 for more about this. LNG-IUS may be used.

86 continued

6.87 CAN COPPER IUDs CAUSE LOCAL OR SYSTEMIC ALLERGIC REACTIONS?

Definite cases have been reported, though they are rare. For instance one case reported in 1976 presented with urticaria, joint pains, and angioneurotic oedema, and positive scratch tests showed a true copper allergy. There have also been reports (and I had one clear case) of marked reversible uterine pain and tenderness plus vaginal discharge, with no evidence of infection, resolving immediately after removal of the device. Referral to a dermatologist for specific allergy tests may be indicated, though most contact allergies to metal bangles or rings are not due to copper.

6.88 IS THERE EVIDENCE THAT ANTIBIOTICS, ANTIPROSTAGLANDIN OR IMMUNOSUPPRESSIVE DRUGS MIGHT IMPAIR THE EFFICACY OF IUDs?

Since there is no evidence that the inflammatory reaction in the uterus and tubes of IUD-users is normally caused by any infective process, the few reports of pregnancy occurring during antibiotic use can be dismissed as coincidences. One study comparing pregnancy rates in IUD users with and without rheumatoid arthritis has shown no evidence that interference with endometrial prostaglandin metabolism by PGSIs can impair IUD efficacy, though this had been suggested in a French study.

There are reports that immunosuppressed transplant patients are more likely to become pregnant if they use IUDs. Probably more important is the risk of severe and silent *infection*. Hence other methods of birth control should be advised if such drugs must be used (not including corticosteroids except in high dose).

6.89 WHAT ARE THE IMPLICATIONS FOR IUD-USERS OF ANATOMICAL LESIONS OF THE HEART?

This is WHO 3. It would definitely be preferable for such women to use another method – because of the increased risk of bacterial endocarditis. The main time of risk for this would be at insertion.

The fitting of an IUD should be avoided if there is a past history of endocarditis already, or of severe pelvic infection; or of cardiac surgery for the lesion if *prosthetic valve(s)* were fitted. Intravenous drug-abusers are also at higher risk of endocarditis if they have a relevant heart lesion.

If the method were selected at all the fitting should be done by an expert, under optimum sterile conditions, with antibiotic cover. Simple insertions with minor heart lesions may be given the minimal regimen of an oral sachet of amoxicillin 3 g, one hour before the procedure. Otherwise the more elaborate recommendations of the British National Formulary for 'special risk' cases should be followed, using intravenous ampicillin plus gentamycin.

Theoretically the LNG-IUS would be preferable to reduce subsequent infection risk (see Q 6.144). The patient would need to be warned even more carefully than other IUD-users to seek prompt medical advice should she develop pelvic pain, deep dyspareunia, or excessive discharge. Any of these might herald a focus of pelvic infection and risk of bacteraemia.

Antibiotic cover for *removal* would only be indicated if it was difficult, and especially if intrauterine instrumentation were to be required.

6.90 A PROPOS OF PROSTHETIC HEART VALVES IN THE LAST ANSWER: WHAT IF A WOMAN HAS ANY OTHER PROSTHESIS WHICH CAN BE PREJUDICED BY INFECTION, SUCH AS A HIP REPLACEMENT?

This in my view is in the WHO 2 category. An oral amoxycillin 3 g sachet one hour prior to the insertion should be more than sufficient cover, however.

6.91 WHAT ARE THE IMPLICATIONS OF DIABETES FOR A POTENTIAL IUD-USER?

It was suggested in a study from Edinburgh that diabetes rendered both inert and copper IUDs less effective. However, other workers, notably in Scandinavian countries, have completely failed to show this association.

More relevant is the fear that diabetes might make any pelvic *infection* more severe than it otherwise would be. However the IUD, or perhaps even better the LNG-IUS remains a valid option, particularly for diabetics at low risk of STDs.

6.92 MAY AN IUD BE USED BY A WOMAN WITH UTERINE FIBROIDS?

The answer is yes, provided the cavity of the uterus is not distorted by any submucous fibroid, and (as will normally follow) she does not suffer from menorrhagia. After careful bimanual examination, and the usual discussion about future fertility, etc., provisional arrangements may be made for the device to be inserted. The woman should be warned that plans may have to be changed if, early in the insertion procedure, the uterine sound detects an obvious submucous fibroid – as in Figure 6.7.

Where the facilities exist, a preinsertion ultrasound scan is crucial, requesting specifically that the uterine cavity be checked for distortion by submucous fibroids. If there is distortion, a GyneFIX™ can still be tried; or to control heavy periods and with warning about increased risk of expulsion and of malposition, the LNG-IUS is usable. (This is where an implantable version of the latter would be so useful.)

CHOICE OF DEVICE

6.93 HOW CAN ONE SELECT THE BEST IUD FOR EACH WOMAN?

Feet come in different sizes and shapes, and shoes therefore come in many different fittings. Even without recognized distortions of the uterine cavity (Fig 6.7), the sizes and shapes of uteruses similarly vary. There is no fixed relationship between total uterine length as measured with a standard uterine sound and uterine cavity length which can comprise as little as one-third of the total (Fig. 6.8). Maximum fundal width also varies between individuals, and is less in vivo than when measured on hysterectomy specimens. The living uterus is a muscular organ, which contracts and relaxes, and whose tonus also varies with the menstrual cycle (Fig. 6.9). Yet traditional framed IUDs come in constant shapes, and sizes which are often too large for the cavity in which they are to be placed.

In earlier editions I asked the manufacturers to produce a wider range of sizes for each design. But that approach has I think now been superseded by the implantable (frameless) technology of GyneFIX™

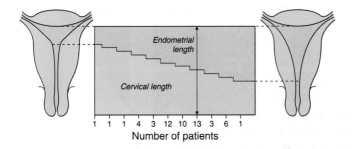

Figure 6.8 Measured endometrial and cervical lengths. Q 6.93. Eleven different combinations were noted in a series of 55 patients, all with the same total uterine axial dimension of 7 cm. (From Hasson H 1982 Uterine geometry and IUCD design. *British Journal of Obstetrics and Gynaecology* Supplement 4: 3, Figure 3)

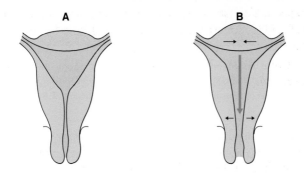

Figure 6.9 Functional changes in uterine shape. A, post-ovulation; B, at menstruation. Q 6.93. From Hasson H 1982 Uterine geometry and IUCD design. *British Journal of Obstetrics and Gynaecology* Supplement 4: 3, Figure 2)

Q 6.139). This must be more logical and I expect it to be applied increasingly, to hormone-releasing as well as to copper devices.

6.94 GIVEN THE RANGE OF IUDS AVAILABLE IN THE UK, WHAT IS YOUR NORMAL FIRST CHOICE (FIG. 6.8) FOR A PAROUS WOMAN?

The main framed devices available are shown in Figure 6.10. See Figure 6.10 and 6.12 for the GyneFIX™.

The Copper T-380: for most parous women I usually (1999) choose this. It is the 'gold standard' for copper IUDs, with one of the lowest cumulative

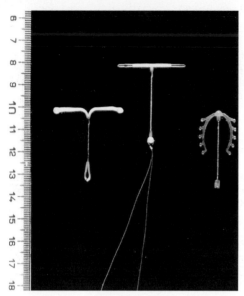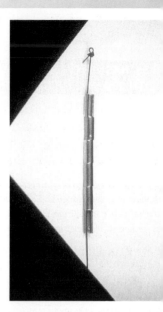

Figure 6.10 The main framed copper IUDs available in the UK (1999) – Nova T, Gyne T-380, Multiload and GyneFIX™. From Kubba A, Sanfilippo J & Hampton N (1999) *Contraception and Office Gynecology: Choices in Reproductive Healthcare.* pp 94–95. London: W.B. Saunders.

pregnancy rates so far reported (Q 6.10) and a UK-approved intra-uterine lifespan of 10 years (*FDA-approved* for 13 years!) – meaning a bargain price of around £1 per year.

The Nova-T has a narrower inserter tube but has the following serious disadvantages in comparison with the Copper T-380:

1 It has definitely a *higher pregnancy rate*, in most studies approaching 1–2/100 woman-years in the first year of use and cumulatively reaching 6 at 5 years – at least 4 times the rate of the copper-banded IUDs including the T-380 and the GyneFIX™ (see Q 6.10).

2 WHO studies suggest it is best *not* used for more than its approved 5 years life, by women under age 40.

3 The *ectopic pregnancy rate* is also much higher than that of the Copper T-380. This suggests it is less effective at blocking fertilization (see Q 6.30).

At MPC for years now our only indication (due to its smaller inserter tube) for the Nova T has been for emergency contraception when required by a nulliparous woman, but then only when it will be removed in the next cycle when the woman is established on another method. It is just not effective enough, even more so in the young.

6.95 HASN'T THE MANUFACTURER PRODUCED A NEW NOVA T WITH 380 mm² OF COPPER WIRE? WILL IT BE MORE EFFECTIVE?

Yes. The Nova-T 380 is more acceptable for use (at least to 5 years) than its predecessor. However I have not seen data showing that its effectiveness or its long-term reliability can quite match those of of the Cu T 380, either against intra- or extra-uterine pregnancy.

6.96 WHEN WOULD YOU RECOMMEND USE OF MULTILOAD IUDs?

Multiloads tend to cause greater cervical discomfort (at removal as well as insertion) and are not so enclosed in a sterile tube while traversing the (always) contaminated endocervical canal. Their efficacy is less than the Copper T 380, and even their expulsion rate does not (as used to be taught) show any comparative advantage in the WHO RCTs.

6.97 WHICH IUD DO YOU SELECT FOR THE NULLIPAROUS WOMAN?

- *If* the method is used at all, and this should be infrequently (see Q 6.86), the choice for long-term use among marketed IUDs still should normally be the *Copper T 380* if it can be fitted – using local anaesthesia and dilatation as required (see Q 6.110).
- The *GyneFIX™* (Q 6.139) with its small physical size (Q 6.61), narrower inserter, and low expulsion rate is also an excellent choice, above all for the tiny or distorted uterus. Its greater price is the main obstacle, so some services use it mainly for nulliparae who need a copper IUD for emergency contraception and then subsequently plan long-term use (the Nova T being cheaper for that-cycle-only use).
- The *LNG-IUS* (Q 6.148) is even more expensive and for the present (see Q 6.145) still has the problems of being on a frame rather than implanted. However some data do suggest it would reduce (not eliminate) the risk of PID, and hence could be a good choice especially if the nullipara has heavy or painful periods. The higher cost may sometimes justify a preliminary ultrasound scan to check first that the cavity is adequate.

The above devices all share the advantage of great efficacy, even in the highly fertile, against both intra- and extra-uterine pregnancies.

By contrast:

- The *Multiload Cu-250 Short* now has very little to commend it for nulliparae aside from price. It was indeed designed for such women with an ultrashort uterine cavity, but it has a small copper load and therefore relatively reduced efficacy compared with banded devices and is only licensed for 3 years' use.

6.98 WHICH DEVICE DO YOU CHOOSE FOR WOMEN WHO HAVE EXPELLED A PREVIOUS IUD?

The GyneFIX™, for obvious reasons (Q 6.139). But the same kind of device as just expelled may be used if it is otherwise the best choice (e.g. LNG–IUS) and there are reasons for believing there was less than ideal placement of the first IUD.

INSERTION PROCEDURE

6.99 WHAT IS THE IMPORTANCE OF CORRECT INSERTION?

This cannot be overstressed. A good 'revision test' is to check for yourself how it can be true that poor insertion technique is capable of producing every one of the eight IUD problems listed above (see Q 6.22).

6.100 WHEN SHOULD ONE PERFORM SO-CALLED INTERVAL INSERTIONS?

- *Copper IUDs, whether framed or frameless.* See Qs 6.15–6.17 for discussion of the optimum time in menstruating women, which is *any time* from around the *end* of the main menstrual flow through to day 14 of a 28-day cycle, normally. But this can be extended for copper IUDs to day 19 (adjusted for cycle length) even if contraception has been effectively non-existent up to that day, using it as a postcoital (anti-implantation) method.

  Thereafter, insertion could be even later if you are confident that there cannot already be an implanted pregnancy from intercourse earlier in the cycle, or up to 5 days after a single act of unprotected intercourse late in the cycle.
- *The levonorgestrel IUS* (see Q 6.143). In brief here, the speed with which this extremely effective method operates is not great enough within the first cycle for it to act as a postcoital method. Therefore in cycling

women it is recommended that insertion is performed within the first 7 days. If any later, there must be 'believable and really effective' contraception up to the day of insertion and condom use thereafter at least for the next 7 days.

6.101 WHEN SHOULD IUDs BE INSERTED FOLLOWING A FULL-TERM DELIVERY?

Postpartum, normal policy in this country is for IUD insertion to be delayed until the postnatal visit, i.e. at about 6 weeks. This is fine for lactating women, but if they are not breastfeeding, the woman will need to use another method of birth control from the fourth week onwards (see Q 4.40). Hence insertion during that fourth week by an experienced clinician may sometimes be contraceptively preferable, depending on the amount of lochia and satisfactory uterine involution (see Q 8.22).

Immediate postdelivery insertion with careful fundal placement, manually or using a spongeholder or ring forceps, and directly after delivery of the placenta, has been shown in several studies to have high (but in some circumstances acceptable) subsequent expulsion rates. The GyneFIX™ is under development for this indication, with a biodegradeable enhancement to its implanted knot (see Q 6.139). The offer of an IUD to a woman who is still in the delivery room may one day be a realistic possibility.

6.102 WHAT IS THE OPTIMUM INSERTION TIME AFTER LOWER SEGMENT CAESAREAN SECTION?

A Copper T 380 can be sutured to the fundus with chromic catgut, by way of the lower segment incision.

However, normal practice is to defer insertion at least to 6 weeks (some would say 8 weeks) to be sure of complete healing of the lower segment scar. Since after involution this potential weakness finishes up very low, at the level of the internal os, there would in fact be no objection to the insertion by an experienced, careful clinician at the same time as for other women (i.e. at about 6 weeks).

- Puerperal infection (with or without operative delivery) would of course indicate postponement – if indeed an IUD insertion were ever to be appropriate.

6.103 WHEN SHOULD IUDs BE INSERTED FOLLOWING ANY KIND OF ABORTION?

Careful studies have shown that immediate insertion at the time of evacuation of the uterus – whether for legal induced abortion, or following an incomplete miscarriage – can be good practice in selected cases. Surprisingly to many, no statistical differences with respect to subsequent infection were found in RCTs comparing two groups of women, one receiving and the other not receiving a framed copper IUD at the time of uterine evacuation in the same service.

The expulsion rate in the above studies was higher than for interval insertions. So the GyneFIX™ has been devised with a slightly larger polypropylene knot, to substantially reduce that risk. It is called the GyneFIX^PT

The studies were performed by experts. There is the fear that in less experienced hands a fragment of products of conception might be retained, and the insertion of a foreign body might then both facilitate infection and render such infection more severe.

In my view, therefore, insertion at the time of the evacuation could be good practice almost routinely in parous women, with:

- preliminary full counselling,
- preliminary microbiological screening (for *Chlamydia* anyway), *and*:
- antibiotic chemoprophylaxis (Q 6.60).

The same protocol could be followed for appropriate nulliparae too, especially using the GyneFIX^PT; but being prepared in cases of any doubt to postpone the insertion for 2–4 weeks.

6.104 DO YOU HAVE ANY PRACTICAL TIPS FOR IUD/IUS INSERTION IN AN OLDER PERIMENOPAUSAL WOMAN WHOSE CERVIX MAY BE TIGHT DESPITE PREVIOUS PARITY – DUE TO HYPO-OESTROGENISM?

This is a very real problem which we have faced at MPC during our (highly successful) studies of the LNG-IUS as the progestagen component of HRT. The solution, which can dramatically improve (soften) the cervix, is to give a good dose of standard HRT oestrogen for one month before the planned insertion, systemically or to the vagina. Vaginal misoprostol is another useful option, the night before. See Q 6.36(3) (and page 507).

6.105 WHAT ARE THE MINIMUM PRACTICAL REQUISITES?

1 A firm couch at a convenient height.
2 A good adjustable light.
3 Sterile equipment, ideally from a central sterile supply department:
   (a) bivalve speculum;
   (b) Stiles or Allis holding forceps, preferably *not* a toothed tenaculum, to reduce cervical pain;
   (c) sponge forceps;
   (d) uterine sound;
   (e) galley pot plus swabs for sterilizing solution;
   (f) scissors;
   (g) sterile gloves (If they are *not* sterile and a no-touch technique is planned, great care must be taken to maintain a 'sterile field' over one side of the trolley, ensuring the handle ends of all instruments which have been touched are systematically placed to the opposite side);
   (h) Spencer-Wells forceps.
4 In reserve:
   (a) local anaesthetic, needles and syringes;
   (b) small cervical dilators up to 6 mm diameter;
   (c) an emergency tray (see Q 6.118).
5 *An assistant* in the room – not necessarily a qualified person, but *someone* (to aid sterile technique and above all to reassure the patient).

6.106 WHAT ARE THE CHARACTERISTICS AND QUALITIES OF A GOOD IUD DOCTOR, WHATEVER THE DEVICES, WHEREVER INSERTED?

1 First and foremost, the clinician should be really well trained, which means excellent bimanual and speculum technique for a start, followed in the UK by the theoretical and practical training now organized by the Faculty of FP&RHC. This is in two stages, with after the basic Diploma a special advanced course leading to the Letter of Competence in intrauterine contraception techniques (including cervical local anaesthesia and the management of 'lost threads'). A separate additional training has been organized for GyneFIX™ since its insertion technique is so different – although not difficult when properly taught. This brief apprenticeship training with a good instructing doctor beats any amount of book learning (as for cap fitting, see Q 3.34).

2   Before attempting insertion in any patient, some initial practice with the same devices using a small plastic model and working through the manufacturer's instruction sheet is, in my view, *essential*. Such a 'dry run' should also never be omitted whenever a new device (e.g. GyneFIX™) or new inserter (e.g. recently for the Copper T 380 and LNG-IUS) arrives on the contraceptive scene.

3   Initial competence with any device should be *maintained* by continuing experience, and this cannot be by the insertion of only one device every 3 months.

4   During both examination and insertion, gentleness as well as competence should be the rule in all manoeuvres, especially when the sound or loaded inserter enter the uterine cavity. (Such gentleness is not the same as hesitancy or being excessively slow.)

5   Last but not least, the clinician should be a good communicator, able to use plenty of that 'aural valium' whose route of administration is the ears!

6.107 HOW DOES THE INSERTION PROCESS BEGIN?

Preferably by a good relationship developed during *earlier counselling* (see Q 6.119). The result of screening for STIs especially *Chlamydia* should be available. If not, there need to be good grounds for *not* giving chemoprophylaxis with e.g. doxycycline (Q 6.57).

1   First, make yourself known to the woman. Even a brief initial conversation helps, followed by a matter-of-fact and informative commentary throughout the insertion procedure.

2   Make it explicit that *she is in control, and that you are primarily her agent.* During the procedure give warning of any actions which might cause discomfort, e.g. the needle for paracervical block or the application of the Allis or Stiles forceps (*not*, without LA, a toothed tenaculum) to the anterior lip of the cervix.

6.108 HOW IMPORTANT IS THE INITIAL BIMANUAL EXAMINATION (BME)?

This is essential. It has two main purposes:

1   First, to ensure that there is *no uterine or adnexal tenderness* especially on moving the cervix. (Check verbally that there is also no dyspareunia.) Positive findings mean that the insertion should be postponed.

2   The second essential purpose is to identify the size, shape, mobility and *direction and position* of the fundus.

6.109 WHICH IS THE BEST POSITION FOR THE PATIENT TO ADOPT DURING THE INSERTION?

Most insertions in the UK are performed with the patient in the dorsal position. Sometimes it radically improves access to use the left lateral position, which after all is equivalent to lithotomy rotated through 90°. This is of particular value if the cervical canal is very flexed and the cervix points directly either anterior or posterior.

The left lateral does lead to loss of eye contact with the woman, which must be replaced by better-than-average verbal communication.

6.110 WHAT ARE THE INDICATIONS FOR PREINSERTION ANALGESIA OR LOCAL ANAESTHESIA (LA)?

Most parous women questioned after an uncomplicated IUD insertion without LA reckon that the needle would have caused more discomfort than it would have removed. However, that is often *not* the view of the *nulliparous*.

At the MPC it is the norm that *all women* are *offered* premedication with a PGSI, normally mefenamic acid 500 mg, half an hour to an hour before the procedure (checking first for contraindications). If they are unusually anxious a short-acting benzodiazepine may be added.

A sizeable proportion, especially of nulliparae, are also helped by a *paracervical block* (about 10 ml of 1% lidocaine injected under the skin of the cervix, first at 12 o'clock intracervically, and then laterally at about 3–4 o'clock and 8–9 o'clock, injecting deep so each dose reaches the level of the internal cervical os.)

After training, this is not a difficult nor time-consuming addition to the procedure.

Another possible and 'non-needle' option is 2% lidocaine antiseptic gel, which usefully also contains 0.25% chlorhexidine. Sufficient (no more than 1.5 ml) of this 'Instillagel' is injected via a special quill to just fill the cervical canal up to the internal os, but there must then be a minimum wait for it to act. A significant benefit was shown in a small trial in 1996 in Leeds after waiting only one minute before passing the sound: we would prefer to wait at least 3 minutes.

6.111 SHOULD TISSUE FORCEPS BE APPLIED TO THE CERVIX, AND SHOULD THE UTERUS BE SOUNDED?

Normally yes: Stiles or Allis forceps cause minimal discomfort, reduced to nil if a little LA is injected at 12 o'clock. X-ray studies have proved that gentle traction straightens the canal and very much assists in passing the sound. The latter is also essential:

1 to confirm the direction and patency of the cervical canal;
2 to estimate the length of the uterine cavity (see Q 6.93);
3 to exclude obvious intrusion of any submucous fibroid or uterine septum. *This should be done in all insertions by gently rotating the handle of the sound through a small arc.*

The sound should be passed with minimal force, rested between the finger and thumb like a loosely held pencil. Note that the anatomy of the cervical canal is variable. Be prepared to repeat the BME, or to withdraw and reinsert the sound if it does not pass readily OR move on to using dilators (Hegar 3–6 should be available).

6.112 WHAT ABOUT ANTISEPSIS?

This is much less important than pre-screening for specific pathogens and, as appropriate, antibiotic cover, see Q 6.56–57. Remember that the flora of the endocervical canal is almost identical to that of the vagina.

All the same, the cervix should be first carefully inspected and, if there is a purulent discharge, swabs (re-)taken (or the patient referred), and the insertion postponed. Otherwise the cervix should be thoroughly cleansed with a gauze swab usually dipped in aqueous antiseptic, concentrating on mechanical removal of any mucus at the external os.

6.113 WHAT OTHER PRACTICAL POINTS SHOULD BE CONSIDERED?

1 Only at the last minute, and after satisfactory sounding, should the device be loaded into its inserter, for fear that it should lose its 'memory'

2 Some devices (e.g. Multiloads) are primarily pushed into the uterus; most are inserted by a 'pull' technique in which the plunger is kept stationary and the inserter tube pulled back over it.

3 We all have a sensible paranoia about perforation, but this leads to a tendency for the Copper T 380, or the LNG-IUS (or Nova T) to be inserted rather low, risking expulsion – or even implantation above the device. I teach that after the side arms of the above-mentioned devices have been released, you have an object which is most unlikely to perforate. Therefore, at that point in the insertion sequence after the arms have just been released from the top of the inserter tube, the latter should be gently advanced towards the fundus. This may mean allowing the cervical stop to be pushed (caudally) by the external os, until the very top of the cavity is reached – always looking at the woman's face so as to be sufficiently gentle throughout.

It has surprised me how often I have found that my initial estimate of the fundal depth was a centimetre or more less than the measurement from tip of tube to stop after this has been done.

4 Take care that the device finishes in the *right plane*, by observing the marker wings on the inserter, as well as in the correct high fundal position. If in doubt the device should be removed and a new one inserted.

GyneFIX™ has a very specific technique which must be taught with the help of the manufacturer's video, polystyrene models and then supervised insertions.

6.114 WHAT ABOUT THE PREVENTION OF THE RARE IUD INSERTION 'CRISES'? ○

1 First, so far as possible, they should be *prevented* by the presence of an assistant, a calm and relaxed atmosphere, combined with obvious competence and teamwork.

2 During the insertion, gentleness and accuracy while passing both sound and loaded inserter along the cervical canal reduce the incidence of vasovagal reactions.

3 Above all, starting at an earlier stage, good counselling and selection of cases, combined with a low threshold for premedication with an analgesic and perhaps a sedative, with or without paracervical block during the insertion; these are the essential prophylactic measures.

6.115 WHAT IF A VASOVAGAL ATTACK FOLLOWS DESPITE EVERY PRECAUTION?

The patient becomes white and may sweat with a slow pulse. Rarely is there no warning – be alert!

1 The first thing to do is to abandon the procedure, stop any cervical stimulation, and remove a partially inserted device (but *not* one that is well placed).
2 The woman's head should be lowered or her feet elevated and, if available, an airway inserted.
    All this takes a bit of time and occupies anxious bystanders, which is excellent because the majority of attacks are self-limiting.
3 At this point, 500 mg of mefenamic acid should be given, if not used as a premed. A non-PGSI such as dihydrocodeine can always be added.

6.116 WHAT SHOULD BE DONE IF THE WOMAN CONTINUES TO SUFFER SEVERE DYSMENORRHOEIC PAINS?

I have no experience of the use of glyceryl trinitrate either sublingually or as a vaginal spray for severe uterine cramps, but it is said this may help (and also as a premedication).

If the woman continues in severe pain with pallor for 30 minutes after the insertion, in my view even a fully inserted device should be removed. The chances of long-term successful use of the IUD/IUS in this situation are too low. If ultrasound scanning were routinely done (see Q 6.93), most such cases would be explained by malposition or because of an unexpectedly small or even distorted uterine cavity. In an occasional case one might also be avoiding the later problems of an incipient perforation.

A subsequent attempt with local anaesthesia, an expert practitioner, and now most commonly using the GyneFIX™ may be successful. Consider also using preliminary exogenous oestrogen to soften the cervix or misoprostol (see Q 6.36(3)).

6.117 WHAT UNUSUAL COMPLICATIONS OF IUD INSERTION MAY OCCUR?

1 *Persistent bradycardia.* If the pulse is persistently less than 40 beats/minute, the slow intravenous injection of atropine 0.6 mg may help. If the

pulse is absent and the patient unresponsive a vigorous thump to the praecordium is more than most clinicians will be called upon to do in a lifetime of inserting IUDs. (Though any competent doctor or nurse ought also to be prepared to initiate cardiopulmonary resuscitation).

Beware of vomiting and the risk of inhalation of fluid when consciousness returns.

2 *Asthmatic attack, laryngeal oedema* or other allergic reaction. Treat urgently with 0.5–1 mg (contained in up to 1 ml) of epinephrine 1: 1000, **intramuscularly**.

3 *Grand mal attack.* This may occur even in the absence of any history of epilepsy or the subsequent development thereof. It is usually self-limiting. Diazepam should be available. A good presentation for this situation is Stesolid rectal tubes; one 10-mg dose is administered rectally, repeatable once if there is no response after 5 minutes.

Epilepsy needs to be distinguished from:

4 *Alkalosis* due to overbreathing, causing paraesthesia and carpopedal spasms. Treatment is by reassurance, and instruction in (supervised) breathing in and out of a plastic bag.

6.118 IN SUMMARY, WHAT SHOULD BE AVAILABLE IN THE EMERGENCY TRAY?

1 A well-fitting facemask and separate Guedal airways.
2 Diazepam 10 mg either for rectal (Stesolid tubes) or intravenous injection.
3 Atropine 0.6 mg for intravenous injection.
4 Epinephrine 1 ml of 1 : 1000 for intramuscular injection.
5 Mefenamic acid oral tablets – dose 500 mg.
6 Dihydrocodeine tablets – dose 30 mg.
7 Short-acting benzodiazepine tablets (temazepam 20 mg) for premedication.
8 Syringes, needles, etc. as appropriate.

NOTE: This is all that is required, and most will never be used.

PATIENT INFORMATION AND FOLLOW-UP ARRANGEMENTS

6.119 WHAT MAIN POINTS SHOULD BE MADE IN ADVANCE, WHEN COUNSELLING ANY PROSPECTIVE IUD USER?

As usual, a balance has to be struck between creating unnecessary fears which may impair the woman's acceptance and satisfaction with the method, and the need to help her reach an informed and valid decision based on the likely benefits and risks for herself. During counselling, often rightly delegated to the family planning-trained nurse:

1 Mention first the many *advantages* of the method (see Q 6.19). Let her see and ideally handle the device she is to receive.
2 The possibility of failure including after unrecognized expulsion should be mentioned, though this is now much less of a problem if we use either of the banded copper IUDs, or the IUS (Q 6.143).
3 Attention should be drawn to *pelvic infection* and *ectopic pregnancy*. Explain how both are linked with sexual transmission of infections. Elicit a careful history of past PID or treatments at a genitourinary medicine clinic. Under age 30, early (under 16) coitarche has been shown to be an excellent surrogate measure for having multiple partners. But there is more to a proper sexual history (Q 0.13–14).

Embarrassment should not stop plain good medicine, which is to go on to say something like:

You know better than I can possibly know, what your likely risk of (sexually transmitted) infection might be. This depends mainly on you and also your partner: stop and think, might he be other than a completely one-girl man?

Stress also the importance of returning promptly to the clinic should relevant symptoms occur (see Qs 6.23 and 6.122).

4 Arrange at least a *Chlamydia* screen if at all possible, and usually antibiotic cover if no result is available (emergency contraception) – see earlier discussion (Qs 6.56–6.57).
5 In my view it should also be pointed out that some discomfort is common during insertion, helped by the use of premedication – with added local anaesthetic perhaps, taking account of the woman's own views about needles.

6 Problems like perforation are rare but should be mentioned with the aid of the leaflet (see 7). Honest and accurate answers should be given to all questions (see Q 4.100).

7 Finally, counselling should be backed up by a user-friendly leaflet, such as the *Choosing and Using* one from the Family Planning Association, '*to be read now before the insertion, but also for you to keep for future reference*'.

6.120 WHAT INSTRUCTIONS SHOULD BE GIVEN TO THE WOMAN AFTER IUD INSERTION?

1 She may be reminded that the method is effective immediately.

2 She should also be reminded/encouraged that if she is ever in future not in a very stable relationship, she should use a barrier (preferably condom) as well (see Q 6.18), thereby reducing both the risk of failure and of infection.

3 She should be carefully instructed in the palpation of her cervical threads, and advised that this check should be done post-menstruation in each cycle before the device is relied on. See Qs 3.44 and 6.171, for some practical points about cervical palpation. If she becomes unable to feel the threads, or palpates the hard end of the device, she should be told to take additional contraceptive precautions and arrange an early examination.

4 Since sperm can be biovectors of STI pathogens and the process of IUD/IUS insertion interferes with protective mechanisms at the cervix (Qs 6.54–6.55) it is now MPC policy to recommend abstinence (or condom use) for the next 3 days.

5 Tampon use is also discouraged for 3 days, hopefully allowing enough time for the cervical barrier to be reconstituted.

6 *Important*: before leaving after the insertion she should be given instructions, preferably backed by a handout, concerning those symptoms which should lead her to contact the clinic/surgery immediately, during the critical next 2–3 weeks (see Q 6.58).

7 If she has neither been pre-screened for at least *Chlamydia* nor is being given antibiotic prophylaxis then it may be safer to arrange a follow-up visit at about 1 week (see Qs 6.52 and 6.121)

Longer term, each IUD-user should be encouraged to report and as appropriate return promptly at any time should any relevant symptom develop – see Q 6.122.

6.121 WHEN AND FOR WHAT PURPOSE SHOULD THE FIRST FOLLOW-UP VISIT TAKE PLACE?

About 6 weeks after the insertion is usual, on a date planned to be after the first expected menses, so as to exclude (partial) expulsion.

However the important data discussed at Q 64 suggest that making the first visit routinely at about 1 week would be preferable, certainly if steps have not been taken to ensure 'a Chinese cervix'! However if they were, the woman should be advised (see Q 6.120 above) to attend as an emergency for examination if she has *pain* or other symptoms which might be PID-related during the first 20 days. Infections are so much (six times) commoner in this post-insertion phase, that this protocol should permit more prompt, possibly tube-saving, antibiotic treatment.

At the routine 6-week visit the woman should be asked about all relevant symptoms (Q 6.107). She should be asked whether she can feel her threads, and retaught as indicated.

On speculum examination the threads should be seen. As a general rule, in my view, but especially if the threads have apparently lengthened, the *lower* cervical canal should be sounded. This can be done with a sterile sound, or very simply using the omnipresent throat swab or even a Cytobrush (not advanced higher than the internal os). In this way partial expulsion of a framed IUD may be detected and the device replaced before an avoidable intrauterine pregnancy occurs. A bimanual examination should also be done to detect tenderness and adnexal or uterine enlargement.

6.122 HOW FREQUENTLY SHOULD SUBSEQUENT VISITS TAKE PLACE?

If the first visit is at 1 week, another at about 6–8 weeks is still logical, since expulsions are commonest in the early months of use. Thereafter, in women without symptoms an annual routine visit is quite sufficient.

1   More important than any routine pelvic examination is *an IUD programme which makes it really easy for a user to obtain medical advice and help at once should a new problem occur*: notably an attack of pelvic infection or an ectopic pregnancy or 'lost threads'. *She should therefore be fully taught with a leaflet about all the symptoms which require prompt action (Q 6.119) and know where to obtain telephone advice (e.g. from the Advice Sister at MPC).*

2 Iron deficiency anaemia is very easy to miss in long-term users with heavy bleeding. This should be excluded or treated if present.

6.123 ARE IUDs ALWAYS EASY TO REMOVE BY SIMPLE TRACTION ON THE THREAD(S)?

Not if the threads are missing (see Q 6.36). But even without that problem the device may be malpositioned or embedded, or there may be a type of partial cervical perforation (Fig. 6.11). In such cases it may sometimes be possible under local anaesthesia to grasp the devices and push it in a cranial direction to disimpact it first. Excessive traction at removal must always be avoided especially under general anaesthesia, for the reason noted at Q 6.47.

GyneFIX™ is removed by simple firm traction, with a pull which has been measured to be no greater than required to remove a Multiload IUD, and causes minimal discomfort.

6.124 DO YOU HAVE ANY TIPS FOR REMOVAL OF IUDs WHICH ARE A BIT STUCK AFTER THE MENOPAUSE? MUST THEY ALWAYS BE REMOVED AT ALL?

This is mainly a problem when removing inert IUDs or Multiloads, 1 year after the last period. A solution is to prescribe natural oestrogen, e.g. one cycle of Premarin 1.25 mg daily beforehand. This will soften the cervical canal. Mefenamic acid 500 mg as a premed also helps. See Q 6.36(3).

A   B

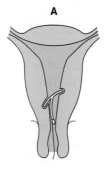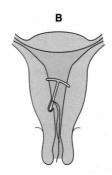

Figure 6.11   Two varieties of partial cervical perforation. Q 6.123. Both of these could cause difficulty in removal. Both are best treated under appropriate anaesthesia by grasping the end of the device, and pushing in a cranial direction before traction.

It is actually a matter of debate whether devices which are very 'stuck' (with or without avulsion of the threads) do necessarily have to be removed, after the menopause or after endometrial ablation. The postulated risk of a pyometrium is small and can be dealt with in the individual case. I would, personally, not now feel the risks of a general anaesthetic were justified for removal of an IUD postmenopausally, and would simply warn the woman to seek advice at any time later if she were to develop an offensive discharge.

6.125 ARE IUDs A GENUINE CAUSE OF MALE DYSPAREUNIA?

Certainly; above all if a framed device is partially expelled so that its end just protrudes from the external cervical os! More commonly, some men notice the threads of the device.

If this problem is not resolved by slightly altering positions of intercourse, the threads should be trimmed – but not to within a few millimetres of the os. This can actually worsen the situation. ... Rather, if necessary, they should be shortened to lie wholly within the cervical canal. Ensure that this is noted in the records and that the woman will report the fact to any future doctor. Long-handled Spencer-Wells forceps should easily retrieve the threads when removal is required.

6.126 IS SHORT-WAVE DIATHERMY TREATMENT CONTRAINDICATED IN IUD-USERS?

This treatment is now rarely given to patients with chronic pelvic pain, in whom removal of the device would normally first be tried. However, if there is an IUD present there is certainly a theoretical possibility that the copper wire might heat up. Experiments with devices in recently excised hysterectomy specimens have shown no obvious damage or charring to the endometrium, and the devices have merely become pleasantly warm. So this treatment is relatively contraindicated (WHO 2).

6.127 ARE MODERN METHODS OF IMAGING DANGEROUS FOR THE IUD-WEARER, SPECIFICALLY NUCLEAR MAGNETIC RESONANCE (NMR)?

Ultrasound is harmless, X-rays have no added risk, and provided the device is non-ferrous NMR would cause no problems. However, with steel devices (e.g. the M-device and Chinese rings) there would be truly be a potential hazard of internal trauma, caused by movement of the ferrous metal caused by the magnetic field.

6.128 ARE IUDs CONTAINING COPPER AFFECTED BY ANY VAGINAL PREPARATIONS?

There is no clear evidence that material from the vagina reaches the copper or affects the biochemical processes which cause the contraceptive effect (see Q 6.5).

DURATION OF USE

6.129 DO THE WHITE DEPOSITS ON IUDs REMOVED AFTER VARYING DURATIONS WITHIN THE UTERUS HAVE ANY CLINICAL SIGNIFICANCE, PARTICULARLY IN COPPER IUD-USERS?

These deposits have been studied intensively. They contain organic material along with calcium, sulphur and phosphorus and other inorganic elements. They are not now thought to be linked with IUD failure. Many women's devices never develop this deposit. When present, if the IUD is copper bearing it seems that sufficient copper can pass through the deposit to continue the contraceptive effect. It is not an important factor in the rate of copper elution (see Q 6.131).

The explanation for failure of modern IUDs which are so effective when correctly located is, nearly always, less than ideal placement within the uterine cavity (see Qs 6.11 and 6.12).

6.130 HOW OFTEN SHOULD INERT IUDs BE REPLACED?

In the few women who still retain these: except for Dalkon shields without special cause they should never be routinely replaced. Possible causes include ALOs (Qs 6.70–6.74).

6.131 HOW OFTEN SHOULD COPPER IUDs BE REPLACED?

All the marketed devices have an officially approved duration, normally 3, 5 or 10 years. The reason for any limit is anxiety that the amount of copper available for release from the device might decline to a level at which the pregnancy rate would increase. Yet the recommended banded copper IUDs show a decline in the annual conception risk for as long as they have been studied.

With copper *wire* IUDs such as the Nova T the annual risk is about the same and may even go up after 5 years in women under 40. Hence the advice below (Q 6.134).

6.132 WHAT ARE THE BENEFITS OF LONG-TERM USE OF IUDs?

Long-term studies (especially the WHO study) have repeatedly shown a steady reduction with increasing duration of use in:

1   pregnancy rates (not Nova T, see Figure 6.2 and Q 6.131);
2   expulsion rates;
3   infection rates (overall);
4   bleeding/pain removal rates.

Exceptions which show a positive link with duration of use are carriage of ALOs (see Qs 6.70–6.74) and ectopic pregnancy (see Q 6.29) – but the latter association is probably confounded by increasing age.

6.133 WHAT ARE THE EXPLANATIONS FOR THE APPARENT IMPROVEMENT WITH DURATION OF USE OF IUDs IN THE RISKS OF PREGNANCY, EXPULSION, INFECTION, AND REMOVAL FOR BLEEDING OR PAIN?

It is too simple to interpret this as a genuine improvement due to the device 'bedding down'. The main point is that the long-term population of IUD-users is highly selected, and in all studies is only a small proportion of those who originally had devices inserted. They are the 'survivors', so to speak. Their success in long-term use has less to do with the passage of time as such, than with selection for features of the individual women themselves as compared with others earlier in the study:

1   They are likely to have been well fitted with an IUD, which was well matched to the particular shape and size of their uterus.
2   They are obviously well distanced in time from insertion-related expulsion, infection and bleeding/pain.
3   *Much the most important factor*: the women with any side-effects or complications severe enough to have their device removed are by definition no longer in the study. For example, the most fertile become pregnant within the first year and have their devices removed, hence the reported pregnancy rates in later years are based on observation of a subgroup of the relatively infertile. Similarly those whose partners are

less likely to transmit a sexually transmitted infection to them are over-represented among long-term users.

4 They are also a little older – see Qs 6.23 and 6.52.

6.134 WHAT THEREFORE IS THE VIEW OF THE UK-FPA AND THE NATIONAL ASSOCIATION OF FAMILY PLANNING DOCTORS (NOW THE FACULTY OF FP&RHC) REGARDING LONG-TERM USE OF COPPER IUDs?

A statement published in *The Lancet* on 2 June 1990 remains substantially in force, except that the Copper T 380 is now fully approved for twice the 5 years mentioned:

> *For routine management the modern copper-bearing IUDs ... should be assumed to have an active lifespan of 5 years. ... Beyond that interval, an experienced doctor or nurse should discuss with the client the option of changing the IUD or leaving it in (it is wise to record this discussion in the notes).*

NOTE: Basically, 'if it ain't broke, don't fix it'. But there is one thing specifically to record, that no promise was made that the device could not possibly fail; only that the failure rate is believed to be no higher than during the preceding years of successful use.

6.135 DO YOU STILL FOLLOW THE NAFPD STATEMENT FOR OLDER, COPPER WIRE IUDs? AND WHAT ABOUT THE LNG-IUS (MIRENA)?

In a word, NO. Studies in Manchester showed that standard (200 mm) copper wire devices begin to lose copper at an accelerated (and linear) rate from an average of 27 months onwards. The rate of copper release was greater than average if the women complained of heavy uterine bleeding. After 4 years' use 28% of removed IUDs show fragmentation of the wire. Silver in the core of the Nova-T wire prevents that occurrence but would not otherwise reduce the rate of copper release. Indeed it might even eventually increase it when silver becomes exposed, by a 'battery effect'.

Clinical studies correlate well with this laboratory work. A review of all the studies of copper wire IUDs *including the Nova-T* suggests that use beyond about 5 years might start to raise the pregnancy risk above the low rate which that (by now highly selected) woman should have. But this is not true of the copper-banded devices, whose upper duration limit is not known but certainly exceeds 10 years (see Q 6.10).

In the light of all this, most authorities would rarely apply the NAFPD *Lancet* advice in the case of young women under age 40, to use of copper *wire* IUDs beyond 5 years. This is because exchange to a more effective banded IUD (Copper T 380, or as appropriate the GyneFIX™) would be preferable.

The LNG-IUS should not normally be left in situ beyond its licensed 5 years, even above age 40, see Q 6.136. After about 7 years the woman will have, effectively, an 'inert' IUD. This is possibly acceptable for contraception from age 47 (WHO 3), but never as part of HRT (Q 6.149).

6.136 WHAT ABOUT COPPER DEVICES WHICH WERE FITTED ABOVE AGE 40?

In a supplementary letter, it was also stated in the *Lancet* 1990 by the Chairman of NAFPD that *any copper device* (even one of the non-banded ones) *which was fitted above age 40 may remain in situ until the menopause* (or until 1 year after for contraceptive safety, see Q 8.34). This is acceptable because with diminishing fertility IUDs so very rarely fail above 40.

The *Lancet* statement, like the later WHO report (see Q 6.64), points out that less frequent replacement would have enormous health advantages, in reducing the insertion-related risk:

- PID (the main time it ever happens!),
- perforation (the only time it ever happens)
- expulsion and
- malposition; not to mention
- inconvenience, pain, upset and costs for the woman!

However for many IUDs and the IUS this policy of long-term use is still unlicensed, so the criteria for Named Patient usage must be observed (page 507).

6.137 HOW REVERSIBLE IS IUD CONTRACEPTION?

Completely, or very nearly so. All prospective studies of the return of fertility after elective removal of IUDs have shown that the subsequent conception rates are indistinguishable from those to be expected in that population. The Oxford/FPA study found that within 2 years 92% had given birth, a similar delivery rate to the ex-diaphragm users.

Clearly, the women whose fertility might be impaired by IUD use are more likely to be those who drop out because of medical complications such as ectopic pregnancy or pelvic infection. Two American case-control studies reported in 1985 that past IUD use was significantly commoner in primary tubal infertility cases than in controls. The effect was less for copper-bearing IUDs and not significant if monogamy was reported. But so far there has been no successful prospective study following up a total (large) population of IUD-users and taking account of removals for medical reasons as well as for intention to conceive.

For the vast majority of acceptors the IUD is a fully reversible method of contraception. Among those who suffer tubal infertility due to PID or ectopic pregnancy, the prime responsibility does not lie at the door of the IUD itself (see Q 6.29). The frequency of this catastrophic outcome can be minimized by careful selection (see Qs 6.83–6.86); careful IUD insertion (see Qs 6.107–6.113), with screening and consideration of antibiotic cover; and the rigorous follow-up of fully informed women.

6.138 ARE THERE ANY SPECIAL CONSIDERATIONS IF A WOMAN WANTS TO CONCEIVE AFTER USING A COPPER IUD?

- It is usually advised that she uses condoms until after the first spontaneous period, to clear the endometrium of copper or levonorgestrel: though there are no data to support or refute that suggestion.
- See Q 6.25 for the implications of *in situ* failure of copper IUDs, and Q 6.145 for the LNG-IUS.
  Given the increased likelihood that IUD-users may have bacterial vaginosis, and the data that this may increase the risk of amnionitis and premature rupture of the membranes: it may be worth at least considering excluding that diagnosis (and treating as appropriate) before IUDs are removed electively to conceive.

GYNEFIX™ AND THE LEVONORGESTREL–IUS

6.139 WHAT IS GYNEFIX™ (FIG. 6.12), AND HOW IS IT INSERTED?

This unique frameless device is the result of some good lateral thinking by Dirk Wildemeersch of Belgium. It is simply a single monofilament polypropylene thread which dangles in the uterine fundus, bearing six copper bands similar to those on the Copper T-380 (Fig. 6.12). A small anchoring loop and knot at the fundal end are inserted a measured distance

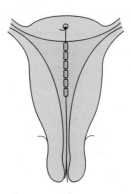

Figure 6.12 The GyneFIX™ IUD *in situ*.

of 9–10 mm into the myometrium by a special stylet, passed through the inserter tube which is first pressed firmly against the fundus.

Special training is vital for safe insertion of this IUD and is available, through the Faculty of FP&RHC (Q 6.114).

It is licensed for 5 years, though this duration is likely to increase as more data are obtained, since it is a banded copper IUD.

6.140 HOW DOES GYNEFIX™ COMPARE WITH THE GOLD STANDARD, THE COPPER T 380?

Initial results are very promising. In short, it seems to be about as good in most respects and better in some:

- Its main advantage after a 'learning curve' for the practitioners is a *lower expulsion rate* (only 0.4% in the first year when inserted by experts).
- *Insertion*, after one sharp sensation as it is implanted, causes appreciably less dysmenorrhoea pain thereafter;
- It *cannot cause uterine pain of mechanical origin from a frame*, since it has no frame. So far there is not RCT proof of this advantage, however:
- Once correctly inserted, *partial expulsion* is almost impossible
- Movement of the device in the uterus to produce *malpositioning* (which is also one cause of lost threads) is also less likely than with a framed IUD.

With regard to *efficacy* when in situ, I expect it to be similar (no good comparative data). The overall efficacy in a population will depend on how many unrecognized expulsions occur (probably fewer of them with GyneFIX™, but there is evidence that they are more easily overlooked when they happen, leaving the woman exposed).

No difference in the rate of *bleeding problems* or *pelvic infection* has yet been established in a large enough RCT. The smaller foreign body might be advantageous for the quantity of bleeding if not its duration (Q 6.78) and maybe for the severity of any infections (Q 6.61) – but we await good data. In the initial European study infections were very rare and there have so far been no ectopics. But all this information is difficult to interpret since it may depend on recruitment of an unusually low-risk population plus unusually high expertise in the research doctors. ...

6.141 WHAT ARE THE LIKELY OR KNOWN PROBLEMS WITH GYNEFIX™?

- *Perforation* is always possible with IUDs and this one has a sharp stylet within a quite narrow firm tube. The rate is unknown but unlikely to be lower than the 1:1000 rate usually quoted for framed IUDs – and it *could* be much higher in the hands of inadequately trained or inexperienced personnel.
- there was no evidence in a very preliminary study of either implantation *endometriosis* or of more than an extremely localized inflammatory reaction at the site of the anchoring knot.

6.142 SO WHAT ARE THE INDICATIONS TO USE GYNEFIX™?

These will relate partly to its cost, which is more than twice that of the Copper T 380, which is also licensed for longer, and on whether its expected benefits above are fully realised. For the time being at the MPC and related services we use it primarily for:

Women at known increased risk of expulsion (past history).
Women with a past history of excessive pain during attempted use of a framed copper IUD (either immediately or in early months of use).
Women with a distorted uterine cavity or sounding to a depth less than 5.5 cm (in whom any framed IUD would be contraindicated).
Selected nulliparae with light or normal periods, not specially indicating use of the LNG-IUS.
Immediate insertion after therapeutic abortion (GyneFIX^PT version with a larger knot).

6 We are also undertaking an RCT to establish whether it may prove to be the most appropriate copper IUD for emergency use, especially if followed by continuing use.

6.143 WHAT IS THE LEVONORGESTREL IUS/LNG-IUS (MIRENA – ALSO KNOWN AS LEVO NOVA)?

This Nova-T shaped device is shown in Figure 6.13. It releases 20 μg/ 24 hours of levonorgestrel (LNG) from its polydimethylsiloxane reservoir through a rate-limiting membrane, over at least 5 years (though initially licensed in the UK for just 3 years).

Its main contraceptive effects are local, by endometrial suppression and changes to the cervical mucus and utero-tubal fluid which impair sperm migration. The blood levels of LNG are about one quarter of the peak levels in users of the POP, and so ovarian function is altered less. Most women continue to ovulate and in the remainder sufficient oestrogen is produced from the ovary even if they become amenorrhoeic as many do: this is primarily a local end-organ effect.

6.144 WHAT ARE THE ADVANTAGES OF THE LNG-IUS?

1 It has unsurpassed efficacy, around 0.2 per 100 woman-years.
2 Return of fertility is rapid and appears to be complete.
3 It is highly convenient, has few adverse side effects and some beneficial effects on the menstrual cycle.

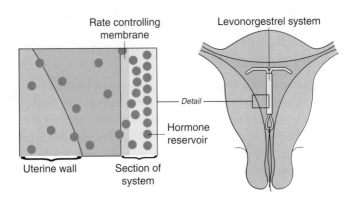

Figure 6.13 The levonorgestrel intrauterine system (LNG-IUS). Q 6.143

It is in short a contraceptive in which the 'default state' is one of contraception, unlike pills and condoms where the default state is the reverse, conception!

The above advantages are of course shared with the Cu T 380, which is the best current copper IUD. However that is where the similarity ends. It fundamentally 'rewrites the textbooks' about IUDs, so that it really deserves a different category of its own (hence 'IUS' for intrauterine system not IUD).

The user of this device can expect a dramatic reduction in amount and, after the first few months (discussed below), in duration of blood loss. Dysmenorrhoea is also generally improved.

The LNG-IUS is now the contraceptive method of choice for most women with heavy menses. It shows promise as a first-line treatment for this problem, and is indeed licensed for this in any woman who needs or may one day need contraception. (Only if she is herself sterilized would use of this IUS for 'menorrhagia' have to be on a 'named patient basis'). It can also provide progestogenic protection of the uterus during oestrogen replacement therapy by any chosen route. For this use the 'named Patient' criteria do need to be fulfilled (page 507).

Though not yet proven in an RCT, the LNG-IUS may reduce the frequency of clinical PID, particularly in the youngest age groups who are most at risk. This should make it possible to offer the device to some young women requesting a default state contraceptive who would not be good candidates for conventional copper IUDs. (ALOs may still be reported, see Qs 6.73–6.74 for management.)

The data on file and published for this device show a definite reduction in the risk of extra- as well as intra-uterine pregnancy, which can be attributed to its greater efficacy by mechanisms which reduce the risk of pregnancy in any site.

6.145 WHAT ARE THE DISADVANTAGES OF THE LNG-IUS?

It has the same risk of *expulsion* and of *perforation* and *malpositioning* as the Nova T, since it uses the same design. It has in short all the disadvantages of a frame, which are minimized with GyneFIX™ (and I am lobbying the manufacturers for some form of hybrid using the same anchoring technique, as soon as can be!)

A more important problem is the *high incidence in the first post-insertion months of uterine bleeding, which though small in quantity may be very frequent or continuous* and can cause considerable inconvenience. This usually settles to a very acceptable light monthly loss, but can take 3–6 months to do so.

- Later in the use of the method amenorrhoea is very commonly reported.

For both of these effects, particularly the first, 'forewarned is forearmed': implying good counselling in advance of the fitting of Mirena. In my experience, women can accept the early weeks of frequent light bleeding as a worthwhile price to pay for all the other advantages of the method, if they are well informed in advance, and coached and encouraged as appropriate while it is occurring. The amenorrhoea can even be explained and interpreted to a woman as a positive advantage of the method, rather than an adverse side-effect.

- Women should also be advised that though this method is mainly local in its action it is not exclusively so: it is a hormonal method. Therefore there is a small incidence of steroidal side-effects such as bloatedness, acne and depression. Blood levels are higher in the first 2 months than later, and women can be informed that the symptoms usually resolve over that time.
- Functional ovarian cysts are also more common, but are usually asymptomatic and if not they should be monitored as they usually resolve spontaneously.
- In the extremely rare event of in situ failure of the LNG-IUS, if the system were not removed well before organogenesis there is real uncertainty that the fetus would not be harmed by the high local concentration of levonorgestrel. There are no data.

6.146 WHAT ARE THE CONTRAINDICATIONS TO THE LNG-IUS?

There are very few absolute contraindications:

1 Allergy to a constituent.
2 Suspected pregnancy.
3 Unexplained uterine bleeding.
4 Current active pelvic infection or pelvic tenderness, or purulent cervical discharge.
5 Recent proven STI, unless fully investigated and treated (can be WHO 3)
6 Severely distorted uterine cavity – though it may be usefully inserted after preliminary hysteroscopic removal of a submucous fibroid, and occasionally after uterine ablation (see Qs 8.60–8.61).

7 Current active hepatocellular disease or liver tumour (possibly WHO 3).
8 Current active arterial disease (this is arguable, probably WHO 2/3 in most cases).
9 Past attack of bacterial endocarditis, or a prosthetic heart valve present.
10 Very severe immunodeficiency (possibly WHO 3 if nil else useable).
11 Current active trophoblastic disease with raised HCG.
12 In addition: the LNG-IUS should not be used as a postcoital intrauterine contraceptive (at least one failure has been reported – it may not act quickly enough).

6.147 WHAT ABOUT RELATIVE CONTRAINDICATIONS TO THE LNG-IUS?

If you look through those listed above (Q 6.86) for copper IUDs, most are irrelevant, or 'weakly' in category WHO 2, and some are indications!

- If there is structural heart disease and this IUS is chosen there should of course be full antibiotic cover for the insertion as at Q 6.89.
- Although enzyme-inducing drugs might theoretically weaken the contraceptive effect there is no evidence so far that they can do this, given the very high local concentration of levonorgestrel.
- It may be used during breastfeeding (like the POP, see Qs 5.55–5.59).

6.148 ARE THERE ANY SPECIAL POINTS ABOUT INSERTION OF THE LNG-IUS?

- It should be inserted by day 7 of the normal cycle, for the reasons explained at Q 6.7. Later insertion is advisable only if there has been excellent contraception up to that time and continued (e.g. condoms) thereafter for a minimum of 7 days.
- The *technique* itself is almost identical to that for the Nova-T: see Q 6.113. However the insertion tube is wider (4.8 mm rather than 3.7 mm), meaning that effective local anaesthesia and dilatation to Hegar 5 or even 6 are not infrequently required (though rarely in multiparae, who are still, as for copper IUDs, the best target population).
- The side-arms need to be positioned so their round ends just protrude from the tip of the inserter tube. Otherwise the edge of the latter may catch, and fail to negotiate the internal os. Kinking of the tube may then also result. A new insertion gadget is expected in 2000.

6.149 WHICH WOMEN MIGHT PARTICULARLY CONSIDER A LNG-IUS?

If it were not for price considerations, the size of its inserter and its initial post-insertion bleeding problems, this method could be selected for almost any IUD-acceptor. It fulfils many of the standard criteria for an 'ideal' contraceptive (Table 6.3). It approaches 100% reversibility, effectiveness and even, after some delay, convenience. This is because, after the initial months of frequent uterine bleedings and spotting, the usual outcomes of either intermittent light menses or amenorrhoea are very acceptable to most women. Adverse side-effects are few and in general they are in the category nuisance rather than hazardous. Evidence continues to accumulate of non-contraceptive benefits, including a useful reduction in symptoms of the premenstrual syndrome in about half of those receiving it.

- Though it may be chosen by some young women with heavy menses or unable to accept alternatives, it is particularly suitable for *women in the older reproductive years* with contraindications to other options, or with heavy periods. There is then the possible option of providing the progestagen component of a most useful form of '*contraceptive and no bleed HRT*' to follow, if they are later prescribed oestrogen by any chosen route. (But see page 507, so long as this remains an unlicensed use; and it *must* be replaced every 5 years, Q 6.135).
- The LNG-IUS can often provide an excellent solution for the contraceptive dilemmas of many women suffering from interacting medical disorders or risk factors, e.g. severe diabetes and SLE (Qs 4.131–4.134).

TABLE 6.3 THE 'IDEAL' CONTRACEPTIVE

1 100% reversible
2 100% effective (with the 'default state' as contraception)
3 100% convenient (and non-coitally-related)
4 100% free of adverse side-effects (neither risk nor nuisance)
5 100% protective against sexually transmitted infections
6 Possessed of other non-contraceptive benefits
7 Maintenance-free (needing no ongoing medical intervention)

CONCLUSIONS

6.150 WHAT ARE YOUR TEN COMMANDMENTS ABOUT IUD INSERTION?

See Qs 6.104–6.113 for more details.

1 Thou shalt never insert any IUD without training, and without first having practised each step of the insertion procedure on a plastic pelvic model – and keeping in practice.
2 All manipulations of the cervix and uterus shall be performed gently – but not tentatively.
3 Thou shalt always consider and *discuss the option* of local anaesthesia – and always *offer* a PGSI, and always use 'aural valium, and vocal local'.
4 Thou shalt ensure the best position of the patient for insertion (consider left lateral), always have an assistant, and use good equipment with a good light.
5 A preliminary BME will never be omitted.
6 The insertion will be postponed, pending diagnosis and treatment, whenever there is the slightest pelvic tenderness or other evidence suggesting infection.
7 The cervix will be thoroughly cleansed by repeated swabbing, and antiseptic technique followed for all objects passed through the endocervical canal into the sterile uterine cavity.
8 Careful sounding of the uterus will not be omitted – to check the direction and patency of the canal and to assess the uterine cavity. Hegar dilators (3–6) will be available.
9 The device if it has a frame will be loaded into its inserter at the last possible moment – to preserve its asepsis and 'memory'.
10 The correct technique will be used to deliver the IUD in the right plane to the correct high fundal position.

6.151 WHAT ARE YOUR TEN RESOLUTIONS FOR THE CONSCIENTIOUS IUD DOCTOR?

1 Remembering that one of the main times of action of IUDs is the last 9 days of the cycle I will follow the 7-day rule for elective IUD removal (Q 6.14), to avoid 'iatrogenic pregnancies'. I will also be prepared to proceed with IUD insertion up to 'day 19' in selected cases (Qs 6.17, 7.15).

2 Since the main IUD hazards and contraindications relate to threats to fertility, I will always make this the main point when counselling the *nulliparous*.

3 Since the rates of *in situ* pregnancy, expulsion and pelvic infection are inversely related to age, I will always make these potential risks the main element when counselling the *young*.

4 Since incorrect insertion/malposition can cause every category of IUD problem, I will ensure that my own insertions are competent, careful and gentle, and use the 'longest lived', appropriate IUD (Qs 6.132 and 6.136).

Subsequent to fitting the right device in the right woman using the right technique, I will remember and (as appropriate) teach my patients the following:

5 That pain and bleeding are serious symptoms until proved otherwise, especially if sustained and intermenstrual.

6 More specifically, that any woman with menstrual irregularity and pelvic discomfort has an ectopic pregnancy until proved otherwise.

7 That 'lost threads' means the woman is pregnant or at risk of pregnancy until proved otherwise.

8 That in any continuing pregnancy the IUD should be gently removed in the first trimester if feasible, to reduce the risks of abortion and preterm delivery.

Moreover, there are two equally important but opposite slogans:

9 'Leave well alone' (often, after counselling, in asymptomatic long-term users). Yet, contrariwise:

10 'When in doubt take it out' when the woman does have troublesome symptoms; and also for her own reasons upon her request, so the method is never one over which (wrongly) only the doctor has control. But then I must not forget to ask about any intercourse in the preceding 7 days, and her plans for future contraception.

6.152 WHAT PROBLEMS OF IUD USE IN BRITAIN SHOULD BE REPORTED TO THE MEDICAL DEVICES AGENCY?

Any problems or complications whether or not in the list at Q 6.22, especially:

1 extrauterine pregnancy (or intrauterine, for the new GyneFIX™);
2 perforation/translocation;
3 severe pelvic infection – most especially actinomycosis (see Q 6.72) or bacterial endocarditis (see Q 6.89);
4 apparent true allergy to any constituent of IUDs (Q 6.87);
5 apparent interaction with a drug or imaging technique (see Qs 6.126–6.128);
6 severe insertion reactions (Q 6.117);
7 any unusual *possibly* related event.

QUESTIONS ASKED BY PROSPECTIVE OR CURRENT IUD-USERS

GENERAL QUESTIONS

6.153 HOW DOES THE IUD/IUS WORK? IS IT OFTEN CAUSING AN ABORTION?

The answer depends on the definition of when pregnancy begins, see Qs 6.7, 7.2 and 7.3. If your own beliefs make you feel that contraception must *never* operate after fertilization, then this method is not for you.

6.154 CAN THE COPPER BE ABSORBED FROM COPPER DEVICES INTO THE BODY?

A tiny amount is absorbed, but very little so it is only just detectable in the blood. By far the majority of the small amount of copper which is lost over the years goes out in the vaginal fluid.

6.155 WHY DOES THE IUD/IUS HAVE A TAIL? CAN I PULL IT OUT MYSELF?

Mainly to check that the device is present, but also to remove it when required. Deliberate self-removal is not recommended, but could be done. . The GyneFIX™ is the most vulnerable to being removed by mistake, when chasing a 'lost' tampon perhaps.

6.156 WHICH IS SAFER, THE IUD OR THE ORDINARY PILL? CAN A WOMAN DIE FROM USING AN IUD/IUS?

Overall, the risk of death or life-endangering disease is very low with both methods, but even lower with an IUD. Deaths have been caused but they are extremely rare.

The problems are focused in the pelvic area and not all over the body, and they can be minimized, see Qs 6.150 and 6.151. The main problems have to do with future fertility (see Qs 6.23, 6.84 and 6.86).

6.157 DOES THE IUD/IUS CAUSE ANY KIND OF CANCER?

There is no evidence for this, whether for copper or hormone-releasing varieties (see Q 6.22).

6.158 IF I GET PREGNANT, WILL THE BABY BE HARMED?

Again there is no evidence of this, even if the pregnancy occurs with a copper device still in position. It should normally, however, be removed in early pregnancy (see Q 6.25 and Q 6.145).

6.159 WHAT HAS USING THE IUD/IUS GOT TO DO WITH THE NUMBER OF SEXUAL PARTNERS I HAVE?

A great deal, since the main problem with IUDs is pelvic infection, and nearly all IUD-linked infections are actually caught sexually. Also relevant is the number of sexual partners of your own partner, even if you are entirely faithful to him. (*See also the question at Q 6.119(3)*).

COUNSELLING AND FITTING OF IUDs

6.160 DO I NEED MY PARTNER'S/HUSBAND'S AGREEMENT TO HAVE AN IUD/IUS?

No, the device can be inserted without his agreement. The threads can be cut off if you so request. However, clearly it is always best if the couple are both agreed, whatever method of family planning is chosen.

6.161 SHOULD I ASK TO SEE WHICH IUD/IUS I HAVE BEFORE IT IS FITTED?

Yes, most certainly. Ideally you should also write down its name and the date of fitting, in case you move to the care of a different doctor or clinic.

6.162 I THINK I AM ALLERGIC TO COPPER; WHAT SHOULD I DO?

First, report the matter to your doctor. It may be possible to do special patch allergy tests.

Since most people who think they are allergic to copper turn out actually to be allergic to another metal, it may be right then to insert the device and see how you get on over the next few days. If you get marked discharge and pain within a very few days of insertion, you should return most promptly for advice (see Q 6.87).

6.163 I AM TOLD I HAVE A CERVICAL EROSION (ECTOPY)/A TILTED WOMB/A VERY TINY WOMB – CAN I HAVE AN IUD FITTED?

If these are the only problems (i.e. there is no infection, or the womb is not distorted congenitally or by fibroids) a device can normally be fitted (see Qs 6.85, 6.97 and 6.142).

6.164 I HAVE HEARD YOU GET VERY BAD CRAMP-LIKE PAINS WHEN AN IUD/IUS IS FITTED? WHAT CAUSES THIS AND WHAT CAN BE DONE ABOUT IT?

The pain people feel at insertion varies a great deal, from nothing to severe, and it is not easily predictable. Part of this is caused by the release of substances called prostaglandins, and you can ask your doctor for a specific painkiller that opposes their action. You should also discuss with him/her the possibility of having a local anaesthetic.

6.165 DOES AN IUD/IUS ALWAYS HAVE TO BE FITTED DURING OR JUST AFTER A PERIOD?

No – not only *may* it be inserted later, there may even be certain advantages to not inserting during heavy bleeding (see Qs 6.15–6.17).

6.166 DOES BEING AN EPILEPTIC INCREASE THE CHANCE OF MY HAVING A FIT DURING THE INSERTION?

Yes it does, and your doctor should arrange to have available the treatment to prevent/stop an attack. See also Qs 6.117–6.118.

INSTRUCTIONS AFTER FITTING

6.167 HOW SOON CAN I HAVE SEX AFTER HAVING THE IUD/IUS FITTED?

The protection from a copper IUD or from the LNG-IUS if fitted before Day 8 of your cycle is immediate, but it is now recommended that you wait for about 3 days to reduce infection risk, or at least use a condom (Q 6.120). You would be advised to use condoms anyway for safety if the IUS is fitted on/after day 8 (Q 6.148).

6.168 IF I USE A SPERMICIDE AS WELL AS MY IUD, WILL IT REDUCE THE CHANCE OF INFECTION AS WELL AS PREGNANCY?

Yes, there is some evidence that spermicides are also germicides, so this may well be a good idea if your lifestyle or that of your partner puts you at risk (see Q 6.18). A condom will be even more protective.

6.169 CAN AN IUD/IUS FALL OUT WITHOUT MY KNOWING?

Yes, this is certainly possible (see Q 6.38). The most likely time is during a heavy period, in which case it may be hidden within a large clot or on a tampon which is then flushed down the toilet.

6.170 HOW OFTEN SHOULD I FEEL FOR THE STRINGS?

Once a month is sufficient; best right at the end of a period. This is so that you do not begin to rely on the method each new month, until you have checked that it is still in position.

6.171 HOW DO I FEEL THE STRINGS OF THE IUD/IUS? WHAT SHOULD I DO IF I NOW CAN'T FEEL THEM?

Either squat down or put one foot on the bathroom stool. Insert both your index and middle fingers into the vagina and feel more in a backwards than an upwards direction until you come across the cervix. This feels rather like a nose with only one nostril, and you should then be able to find emerging from the opening one or two little threads feeling like ends of nylon fishing line. If that is all you feel, well and good.

If, however, you feel something hard like the end of a matchstick, this could mean that the device is on its way out. In that case, or if you can no longer feel the threads at all, you must assume that you are no longer protected and start using another method (e.g. condoms). Contact your family doctor or clinic urgently in case 'emergency contraception' is required – most likely by urgent reinsertion (see Q 7.23).

6.172 CAN MY IUD/IUS GET LOST IN THE BODY (PERFORATION)?

Extremely rarely. It is 999 : 1 against this happening in your case. It is a rare cause of the problem of lost threads (see Q 6.42). Should it happen, the most that is normally required is a minor operation called a laparoscopy to retrieve it.

While your lost threads problem is still being sorted out, and you are perhaps waiting for a hospital appointment, make sure that you use another method of family planning (since the womb itself may be empty) and also take immediate medical advice if you get any pain in the abdomen.

6.173 CAN I GO BACK TO USING AN IUD OR IUS AFTER A PERFORATION?

This depends on the cause; but an IUD can often be reinserted with success, since the tiny hole in the womb heals up so completely.

QUESTIONS ASKED BY CURRENT USERS

6.174 DO WOMEN HAVE MORE VAGINAL DISCHARGE WITH AN IUD?

Yes. Sometimes the discharge has a specific and treatable cause, so it should always be reported to your doctor. If testing shows nothing specific and treatable, like bacterial vaginosis or thrush, then it is probably caused by an increase in the usual vaginal fluid (which includes mucus, the fluid of sexual arousal and even semen). That needs no treatment.

6.175 SOMEONE HAS TOLD ME THE IUD CAN BREAK INTO PIECES INSIDE YOU, IS THIS SO?

Years ago there was one dud batch of Lippes Loop devices which were distributed worldwide and were liable to fracture. No modern device will break up, except very rarely if removal is difficult. In that case a minor hysteroscopy operation might rarely be necessary to retrieve the missing portion.

6.176 MY LAST PERIOD WAS VERY LATE AND HEAVY; DOES THIS MEAN I MIGHT BE MISCARRYING AN EARLY PREGNANCY?

Most probably not – heavy periods are not uncommon in regular use of an IUD, and the period could have been late just because your egg was released late in that cycle. However, you should visit the clinic for an examination and advice, partly in case your device was dislodged by the heavy flow. You might also ask about the LNG-IUS ('Mirena').

6.177 CAN MY PARTNER REALLY FEEL THE IUD/IUS DURING LOVEMAKING AS HE SAYS, AND WHAT CAN BE DONE ABOUT IT?

Some men notice the threads, depending on which way the cervix points and perhaps on the position of intercourse. Many couples just adapt their sex lives accordingly, but otherwise it is possible to have the threads cut right off (see Q 6.125).

6.178 CAN I USE A SUNBED WITH AN IUD IN PLACE, OR HAVE VIBROMASSAGE?

Neither of these can affect your IUD in any way.

6.179 IF MY IUD CONTAINS METAL, WILL IT MAKE AN EMBARRASSING 'BLEEP' WHEN I PASS THROUGH SECURITY DEVICES AT AIRPORTS OR LARGE DEPARTMENT STORES?

Despite rumours, this does not appear to be a problem either with copper-bearing or steel devices – presumably because the amount of metal is too small. Another rumour which can be discounted is the one that was started by the woman who accused the magician Yuri Geller of causing the failure of her copper IUD. She claimed that the pregnancy was conceived when she made love on the hearthrug during a television demonstration by the above-mentioned showman of his metal-bending skills!

6.180 CAN I CAUSE MY IUD/IUS TO BE EXPELLED BY VIGOROUS AEROBIC EXERCISES OR INTERCOURSE IN ANY UNUSUAL POSITIONS?

There is no evidence for this, and plenty of ordinary and sexual athletes use the method with success.

6.181 MAY I USE INTERNAL SANITARY PROTECTION AFTER BEING FITTED WITH AN IUD/IUS?

The usual advice is to use only a sanitary towel at first, for the bleeding which follows immediately after IUD insertion until 3 days have elapsed. Subsequently sanitary protection can be entirely at a woman's choice.

Prolonged use of the same tampon (more than 12 hours) is always a bad idea, for fear of toxic shock syndrome (TSS).

6.182 ARE THERE ANY DRUGS THAT MIGHT INTERFERE WITH THE ACTION OF MY IUD/IUS?

Tell your doctor about the IUD if you are to receive any treatment. Should this be a corticosteroid or other drug which may interfere with immune responses, it may be better for you to transfer to another method of birth control. However, there is no current concern about either antibiotics or painkillers (see Qs 6.86(12) and 6.88), or other treatments (Q 6.126).

6.183 DO I REALLY HAVE TO HAVE MY COPPER IUD CHANGED AT A SET TIME, WHEN IT IS SUITING ME WELL?

Nowadays this is becoming less and less necessary, and definitely not if your device was fitted above the age of 40. See Qs 6.129–6.136 for a full answer to this most important question.

6.184 HOW IS AN IUD/IUS REMOVED? IS IT EVER DIFFICULT?

Normally there is no problem; there is much less discomfort than having the device fitted in the first place. However, there are some situations in which it is more tricky and uncomfortable (see Qs 6.36 and 6.123).

6.185 IF MY IUD/IUS IS REMOVED SO THAT I CAN TRY FOR A BABY, SHOULD I WAIT, USING ANOTHER METHOD FOR A SET TIME?

It is recommended that you wait for one period to 'clear the womb' first. But this is not vital. Even women who conceive immediately the device comes out (so it was still in place during the last period before the pregnancy) seem to be as likely as anyone else to have a normal baby.

7 Emergency (postcoital) contraception

BACKGROUND AND MECHANISMS

7.1 WHAT IS THE DEFINITION OF POSTCOITAL EMERGENCY CONTRACEPTION (EC)?

In current usage this is any female method which is administered after intercourse, but has its effects prior to the stage of implantation. The latter is believed to occur no earlier than 5 days after ovulation. Any method applied after intercourse which acts after implantation, even if this is before the next menses, should properly be called a *post-conceptional* or *contragestive* agent.

   The lay term 'morning after pill' is not ideal, since it may actually cause pregnancies by preventing women from realizing they can present many hours later than the 'morning after' (see Q 7.5). We now prefer to say 'the emergency pill'. Yet efficacy is greater the earlier hormone regimens are commenced (Q 7.6).

Yes. Though the methods usually work by preventing fertilization, it is undeniable that the mechanism may often be through blocking implantation. The question is whether the prescriber and the woman concerned are happy to accept the view of most modern biologists and ethicists, that '*conception*' is a *process*, which certainly begins with the fusion of sperm and ovum, but is not complete until implantation.

The situation is clarified by considering the *status of the unimplanted blastocyst* (Fig. 7.1). If it stays where it is in the cavity of the uterus it is in a 100% 'No-Go' situation – unless and until it can stop itself being washed away in the next menstrual flow by secreting enough human chorionic gonadotrophin (hCG) into the mother's circulation to maintain the corpus luteum. The all-destroying menses cannot be prevented without successful implantation.

A second feature of the unimplanted situation is, the mother's physiology does not 'know' the blastocyst is present, yet. Only after

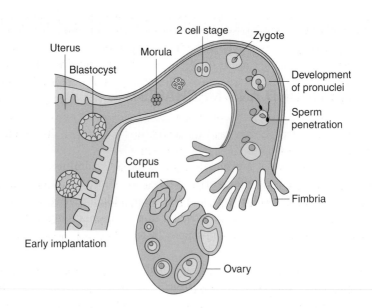

Figure 7.1 Ovulation, fertilization and early development to the stage of implantation. Q 7.2 considers the *status* of the unimplanted blastocyst, labelled above.

implantation is there a two-way relationship, and for the first time 100% 'No Go' for the blastocyst becomes 'Go'. Now there is 'carriage'. As has been well said, at the earlier stage, when there is not yet 'carriage' how could application of any method of birth control be 'procuring a miscarriage'?

Finally, with at least 50% of blastocysts regularly failing to implant there seems little logic in putting a high value on something with which Nature itself is so prodigal.

Prescribers must of course respect the views of their patients, and EC methods should not be used for any who are unhappy with the above interpretation. They should then, however, also understand the implications in relation to other methods (see Qs 6.7 and 7.3).

7.3 WHAT ARE THE IMPLICATIONS OF REJECTION OF EC METHODS ON ETHICAL GROUNDS?

In the main, this means that the woman concerned should also not use either IUDs or IUSs, or the progestagen-only pill (see Q 5.76). All these methods may operate in a minority of cycles, but sometimes, by blocking implantation.

7.4 WHAT IS THE HISTORY OF EMERGENCY CONTRACEPTION?

This is probably almost as old as the first recognition that semen is in some way responsible for pregnancy. Douching has been used since ancient times and remains in use today; 25% of women presenting for EC treatment in one UK study had first used a shower attachment, flannel or paper tissues, with or without a spermicide or household germicide. These methods are doomed to frequent failure, because sperm have been found in cervical mucus within 90 seconds following ejaculation.

The Persian physician Al-Razi suggested: 'first immediately after ejaculation let the two come apart and let the woman arise roughly, sneeze and blow her nose several times and call out in a loud voice. She should jump violently backwards seven to nine times'. Jumping backwards supposedly dislodged the semen, while jumping forwards would assure pregnancy.

A range of EC pessaries and douches have been described over the years, including wine and garlic with fennel, used in Egypt as early as 1500 BC; ground cabbage blossoms in the 4th century; and culminating in Coca-Cola in some developing countries even today. The modern mythology says that Diet Coke works best!

The history of more effective methods begins in 1963 with trials of diethylstilboestrol (DES) at Yale University (USA). Because of the risks to any pregnancy should the method fail, DES should now never be used. After the mid-1970s the Yuzpe method (devised by a Canadian gynaecologist) became the first-choice method, using much less EE in combination with levonorgestrel (LNG). But it is now likely to be supplanted by progestagen-only emergency contraception (POEC), using levonorgestrel.

Immediate insertion of a copper intrauterine device (IUD) is an alternative method first reported in 1972 and appropriate in some cases (see Q 7.33).

7.5 WHAT ARE THE CURRENTLY ACCEPTED REGIMENS OF EC TREATMENT?

See Tables 7.1 and 7.2.

1 *Immediate insertion of a copper-bearing IUD* (NB, NOT the LNG-IUS), no more than 5 days after the most probable calculated date of ovulation, even if there have been several acts of unprotected intercourse; or 5 days after any single exposure.

2 *The Yuzpe method.* This is commenced within 72 hours of the earliest act of unprotected intercourse, its efficacy being greatest in the first 24 hours and declining thereafter (though not to nil after 72 hours). Two tablets of a contraceptive containing 250 µg of LNG with 50 µg of EE (Schering PC 4 or Ovran) are given at once, followed by a further two tablets 12 hours later

3 *Use of levonorgestrel (LNG) alone.* This is referred to below as POEC (progestagen-only emergency contraception). If started within 72 hours of the earliest exposure it again has its greatest efficacy in the first 24 hours, declining thereafter but not to nil at 72 hours (Table 7.2). It requires 750 µg LNG stat, repeated in 12 hours (or within 24 hours; Q 7.9). In a large multicentre RCT of 1998 women by WHO (*Lancet* 1998;352:428–33) it proved to be more effective, with fewer side-effects (especially vomiting) and there are also fewer contraindications. At the time of writing (1999) it is an unlicensed use of a licensed substance (see Appendix 1 for 'named patient use'), though an application for licensing is being processed.

Other methods previously in use are now of historical interest only. See also Q 7.7 for variants and Q 7.48 about methods being researched.

TABLE 7.1   CHOICE OF METHODS FOR POSTCOITAL CONTRACEPTION – A BRIEF SUMMARY

Combined hormone method	Levonorgestrel method	Copper IUD
PC4 or Ovran: two pills stat, two pills 12 hours later	Levonorgestrel 0.75 mg stat 0.75 mg 12 hours later	
Normal timing after intercourse		
Up to 72 hours	Up to 72 hours	Up to 5 days after earliest calculated day of ovulation or 5 days after any isolated exposure in that cycle
Efficacy (overall)		
97%	99%	Almost 100%
Side-effects		
Nausea 51% and vomiting 19%	Nausea 23% and vomiting 6%	Pain, bleeding, risk of infection
Contraindications (WHO 4)		
Pregnancy *Current* focal migraine, jaundice, active acute porphyria, sickle-cell crisis, severe liver disease or serious past thrombosis (see text) Allergy to a constituent	Pregnancy Active acute porphyria Severe liver disease Allergy to a constituent	Pregnancy and as for IUDs generally

Reference: WHO (1998) *Lancet* 352: 428–33.
Numbers rounded to nearest integer.

7.6 WHAT IS THE MECHANISM OF ACTION OF EC CONTRACEPTIVE METHODS?

The IUD operates here mainly by blocking implantation (see Q 6.7), since it is usually inserted after ovulation; though if applied earlier in the cycle it can also block fertilization.

The action of the hormonal methods will depend on when in relation to ovulation they are administered. It is important to remember that this could happen to be sufficiently early to prevent or *postpone* ovulation in that

TABLE 7.2 EFFICACY OF YUZPE (COMBINED OESTROGEN–PROGESTAGEN) COMPARED WITH POEC (PROGESTAGEN-ONLY EMERGENCY CONTRACEPTION) WHO FINDINGS (1998)

Coitus-to-treatment interval	Pregnancy rate (95% CI)
72 h or less	
Combined oestrogen–progestagen	3.2 (2.2–4.5)
Progestagen-only	1.1 (0.62–2.0)
24 h or less	
Combined oestrogen–progestagen	2.0 (0.9–3.7)
Progestagen-only	0.4 (0.1–1.6)
25–48 h	
Combined oestrogen–progestagen	4.1 (2.3–6.6)
Progestagen-only	1.2 (0.3–3.0)
49–72 h	
Combined oestrogen–progestagen	4.7 (1.9–9.4)
Progestagen-only	2.7 (0.9–6.1)

cycle (hence the requirement to use a method such as the condom until the next period). It is probable that the uterine fluid/genital tract mucus may also be rendered hostile to sperm or blastocyst.

If, however, the hormones are given after ovulation, the method relies mainly on blocking implantation. The precise mechanism is uncertain, but desynchronization of the histology of the secretory endometrium has been observed along with blockage of oestrogen and progesterone receptors. The agents may also operate indirectly by impairing luteal function.

7.7 MIGHT OTHER REGIMENS WORK?

A very wide range of alternatives has been proposed and there are anecdotal reports of success. These are very difficult to assess, because pregnancy is certainly not inevitable after a single act of intercourse, even if the woman were untreated (see Q 7.13). However, the variants below may be considered even though their efficacy has *not* been established in rigorous trials.

7.8 WILL EITHER OF THE HORMONAL METHODS WORK IF GIVEN LATER THAN 72 HOURS?

Though many prescribers have treated it as such, *the 72-hour time limit has never implied an absolute contraindication*. It does now seem that both hormone methods work best if started in the first 24 hours. But it would not be biologically plausible that either method would lose all efficacy precisely at the end of the tested 72-hour period. Hence if a woman presents later and will not accept the copper IUD alternative, one of the hormonal methods can be given. If so, three things are important:

- It should be explained to her and recorded that such late treatment ought to be usefully better than nothing (working primarily by its implantation blocking mechanism); no one knows how much of its efficacy remains with later use – and much will depend on how much later too, of course.
- Care should be taken, as with similar late use of a copper IUD (Q 7.15), to question her about any possible earlier exposure so that you then proceed in good faith, in the belief that you will not be disturbing an already implanted pregnancy. This means no later than 5 days after calculated ovulation (Q 7.15).
- As it is unlicensed, this late use would have to be on a 'named patient' basis (see Appendix 1, page 507).

7.9 DOES THE SECOND DOSE HAVE TO BE GIVEN ACCURATELY 12 HOURS AFTER THE FIRST?

In some Centres in the 1998 WHO trial the method seemed not to lose significant efficacy if the second dose of either hormonal method was given within the next 24, rather than precisely at 12 hours. This needs confirmation, but allows a young woman first seen in the afternoon to take her second dose at a less unsocial hour (i.e. early next morning, instead of risking waking up her mother by her alarm going off in the middle of the night ...).

7.10 HOW ARE THE REQUIRED HORMONE DOSES GIVEN OR CONSTRUCTED?

Clearly if single tablets with all (or a large proportion) of the required hormones are not marketed or are more expensive, there are various ways of putting together similar doses of the hormone methods.

- *For the Yuzpe method*, seven tablets of Microgynon 30/Ovranette in divided doses will provide 210 µg of EE (instead of 200) and 1050 µg of LNG (instead of 1000) – though more usually the slightly higher dose, eight tablets in divided doses, is actually used for simplicity. Alternatively, four tablets of Ovran provide precisely the same dose as Schering PC4.
- *For POEC*, two tablets each containing LNG 750 µg, marketed as 'Postinor' by Gedeon Richter in Hungary and other Eastern European countries, were used in the WHO and earlier trials; and licensing in the UK is expected in the near future. Until then (and in many countries abroad) the dose may often have to be constructed, with the patient being reassured (sometimes with difficulty!), that a total of 50 tablets of Microval or Norgeston – or 40 tablets of Neogest – is not an overdose.

See the (photocopiable, not copyright) text of our MPC patient information leaflet, reproduced as Figure 7.2 – the section about taking 50 tablets should of course be deleted in services where the single 750 µg tablet is available.

7.11 MIGHT OTHER PROGESTAGENS BE EFFECTIVE?

Other progestagens may well be effective, such as desogestrel or gestodene or even DMPA by injection; but neither their efficacy nor the best doses have so far been evaluated in proper trials.

EFFECTIVENESS

7.12 WHAT IS THE OVERALL EFFICACY OF THE THREE MOST COMMONLY USED EC METHODS?

1   *For the IUD method* the failure rate is very low indeed. We have reported one failure with the device still in situ at the Margaret Pyke Centre (MPC), and there was another, with partial expulsion of the device, reported from elsewhere. This represented two failures in about 1300 insertions reported in the literature to that date. Considering that in this context the risk of pregnancy only applies for the cycle of insertion, this is a rate of 1–2 failures/1300 cycles; entirely compatible therefore with the usually quoted failure rate of the IUD at that time of about 1/100 woman-years (100 woman-years equals 1300 cycles).

2 Reported failure rates for the *Yuzpe combined regimen* vary enormously, depending very much on factors such as the likely fertility of the women, when they were exposed, other acts of intercourse both before and after the treatment and completeness of follow-up. Rates range from 1% for cases with exposure at any time of the cycle, to 2–5% for exposure at around midcycle.

3 Table 7.2 summarizes the basic data on efficacy from the 1998 WHO study, a randomized comparison after single exposure of the combined versus the levonorgestrel-only method. Note the greater efficacy of early presentation within the 72 hours, for both methods. Indeed WHO stated that each 12 hours delay raised the pregnancy risk by almost 50%. *NB, Table 7.2 presents the data as pregnancy rates among all-comers. Yet:*

4 One should really consider in the denominator only those who would actually have become pregnant without treatment (Q 7.13). The WHO did this, based on earlier work showing the risk of conception on each cycle day (an update by Wilcox *et al.* of the Barrett and Marshall work described at Q 1.15). The 'true' failure rates were then considerably higher. In an analysis based on the 1157 women randomized to the two methods who abstained from intercourse until the next menses, the Yuzpe method prevented 74% and the POEC method prevented 89% of the conceptions that would have otherwise been expected.

A useful summary is to say that out of every eight conceptions that would really happen after a single coital exposure, Yuzpe will prevent six and POEC will prevent seven.

7.13 WHAT IS THE LIKELIHOOD OF PREGNANCY AFTER A SINGLE ACT OF INTERCOURSE IN THE ABSENCE OF EC TREATMENT?

See Figure 1.1 at Qs 1.14 and 1.15. If a single exposure is around mid-cycle (days 10–14, corrected to a 28-day cycle) the risk is roughly 20%, peaking at about 30% on the day of maximum risk. At other times during the cycle the risk is somewhere between 0 and 10%.

The probability of conception is lowest in the days before the expected date of the next menses; though the possibility that the cycle in question might be unusually long must always be considered. There is a significant risk from day 7 to about 17 of a 28-day cycle – or the equivalent 10 days after correction for cycle length.

What is emergency contraception?

Emergency contraception is a term used for treatment preventing conception after sex without causing an abortion. Any queries or concerns should be discussed with one of our nurses or doctors. Following treatment we would like to see you again either for ongoing contraceptive care or if you have any worries after taking emergency contraception. In an emergency please contact your GP if the Centre is closed.

What is progestagen-only emergency contraception?

In August 1998 the World Health Organisation (WHO) published some well conducted research showing that the progestagen-only emergency contraception method is highly effective.

- This treatment should be started within 72 hours of the unprotected sex.
- There must be no previous episodes of unprotected sex since your last period.

Is it licensed in the UK?

The hormone it contains (levonorgestrel) certainly is. It is part of many of the most commonly used contraceptive pills. But at the time of writing the relevant government committee has not yet licensed it for the purpose of emergency contraception. Many experts including the Faculty of Family Planning (of the Royal College of Obstetricians & Gynaecologists) and the Family Planning Association strongly support its use, and there is every reason to expect that it will be licensed without undue delay.

Is it legal and safe to use it before licensing?

Yes, but you have to read, understand and accept everything in this leaflet, especially:

- the fact that it is not licensed.
- that a doctor must see you to decide whether this is the best treatment to prescribe for you – and this may involve a longer wait.

How do I take it?

The treatment consists of two doses. The first must be taken within 72 hours of the unprotected intercourse although research shows it is more effective if taken within 24 hours.

You take 25 tablets of Microval – they are small tablets so several can be taken with each mouthful of water – and **then a further 25 tablets 12 hours later.**

NB. This means that from each packet you are given you will have to throw away the 10 remaining tablets.

Is that right, 50 tablets altogether??

Yes: this is still not an excessive dose. It is only because a single pill with the right dose is not yet licensed and marketed in the UK. In some other countries the right dose is available in just one tablet, as we hope it will be one day here.

Figure 7.2 Patient information leaflet re Progestagen-Only Emergency Contraception (POEC

How effective is it?
Studies have suggested that this method works very well i.e. 98–99% effective. The insertion of an IUD is more effective than any hormonal methods. Following the use of any method of emergency contraception, failure is possible. Abnormalities occur in about 2% of all births irrespective of whether the woman has taken hormonal treatments. There is, as yet, no research to show if there is any increase in the risk of having an abnormal baby, but from theoretical knowledge we believe this is very unlikely.

Are there any side-effects?
As with any medicine a minority of women experience side-effects. You may feel sick or very rarely be sick. **If you vomit within 2 hours of taking the pills, please contact the clinic or seek medical advice at the earliest opportunity.** No serious side-effects have occurred in the studies of the method so we feel it is very unlikely to cause any problems.

Should I be seen again?
We suggest you return again when suggested, usually in 3 or 4 weeks – even if all is well. Please make an appointment as you leave.

Future contraception?
Emergency contraception will not prevent a possible pregnancy from unprotected sex earlier in your cycle, nor will it prevent a pregnancy if you have unprotected sex after the treatment. This will be discussed with you by the nurse and/or doctor and interim supplies of condoms can be issued. If you plan to use the combined pill you should start it when your next period begins (no further contraceptive precautions are required if this is by the second day of your next period).

What I should look out for in the meantime?
Your period is likely to come on time (although it may be a little early or a little late). If there is anything you are concerned about you should return to the clinic before the 3-week appointment. Following any emergency contraception that fails, an ectopic/tubal pregnancy (a pregnancy in the wrong place) is a rare but serious occurrence. (This is actually more likely if you do *not* take emergency contraception.) You should go to your nearest Casualty Department in the unlikely event that you get severe pain in the lower abdomen.

Please be straight with us
Finally, we can only help if you are entirely straight with us. Please give us all the facts, particularly if you have taken a risk of pregnancy earlier in your menstrual cycle, or if you might even already be pregnant (e.g. because your last period was not a normal one).

Professor John Guillebaud (Medical Director, Margaret Pyke Centre)

7.14 SHOULD ONE BE PREPARED TO WITHHOLD EC TREATMENT?

This can be a tricky decision. Although the risk of conception is very low if exposure was actually during the menses, or during what are believed to be the very last days of the cycle, the decision to treat depends on many factors: not least the amount of anxiety present. The treatment is very safe, if not entirely risk free.

In future it may be possible to discover, simply and accurately in the clinic, what stage of the menstrual cycle the woman has reached. At present, although treatment is not always indicated, it is not easy to be sure that ovulation will not occur on an atypical day in that particular cycle. Your patient could be having an amazingly short, or long, menstrual cycle out of the blue.

So when in doubt, treat.

7.15 WHAT ARE THE TIME-LIMITS FOR SUCCESSFUL TREATMENT?

1   *The IUD method.* Here the time limit of 5 days relates to the *most likely* expected day of ovulation: i.e. expected date of next menses, subtract 14 days and add 5. This is calculated in good faith from the menstrual data given by the woman, and *applies irrespective of the number of earlier acts of unprotected intercourse.* Five days is well within the time limits from intercourse to implantation, according to the consensus of medical opinion. It will not be construed in law as possibly procuring an abortion.

Though some would play safe and say that the calculation should begin from *the earliest* calculated day of ovulation based on cycle lengths, my view is that, depending on the woman's own views about the ethics of the situation, it should be based on the *shortest likely* cycle. This is strengthened by a recent judgment which suggests some leeway:

Regina v Dhingra, 24th January 1991. Mr Justice Wright did not convict a general practitioner accused of illegal abortion achieved by inserting an IUD 11 days after intercourse, because it was day 18 and thus prior to implantation. 'I further hold, in accordance with the uncontroverted evidence that I have heard, that a pregnancy cannot come into existence until the fertilized ovum has become implanted in the womb, and that stage is not reached until, at the earliest, the 20th day of a normal 28-day cycle, and, in all probability, until the next period is missed.'

2 *Single act of intercourse.* If this was *after* calculated ovulation, *the copper IUD method* may be inserted (if indicated at all) up to 5 days after that act. But exposure once only at say day x − 4 *before* ovulation occurring on day x, allows treatment at x + 5 days. (See 1 above).

3 *The Yuzpe and POEC methods.* There is an increase in the failure rate if treatment is initiated more than 72 hours after exposure. This does not mean the method is *absolutely* contraindicated later (see Q 7.8).

7.16 IS IT ALWAYS PREFERABLE TO TREAT AT THE EARLIEST POSSIBLE MOMENT?

1 *The IUD method* is so effective that delay (any time up to 5 days after ovulation) is unlikely to lead to failure, but would give no advantage.

2 *The Yuzpe and POEC hormonal methods.* Here the answer might be different according to whether the mechanism of action were by the blocking of ovulation or of implantation: but no study to date has disentangled the two mechanisms.

*Given the WHO data (Q 7.12(3)) it is best practice to **start** treatment as soon as the women presents. But there remains some flexibility according to the circumstances of presentation and the woman's own views (see Qs 7.8 and 7.9).*

7.17 WHAT REASONS MAY ACCOUNT FOR 'FAILURE' OF THE ORAL HORMONAL PREPARATIONS?

1 Treatment initiated *more than 72 hours after intercourse.*

2 *Unasked-about or unadmitted other exposure, earlier in the cycle.* It is essential always to question each woman most closely about the possibility of inadequate contraception during intercourse at any time *earlier* than the index event.

3 *Vomiting within 2 hours of tablet-taking.* This is an obvious *efficacy* as well as comfort advantage of POEC.

In practice it is a relatively rare cause of failure. Some authorities argue that there is no need to replace the second two tablets if they are vomited back, since the occurrence of vomiting implies a particularly strong pharmacological effect. Again, there are no data to support or refute that view.

Women should be instructed to contact the clinician for consideration of some action, particularly in a high pregnancy-risk case. Such action could be the provision of further tablets (as appropriate these may be given in advance), or rarely the insertion of an IUD.

4   *Non-compliance* leading to inadequate dosage. For this reason some clinicians prefer to see the first dose swallowed in their presence.

5   *Unprotected intercourse* subsequent to the treatment, which may simply postpone ovulation (see Q 7.6). In the real world, this raises the important question: should a planned long-term method, such as the COC or injectable, more often than currently be rightly started *immediately* after the emergency method? (See Q 7.40).

Points 2 and 5 are probably more common explanations than true method failures.

7.18 WHAT ARE THE RISKS IF THE EC TREATMENT FAILS?

This is a vitally important aspect of counselling, dealt with here and in Qs 7.19 and 7.20.

Ectopic pregnancy should be mentioned. Whenever any of the three methods operate at the uterine level, if the woman has pre-existing tubal damage (known or unknown), tubal implantation will clearly not be prevented. Additionally, there is the small possibility that the hormonal methods might interfere with tubal transport. This is disputed.

On the other hand, all the methods reduce the chance of fertilization, so the overall number of ectopics will certainly be reduced, even if the percentage among the pregnancies goes up (see Q 6.30).

Any woman may have tubal damage and since *she will be at risk with or without treatment*, it is safest to warn her to seek prompt advice if any pelvic pain occurs.

7.19 IF THE PREGNANCY IS IN THE UTERUS, WILL IT BE HARMED IN ANY WAY (HORMONAL METHODS)?

A small teratogenic risk cannot be ruled out since insufficient pregnancies have gone to term after hormonal EC treatment failure. In a series collected in the early 1990s by the UK National Association of Family Planning Doctors/Faculty of FP&RHC, there were 178 full-term pregnancies whose outcome was known. The rate of and distribution of abnormalities was reassuringly not different from what would be expected in a normal population, delivering without the previous (Yuzpe) EC therapy (G. Cardy, personal communication). Spontaneous reports to drug regulatory authorities similarly do not suggest any consistent teratogenic effect.

1   Moreover, even if there were a potential adverse effect, exposure will be negligible: if the hormonal methods are correctly used very little if any of the artificial hormone(s) could reach the blastocyst via the uterine secretions since it is not yet implanted. Also:
2   The blastocyst is very resistant to partial damage by noxious agents. Research in animals suggests that it is either destroyed or else, since its cells are 'totipotent', it can recover and develop entirely normally.
3   It is very much accepted clinical practice for women to continue to full term when they have taken the combined or progestagen-only pill for several weeks during organogenesis: a more critical time, and there would also be more exposure (see 1 above). Yet meta-analyses and registers of fetal abnormality have failed even in those circumstances to show any significant increase in major fetal abnormalities.

In practice, the woman can be told:

The risk of a pregnancy being harmed is believed to be extremely small, less than that when the ordinary pill is inadvertently taken in early pregnancy – but no one can ever be promised a normal baby (1 in 50 have an important birth defect). Research so far looking at babies born after failure of the emergency pill has not proved any harmful effects. The risk is so low that after failed EC an abortion should never be recommended solely on fetal grounds.

The circumstances of the failed postcoital conception mean that in practice most women request a therapeutic abortion. If a woman wishes to continue to full term, very detailed records should be kept to the effect that she has fully understood the arguments presented here and realizes that no guarantee can be given that the baby will be normal.

7.20 WHAT ABOUT FAILURE OF THE COPPER IUD METHOD?

In the ultra-rare event of continuing pregnancy following EC insertion of an IUD, management should normally include removal of the device after a preliminary ultrasound scan, as discussed at Q 6.25.
See also Qs 7.36 and 7.38.

INDICATIONS AND ADVANTAGES OF POSTCOITAL CONTRACEPTION

1   It provides a way of escape from an unwanted pregnancy at a time of high motivation after (for whatever reason) unprotected intercourse has taken place.
2   By definition it is non-intercourse-related.
3   All three methods are effective; the copper IUD most.
4   The methods can be applied well after exposure to the risk with a good chance of success: 3 days after if the hormone method is used, and in an extreme case up to 12 days (after exposure on, say, day 7), if an IUD is employed.
5   The methods are safe, though sharing the potential hazards of hormonal/intrauterine contraception respectively. No deaths have been reported.
6   Presentation for the EC treatment gives a welcome opportunity to discuss future contraception; in the case of the IUD, solving the woman's immediate problem can also provide for her long-term needs.
7   The method is under a woman's control (i.e. its use cannot be prevented by her partner, if she can find a sympathetic doctor).
8   The method can be prescribed in advance in many cases: for example, a young woman about to travel abroad and anxious about rape or other circumstances of unprotected intercourse in foreign parts.

Indeed if the POEC method is one day made 'over-the-counter', as I believe (with appropriate protocols and privacy) the evidence justifies, I am sure many women will sensibly ensure they have a course in advance of actual need.

NOTE: However: the present hormonal methods are not yet advised for regular ongoing use, for several reasons (see Q 7.44).

On presentation, depending on time of the cycle that exposure took place (see Q 7.14), whenever the clinician feels that the small risks of the metho are outweighed by the risks of pregnancy and other relevant factors such as the woman's level of anxiety.

7.23 HOW DO WOMEN PRESENT FOR TREATMENT?

No method used

1 '*Moonlight and roses*' summarizes the commonest presentation in this category, where intercourse was unpremeditated. It is often with a new partner, especially first-time ever intercourse or extramarital affairs (e.g. where the husband has had a vasectomy). Or there could have been an unexpected reconciliation with an ex-partner. Bound up in these situations is that saying 'sex is hot but contraception is cold'; something which if discussed would, the woman feels, make her out to be unromantic at best and at worst a slut. Even today and worldwide, far too few men consider that birth control is any of their business whatsoever.

2 Intercourse under the influence of *alcohol* or *drugs*.

3 Total misunderstanding of the '*safe period*' approach, or disregard of the mucus signs (or red light of Persona®, see Qs 1.28–1.29, and 7.33(7) below): these likewise equate to no method used.

4 Special situations:
   (a) *Rape and sexual assault.* Here counselling and management must be even more sensitive than usual and continuing emotional support is likely to be required. Involvement of the nearest Rape Crisis Centre and the local police force may be necessary. Avoid destroying forensic evidence if an accusation is to be made, and arrange tests and prophylaxis (and follow-up) for STIs.
   (b) *Incest.*
   (c) *Women with learning disorders* (taken advantage of).
   (d) *Recent use of teratogens* – drugs, or live vaccine such as polio or yellow fever.

Contraceptive failure (of the method or of its use)

1 The commonest category here is the *split or slipped condom.* In a study from the West Midlands no fewer than 48 out of 80 women reported a broken sheath. In more than one case a fragment of rubber was retrieved from the upper vagina, proving that not all such reports are fictions to appear respectable in the eyes of the provider.

> **NOTE:** In such cases always discuss whether the (rubber) condom might have been exposed to any mineral or vegetable oil (see Q 2.21)

2 Complete or partial *expulsion of an IUD*, identified midcycle. Here careful reinsertion of another IUD is preferable, especially if there has been repeated intercourse since the last menstrual period. But occasionally a hormone method might be preferred.

3 If there has been recent intercourse and deliberate *removal of an IUD* at midcycle is essential as part of therapy for infection (see Q 6.14).

4 *Errors of cap use* – e.g. the discovery after intercourse that it was in the anterior fornix; or its too-early removal.

5 Gross *prolongation of the pill-free week* in a COC-user. Normally through the pill-cycle, when intercourse has continued and pills are missed the woman should simply follow the 7-day rule at Qs 4.16–4.17. *However*, if the pill-free week has been extended to 9 or more days, or the equivalent, *meaning the prescriber evaluates the effect of some combination of missed pills during the first 7 days of a new pack as equivalent to such a 9-day PFI:* I recommend hormonal EC treatment, followed by immediate return to pill taking; and *also* the use of a condom for the next 7 days. (see Qs 4.15–4.25).

   What about midcycle or end-of-pill-cycle omissions?

   (a) Extra hormonal EC treatment is usually redundant for midcycle pill omissions, provided at least seven tablets were correctly taken; though the Faculty of FP&RHC suggests it be given empirically if four or more tablets were missed.

   (b) At the end of the pill-cycle the standard advice to run on to the next pack will nearly always make the woman contraceptively even safer than usual: having only had 'her own' PFI. However the history of missed pills (e.g. through a severe vomiting attack) may sometimes not emerge until after the next PFI has already been taken on top: and this *does* justify proceeding as at (5) above. See also Q 4.22.

6 *In a POP-user:* sexual exposure, any time from the first missed tablet (by 3 hours) until the mucus effect is expected to be restored after 48 hours, justifies hormone EC treatment, followed by 7 days' condom use. But not during full lactation (Q 5.24).

7 *Other contraceptive accidents* involving, for example, spermicides or unsuccessful withdrawal. Also if *injectables* have to be given late – see Q 5.133.

DISADVANTAGES OF POSTCOITAL CONTRACEPTION

7.24 WHAT ARE THE DISADVANTAGES?

The hormonal methods
1 Nausea, and vomiting (see also Q 7.27).
2 Failure rate (1–5%).
3 Contraindications – very few, see Q 7.28. *There is no age limit.*
4 Further unprotected intercourse following therapy must be avoided, in case of postponement of ovulation (see Q 7.6).
5 The next menses may sometimes be delayed (see Q 7.43).

Copper IUD
1 'A surgical' procedure involved – when what the woman is primarily requesting is a quick medical 'fix it'.
2 Pain may be caused to the woman at insertion or subsequently.
3 Risk of causing or exacerbating pelvic inflammatory disease (PID). Where the method must be used and the risk is high because of past infection or the circumstance of exposure (e.g. rape), then after the relevant tests – appreciating that the latter cannot identify *Chlamydia* for a minimum of 5 days after first exposure – antibiotic cover should be given (as at Qs 6.56–6.57).
4 There is a risk of causing all the other known complications of IUDs, since these are so often insertion-related (see Qs 6.22, 6.23 and 6.99).

7.25 WHAT IS THE INCIDENCE OF NAUSEA AND VOMITING AFTER THE CURRENTLY-USED HORMONAL METHODS?

With the Yuzpe hormonal method the frequency of nausea is high, 60% of 168 women studied at the MPC, though it was only slight or moderate in three-quarters of those with the symptom. It was also never prolonged beyond 36 hours, and usually lasted for less than 24 hours. Vomiting (most commonly once only) occurred in 24%, in the MPC study.

In the WHO 1998 study the incidence of these symptoms was as follows

Nausea:	Yuzpe 50.5%	POEC 23.1%
Vomiting:	Yuzpe 18.8%	POEC 5.6%

The POEC advantage here will promote effectiveness as well as the wellbeing of the client!

7.26 WHAT CAN BE DONE TO MINIMIZE THE NAUSEA/VOMITING PROBLEM? SHOULD ONE GIVE ANTIEMETICS?

1 In the first place, forewarned is forearmed; and we will I am sure increasingly be using POEC when other things are equal.
2 Where the timing of intercourse and presentation permit, the second dose should be followed by sleep if possible.
3 Some authorities have recommended the use of antiemetics (domperidone 10 mg with each Yuzpe dose is now proposed). It does not always successfully eliminate the symptom, which is also much rarer with POEC. Hence at MPC antiemetic treatment is given selectively, not routinely.

7.27 WHAT OTHER SYMPTOMS ARE ASSOCIATED WITH EC TREATMENT?

'Fatigue' was reported in the WHO 1998 study. Fairly commonly reported is breast tenderness, plus a range of other symptoms including dizziness, headaches, eye symptoms, etc. The association with therapy is not necessarily causal.

A few women report a 'withdrawal bleed' following treatment and the woman should be instructed not to assume that this is her next period (unless she was treated very late in the cycle), but to take advice.

PATIENT SELECTION AND CHOICE OF METHOD

7.28 WHAT ARE THE ABSOLUTE CONTRAINDICATIONS (WHO 4) TO EC CONTRACEPTION?

See Table 7.1 (page 431).

All methods

• *Pregnancy.* The presence of an early implanted pregnancy may be difficult to eliminate; but every effort should be made by taking a careful history, doing a vaginal examination and where indicated the most sensitive pregnancy test available.

- *Allergy to a constituent*: i.e. levonorgestrel, or ethinyloestradiol or an excipient in the tablets, or to copper (Q 6.87).
- *Patient's ethical objection (if present) to a method possibly operating post-fertilization*. **NB** This need not apply if she presents at risk early in the cycle.

Hormonal methods
POEC
1 Acute porphyria, with past attack (WHO 4). Predisposition is WHO 3 (Qs 4.218–4.219). Other porphyrias are WHO 3 or 2.
2 Severe liver disease with abnormal function tests (WHO 3).

YUZPE
All of above, including porphyrias, are WHO 4 – plus:
3 Current headache in a sufferer from migraine with focal aura.
4 Past significant venous or arterial thrombosis.
5 Current sickle cell crisis.

There is no upper age limit (given sufficient risk of conception) – *either method*.

Non-hormonal method – IUDs
a *The three bullets above* apply.
b The majority of both the temporary and permanent *absolute* contraindications listed at Qs 6.84–6.85 would also be held to apply. However, it is acceptable practice in selected cases to insert a copper IUD with screening and full antibiotic cover (see Q 7.24) when PID has not been excluded; or in women at high risk (especially after rape).

If the IUD method is thought inappropriate for long-term use (e.g. in a nullipara who has had a previous ectopic pregnancy), it can always be removed following the next period.

For long-term use by a young woman, the Nova T would not be a good choice (Q 6.94).

7.29 WHAT ARE NOT CONTRAINDICATIONS TO THE USE OF THE HORMONAL METHODS?

1 Presentation *more than 72 hours* after unprotected intercourse. This is still an option since self-evidently the hormonal method's efficacy does

not disappear precisely at 72 hours. These methods are usable (though with less efficacy) on the same basis as the copper IUD, i.e. up to 5 days after calculated ovulation. NB. But see Q 7.8.

2   *Previous ectopic pregnancy* (see Q 7.18).

3   *Postpartum:* if there exists an ovulation risk, which may anyway be negligible if the LAM criteria apply (Q 1.36), there need be no worries about increased risk of thrombosis with the Yuzpe combined method by that time (see Q 4.49). Either method is also usable (WHO 3) if hCG is persistent following trophoblastic disease (Q 4.75).

The woman can be reassured that the short-term hormonal methods should not impair *lactation*. She maybe concerned to avoid the vanishingly small but unquantified risk through the artificial hormones entering her breast milk (and a female infant might get a withdrawal bleed with the Yuzpe method). This can usually be done without prejudicing lactation by expressing the breast milk and bottlefeeding the infant for 24 hours.

7.30 WHAT IF A WOMAN TAKING AN ENZYME-INDUCING DRUG SHOULD REQUIRE HORMONAL EMERGENCY CONTRACEPTION?

See Qs 4.34–4.36 for a full discussion of this important question in relation to regular use of the COC. The solution here according to Professor Back is simply to increase the dose of either method by 50%. In other words, six tablets of PC4 or Ovran would be taken in divided doses 12 hours apart; or three tablets of 'Postinor'; or no less than 75 tablets of Microval/Norgeston in similar divided doses!

7.31 WHAT IF SHE IS ON A NON-ENZYME-INDUCING ANTIBIOTIC?

Obviously there is not even a theoretical problem if she has taken it for more than 2 weeks, because of antibiotic resistance (see Qs 4.34–4.35), or with POEC. But Professor Back advises no action even if that treatment started more recently: the sheer size of the dose of the combined EC method will compensate in his view for any tiny effect of the antibiotic.

7.32 WHAT ARE THE RELATIVE CONTRAINDICATIONS TO EC IUD INSERTION?

1   All the relative contraindications listed at Q 6.86 might apply if it is intended that the method will be used long term, but some (e.g. history of dysmenorrhoea or menorrhagia) are irrelevant to the very short-term

option, just until the time of the next period with initiation of a different long-term method thereafter (see also Q 7.28).

2 *Past ectopic pregnancy*. Even in nulliparae this is only a weak relative contraindication (WHO 2) to very short-term use in selected cases (Q 7.18) – and only WHO 2 or 3 for long-term use of *banded* copper IUDs (Q 6.33).

7.33 SINCE THE MAJORITY OF WOMEN PRESENTING FOR EC PREFER AND EXPECT ORAL TREATMENT, WHEN SHOULD THE INTRAUTERINE METHOD BE OFFERED INSTEAD?

As the question implies, one of the hormonal methods is the normal first choice *except* where there are special reasons for a copper IUD. These are:

1 *The woman's desire to use the IUD as her long-term method* – could be a very good indication in an older ± parous woman for instance. However it is always permissible and sometimes to be recommended that the device is used purely to solve the immediate problem, and removed at the next menses: (this also means screening and antibiotic cover, see Q 7.28(b)).

2 Where she desires the *most effective* available option, which this is.

3 Where there is an *absolute contraindication to oestrogen* (only applies to Yuzpe – POEC usable), or *progestagen* (i.e. allergy, acute porphyria, very severe liver disease).

4 Where there has been *multiple exposure*, and the clinician inserts the device in good faith no more than 5 days after the most probable calculated ovulation date (see Q 7.15 and below).

5 Where presentation is *more than 72 hours* since a single episode of unprotected intercourse (the upper time-limit being 5 days – but it could be considerably longer so long as the calculation for the day of implantation (length of shortest likely cycle, subtract 14 and add 5 days) does not mean the treatment might be given to an implanted pregnancy).

(In cases 4, 5 above a hormonal method might also be used, relying solely on the anti-implantation effect therefrom: but with much less assurance of efficacy – see Q 7.8).

6 Rarely, after *vomiting of the tablets* when either the Yuzpe or POEC regimen was initially selected. IUD insertion is only indicated if she is a high pregnancy risk case and if the vomiting occurs within 2 hours of the woman ingesting a dose, especially the first dose. Otherwise additional tablets may be given, *maybe along with an antiemetic* (Q 7.26).

7 Rarely, in a woman who has taken a risk but wants to go back to *using Persona®* – and does not wish to wait the added 2 months-plus after taking hormones before she can return to use of that method (Q 1.29).

COUNSELLING AND MANAGEMENT AT THE FIRST VISIT

7.34 HOW IMPORTANT IS COUNSELLING FOR EC?

The treatment is simple and very safe (especially POEC, which has almost no contraindications). Obviously if there has been a simple condom rupture or dislodgement occurring in a stable relationship the amount of emotional support required will be far less than in cases of rape or incest – although the availability of such support should always be clear.

Every woman in this situation is under some stress, and needs information and clear instructions sympathetically given. In practice much of the information can be conveyed by a good leaflet and the counselling – including on the crucial subject of future contraception – most appropriately delegated to a family planning-trained nurse.

With Group Protocols, nurses including School nurses, are at last being enabled to take on the whole emergency contraception workload, which indeed they usually do better than doctors.

In future non-doctor supply (possibly over-the-counter) may be approved, increasing availability and uptake. Even so certain specific safeguards will be important (Q 7.44).

7.35 IN SUMMARY, WHAT ASPECTS SHOULD BE COVERED IN TAKING THE MEDICAL HISTORY?

1 Date of the last menstrual period, and whether it was in any way abnormal.
2 Details of the patient's normal menstrual cycles – shortest, longest and most usual lengths.
3 The calculated date of ovulation.
4 The day(s) in the cycle of *all* unprotected intercourse.
5 The number of hours since the *first* episode of unprotected intercourse.
6 The current method of contraception – Persona® is particularly relevant (Qs 7.129(3) and 7.33). In pill-takers who have missed pills the timing relative to the PFI is critical (Q 7.23(5)).

7 Any contraindications (from the history) to either type of EC treatment (see Qs 7.28–7.33). The past history should include use of enzyme inducers (Q 7.30), all risk factors for the COC since it may be going to be used in future, and any past PID or ectopic pregnancy.

It should be stressed to the woman that the whole 'contract' to give this kind of treatment depends on utmost mutual good faith and honesty, especially concerning the menstrual/coital history.

7.36 WHAT ARE THE TEN MAIN POINTS TO COVER IN COUNSELLING FOR EMERGENCY CONTRACEPTION?

1 Assess the menstrual and coital history as in Q 7.35, and hence whether any treatment is necessary.
2 Discuss the methods available and their mode of action and medical risks.
3 The failure rate of each method, and the implications: i.e. the (almost non-existent) risk of fetal abnormality (see Q 7.19), and of ectopic pregnancy (see Qs 7.18 and 7.29).
4 Explore her attitudes to possible failure of the regimen and continuance of the pregnancy.
5 Discuss the consequential importance of follow-up – and the possibility that her next period might require medical assessment. Suggest that she brings an early morning urine sample if it is surprisingly light or absent.
6 Make the final decision about whether to use EC treatment, and which method, only after full discussion with her.
7 If a hormonal method is selected advise her regarding nausea and vomiting. She should telephone the clinic or surgery for advice if she vomits within 2 hours of either dose. (Or she may be given extra tablets in advance). Consider domperidone (Q 7.26).
8 Discuss contraception in the current cycle (see Q 7.6) – not a problem if the IUD is used.
9 Discuss long-term contraception. See Q 7.39 for the advice to be given if the combined pill is selected.
10 Keep an accurate record, written at the time, dated and signed, especially if unlicensed use (e.g. POEC treatment at all, use of either hormone method more than once per cycle or beyond 72 hours).

7.37 SHOULD THESE WOMEN ALWAYS BE EXAMINED VAGINALLY?

In my view the answer is *normally* 'no', the anxiety so caused for example to a young teenager presenting after her first-ever sexual experience rules it out. But there may be a clinical indication:

1 To exclude a concealed (advanced) clinical pregnancy.
2 Pelvic tenderness or a purulent discharge suggestive of infection may be discovered.
3 Microbiological samples can be taken, especially for *Chlamydia*.
4 Suitability for an IUD can be assessed.
5 Finally, *a baseline is established*: e.g. if an irregular outline of the uterus is noted (suggesting small fibroids) this will assist any follow-up examination. The latter also is only required if clinically indicated (see Q 7.42).

Women receiving a hormonal method should normally also have their baseline blood pressure measured.

7.38 SHOULD THE WOMAN BE ASKED TO SIGN ANY TYPE OF CONSENT FORM?

This is unnecessary provided accurate contemporaneous records are kept, the clinician asserting that the woman gave verbal informed consent. It is most helpful to supplement the counselling with an appropriate leaflet (see Q 4.101 and Fig. 7.2, page 436–7).

FOLLOW-UP

7.39 IF THE WOMAN SELECTS AN ORAL CONTRACEPTIVE SUBSEQUENT TO EC TREATMENT, WHEN SHOULD SHE TAKE THE FIRST TABLET?

It is usual for both the COC and the POP to be commenced on the first day of the next menses. However, there is sometimes a light (and not relevant) withdrawal bleed just after the Yuzpe hormones, and a light 'threatened abortion' loss may also occur very early in pregnancy. It has been MPC practice, therefore, that both the COC and POP should be started on about the second day, when the woman is convinced that the flow is within her own normal range. This slight delay still allows the woman not to be required to use extra contraceptive precautions (see Q 4.49 (Table 4.4) and Q 5.26).

It is important however to ensure this advice does not make her delay beyond Day 3 before starting the COC or POP without extra condom use for 7 days.

7.40 MIGHT SHE BE INSTRUCTED TO START THE COMBINED PILL OR INJECTABLE IMMEDIATELY FOLLOWING PC TREATMENT?

This may indeed be acceptable. There is a medicolegal concern: if the woman were to conceive, and the baby have an important fetal abnormality (as occurs in 2% of cases), a legal claim that the abnormality was caused by the extra packet of combined pills being given after implantation might be submitted. It would, of course, be highly unlikely that such an abnormality was truly caused by the COC (see Q 4.222) or injectable. However, it would be less unlikely than teratogenesis caused by the Yuzpe or POEC regimens alone, given, as they should only be, pre-implantation (Q 7.19).

There are certain circumstances in which this may be acceptable management, provided there has been a thorough and documented discussion of all the implications with the woman concerned – especially in a case where the risk of EC treatment failing is considered to be particularly low. According to the WHO 1998 study, POEC when given in the first 24 hours only has a 0.4% failure rate. One could argue in many cases, therefore, that the risk of conception through poor condom use before the next period easily outweighs the tiny risk of teratogenesis from one course of contraceptive hormone treatment (COC or DMPA) in early pregnancy, when conception using that immediate start policy is so very unlikely.

We need a proper RCT of this, though, comparing (for all relevant outcomes) immediate starting versus starting at the next menses!

See also Q 7.23(5): if the PFI has been lengthened an immediate (re-) start of the COC would already be the normal proposal: so long as it has not been so prolonged as to risk an implanted pregnancy already being present.

7.41 WHAT SHOULD BE DONE IF A WOMAN HAS ALREADY RECEIVED EC TREATMENT AND RETURNS 3 OR 4 DAYS LATER REPORTING CONDOM RUPTURE DURING THE LATEST INTERCOURSE? MAY ONE USE THE HORMONE EC REGIMENS MORE THAN ONCE IN A GIVEN CYCLE?

Yes. Since in clinical practice we cannot be sure when ovulation occurs, and it may have been postponed by the earlier treatment, it may well be right to represcribe, for a second or even a third time. Even three Yuzpe treatments in a month is only the same as one packet of Microgynon; and as used in Hungary Postinor has for many years been recommended for use postcoitally up to four times per month.

The main problem is attempting to exclude the possibility of early conception already present (implantation having already occurred through exposure earlier in the cycle). Irregular bleeding may also follow. And once again this is an unlicensed use (Appendix 1, page 507).

7.42 HOW IMPORTANT IS IT TO FOLLOW-UP EC WOMEN AFTER TREATMENT?

A defined follow-up visit is ideal, normally set for 3–4 weeks post-treatment, but not now insisted on after hormonal EC if the next period comes on normally.

Advice should be given, backed by a leaflet, that the woman should be sure to return:

- if her menses are delayed by more than one week. A pregnancy test may then be necessary and, if there is any clinical doubt, especially concerning an ectopic, a pelvic examination;
- if she has any worrying symptoms, particularly pain or irregular bleeding;
- to continue ongoing contraceptive care – in all cases if she has been fitted with a copper IUD. Beware of the pressure that there may sometimes be to 'leave well alone' in circumstances in which the IUD is a poor choice for long-term use (see Qs 6.83–6.86 and 7.28(b)). The original and better plan to transfer to another method (such as DMPA) may need to be encouraged.

If the method fails, good pregnancy counselling should follow. There is no real difference in the content of this counselling from that when any other method of birth control has failed (see Q 7.19). Unless the woman is having a termination, if she is pregnant with an IUD in position the device should normally be gently removed (see Qs 6.25 and 6.26).

Most important, the woman must be clear that she is free to return without an appointment should an untoward symptom arise, particularly low abdominal pain or heavy bleeding.

7.43 WHAT IS THE USUAL TIME OF ONSET OF THE NEXT PERIOD AFTER EC TREATMENT?

This is variable with the Yuzpe regimen. Among 45 women treated successfully at the MPC, the next period began on the expected date (± 1 day) in 22% and was up to or more than a week early in 62%. Only in 16% of women was the next period 2–6 days late. It is believed that late onset is more likely when treatment was early enough in the cycle to postpone ovulation. When it acts to block implantation the method tends to bring the next period on early, whether or not there is withdrawal bleeding immediately after the treatment (the latter being quite uncommon). It is useful to be able to tell the woman that her next period is likely to be on time or early, so she will not need to be in suspense for too long.

No obvious impact on cycle length has been reported following postcoital IUD insertion.

7.44 WHAT ARE THE OBJECTIONS TO THE POEC OR YUZPE METHODS BEING AVAILABLE IN ADVANCE FOR USE ON A REGULAR BASIS?

1 The treatment would have to be given after each act of intercourse and many women could finish up having taken more hormones than if they simply took the COC daily for 21 days. But repeating either hormonal regimen is certainly acceptable as a short-term expedient (see Q 7.41); also advance prescription of one-off treatment may often be justifiable (see Q 7.21(8)).
2 The concern that this would lead to non-use of regular contraception has been to some extent allayed by a randomized comparative study headed by Dr Anna Glasier in Scotland, and reported in 1998. Very few of the treatment group given a replaceable supply of the Yuzpe regimen used it more than once, and during the one year of study similar numbers in each group transferred to using more reliable oral contraception.
3 Neither hormone method is effective enough to be recommended for use on a regular long-term basis. Even the POEC method only stops seven out of eight of the pregnancies that would otherwise happen every month.

Nevertheless, many women who request regular emergency contraception are those who have intercourse once a month or less, on a rather unpredictable basis. Increasing availability should reduce the unacceptable continuing high rate of unplanned pregnancies.

7.45 SO WHAT IS YOUR VIEW ON EC BEING AVAILABLE OVER THE COUNTER?

Especially with the arrival of POEC, having fewer side-effects than the Yuzpe method and almost no contraindications, I consider that the advantages of over-the counter supply of EC would definitely outweigh its risks.

But the following should be ensured, as minimum requirements:

- Excellent user-friendly labelling/leaflet and check-list of important information for the client.
- A good protocol, for the pharmacist to follow (after training).
- Adequate privacy.
- Easy arrangements for transfer for the insertion of a copper IUD as sometimes indicated.
- Easy arrangements for long-term contraceptive follow-up (via clinic, or family doctor) and to investigate STIs as required.
- A 24-hour telephone hot-line for clients' queries.
- Parallel free NHS supply for those who might not be able to afford the retail product.

7.46 WHAT WOULD BE THE FEATURES OF AN IDEAL EC?

These would be similar to those of any reversible birth control method (see Q 0.15), but the following aspects would require particular emphasis. The ideal EC treatment would:

1 be so effective each month that on a cumulative basis the annual rate of failures was less than 1/100 woman-years (cf. Q 7.12);
2 be effective for the remainder of each cycle as well as in relation to the particular act of intercourse (see Q 7.6);
3 require only a single dose;
4 have no contraindications (at all) – POEC gets very close!
5 have a very low incidence of side-effects, whether dangerous or annoying (such as nausea);
6 cause no disturbance of the menstrual cycle;
7 be free of teratogenic effects.

7.47 WHAT ARE THE PROSPECTS FOR THE FUTURE OF EC?

A really reliable post-ovulatory contraceptive agent with the features in Q 7.46, coupled with a simple and reliable method of determining whether the exposure had been before or after ovulation, would be a considerable advance. Indeed, in the distant future it might be possible for regular release of an EC agent (e.g. from an implant) to be actually triggered by a biological event such as the LH surge.

Another potential approach, though one fraught with ethical and legal difficulties, is the regular use of a post-conceptional or *contragestive* agent to be administrated only when the woman is just overdue her period. Given average fertility this approach would mean exposure to the potential systemic risks of the agent only on a few (4–6) occasions each year; but it would be out of order for many, through being a regular early abortion.

7.48 SPECIFICALLY WHAT AGENTS ARE BEING STUDIED?

1   The greatest current interest is in progesterone receptor blocking agents, such as *RU 486* (*mifepristone*). A single 10 mg dose proved as effective as the 600 mg medical termination of pregnancy dose, when given up to 5 days after a single coital exposure (RCT by WHO, Lancet 1999). Vomiting occurred in only 1.7%. The main problem was postponement of (potentially fertile) ovulation, with 7+ days of delay in the next menses in 18% of cases.

2   Single dose POEC is therefore being tested in an RCT against 10 mg mifepristone.

3   Many of us would be particularly interested in a product, perhaps an injectable, able to be applied up to implantation, which also gave ongoing long-term contraception thereafter (on the model of copper IUD insertion).

QUESTIONS ASKED BY PROSPECTIVE USERS OF POSTCOITAL CONTRACEPTION

7.49 IS THE 'EMERGENCY PILL' THE SAME AS THE 'MORNING AFTER PILL'?

Yes, it is. The reason for the new name is that the treatment (though best started in the first 24 hours) can be given much later than the morning after – at least 72 hours, and after many days if the IUD method is chosen. So the old name was extremely misleading. It should be abandoned!

7.50 ISN'T THE EMERGENCY PILL JUST THE SAME AS THE CONTRACEPTIVE PILL?

One emergency pill contains the same two hormones as in a combined pill, the other is the same single hormone as one of the POPs. But both are given in a different way, i.e. in two larger doses, 12 hours apart, following intercourse.

7.51 IF IT IS SO SIMILAR, WHY DO DOCTORS KEEP THE TREATMENT HIDDEN AWAY? IF MY SEX LIFE IS ERRATIC, WHY CAN I NOT BE GIVEN PILLS IN ADVANCE FOR USE ON A REGULAR BASIS?

An answer to this common question is given at Q 7.44 and 7.45. There are some special reasons it should not be used at all by some women, or why the alternative IUD method would be medically preferable (see Qs 7.28 and 7.33).

However, since the POEC pill method, especially, is so remarkably safe, and there is such an epidemic of unplanned pregnancies in many countries, the benefits would outweigh the risks if it were much more available, e.g. over the counter, supervised by pharmacists. I have a lot of sympathy with this idea, given definite safeguards and the availability of medical back-up (Q 7.45).

7.52 I SHALL BE TRAVELLING ALONE IN THE FAR EAST AND SOUTH AMERICA FOR THE NEXT 6 MONTHS. COULD I TAKE A SUPPLY OF EC TREATMENT FOR EMERGENCY USE?

In this situation, providing there are no contraindications for you to use the method at all, it would certainly be appropriate for you to be prescribed a supply in advance (see Q 7.44). You might, alternatively, consider arranging first a regular method like the pill or even an IUD.

7.53 CAN I WAIT A FEW HOURS FOR MY OWN OR THE DOCTOR'S CONVENIENCE, OR SHOULD I BE TREATED JUST AS SOON AS POSSIBLE?

There should not be any undue delay; treatment in the first 24 hours is best. Certainly there is no need to disturb the doctor within a few minutes or an hour of intercourse! See also Q 7.9 regarding the timing of the second dose.

7.54 SHOULD I MENTION ANY EARLIER TIMES WHEN WE MADE LOVE (SINCE MY LAST PERIOD), WHEN I ATTEND THE DOCTOR FOR MORNING-AFTER TREATMENT?

Yes this is essential. The decisions as to whether to treat and how to treat successfully all depend on your being entirely forthcoming about every relevant fact. This also includes telling the nurse/doctor the correct date of your last period. The whole 'contract' between you and him/her depends on what is called 'utmost good faith'.

7.55 WILL I NEED TO BE EXAMINED BEFORE EC TREATMENT?

Usually not – see Q 7.37.

7.56 WHY MIGHT THE DOCTOR DECIDE NOT TO TREAT ME, IF I ATTEND FOR EC TREATMENT?

The main reason might be that, after considering the time of the month and every other aspect, your doctor judges that there is an almost-nil risk of conception occurring; and that this does not justify the (small) risks of the EC treatment. This would apply especially when COC pills have been missed in the middle or at the end of a packet.

7.57 WHAT SHOULD I DO IF I VOMIT WITHIN 2 HOURS OF EITHER OF MY DOSES, ESPECIALLY IF I ACTUALLY BRING BACK SOME OF THE PILLS?

Take the urgent advice of your doctor. If he or she thinks that there is a high risk of conception in your case, it may be right then to insert an IUD. But more usually it will be enough just to give you additional tablets, or even no special treatment at all (see Q 7.17).

7.58 WHY DID THE DOCTOR/NURSE RECOMMEND A COPPER IUD FOR ME WHEN I REALLY WANTED PILLS?

For one of the reasons in Q 7.33. This could then be a good method for you to continue using long term; but remember that you can instead have it removed after your next period, if you then plan perhaps to transfer to another effective method such as the combined pill.

7.59 WHY SHOULD I USE ANOTHER METHOD OF FAMILY PLANNING BETWEEN EC TREATMENT AND THE START OF MY NEXT PERIOD?

The reason is that sometimes the method may be working not by blocking the fertilized egg from establishing itself in your womb, but instead by blocking egg release. There is then the risk of fertilizing that later egg if your partner does not use another method such as the condom.

7.60 SHOULD I EXPECT A PERIOD IMMEDIATELY AFTER USING EC PILLS?

A few women get what is known as 'a withdrawal bleed' within a day or two of the treatment. This will not seem like a proper period and, unless you were due one, it is important to continue using the condom or any other effective method you were recommended to use, until you have a definite period – or until you are seen for follow-up at the clinic. Fortunately, your proper period normally arrives either on time or a little early. It is still best that you keep your follow-up appointment(s), and this is even more vital if the next period is delayed or unexpectedly light.

7.61 FOR WHAT REASONS SHOULD I SEE THE DOCTOR SOONER THAN ARRANGED, FOLLOWING EC TREATMENT?

The main reason would be because of any pain in your abdomen, because of the small risk of pregnancy in your tube (see Q 7.18).

7.62 DOES MORNING-AFTER TREATMENT CAUSE AN ABORTION?

No, not according to the modern view of when pregnancy starts (see Q 7.2 and Fig. 7.1).

7.63 MUST I HAVE AN ABORTION IF EC TREATMENT FAILS?

Not necessarily. It is thought that this treatment will not significantly increase the risk of an abnormal baby above the surprisingly high 2% risk that all women run. So the decision (always very difficult) about what to do about the unplanned pregnancy is really just the same as it would be if an other method of family planning were to fail, such as the pill (see Q 7.19).

8 Conspectus: present and future

As intended, and mentioned in the Preface, this book has been primarily about how best to select and use the existing reversible birth control technology. *The rather brief discussion of related subjects does not imply that they are unimportant.* See also Further Reading!

This chapter includes much that is useful revision of the information elsewhere in the text. I am particularly indebted to Toni Belfield, Director of Information of the UK Family Planning Association (FPA). She has allowed me to use sections of her own text from a 1992 article in the *British Journal of Sexual Medicine*, but supplemented and much rearranged in this book's question-and-answer style.

8.1 WHAT FACTORS INFLUENCE THE OBSERVED GREAT VARIABILITY IN THE CHOICES OF CONTRACEPTIVE METHODS ACTUALLY MADE BY COUPLES?

Please refer to Figure 8.1 and Table 8.1, along with Tables 0.1 (see Q 0.16) and 0.2 (regarding failure rates).

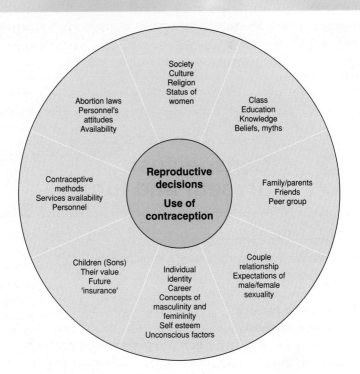

Figure 8.1 Reproductive decisions – The Factors Wheel. (Courtesy Elphis Christopher). See Q 8.1 and Appendix 2.

The relative importance of the two main factors – maximum *health safe* as opposed to maximum *effectiveness* and independence from *intercourse* – and hence the appropriateness of different methods, varies greatly according to all the factors shown in Dr Christopher's 'Factors Wheel' (Figure 8.1 and see also Appendix 2).

Choice, it seems, is seldom based on rational or objective information – the fact that a friend had a dreadful time with an IUD will weigh far more heavily than any amount of statistics that show this is not usually the case. It is also influenced by age and stage during an individual couple's reproductive lifetime. Decisions are made at specific times:

- At the beginning of sexual experience.
- After an accidental pregnancy or 'near-miss'.
- With life changes, e.g. a career change.

TABLE 8.1 THE SEVEN CONTRACEPTIVE AGES OF WOMEN

Age	Suggested method
0 Birth to puberty	No method required. Responsible sex education is essential
1 Puberty to marriage	Either (a) a barrier method; (b) the combined pill/new male or female hormone or peptide options/injectable/implant, but often with a condom or, if available, an effective chemical virucide as well; or, if acceptable; (c) abstinence until the final life-partner is found The choice depends on factors like religious views, perceived risk of sexually transmitted diseases, the steadiness of the relationship, and frequency of intercourse
2 Marriage to first child	First choice probably a pill, but could be one of various injectables/implants followed by a fertility awareness/barrier method for some months before 'trying' for the first child
3 During breast-feeding	Either lactational amenorrhoea method or any progestagen-only method or reversible male method with breastfeeding or a simple barrier method. Intrauterine device or system, male or female injectable or implant likely to be appropriate only if a long gap is expected between pregnancies
4 Family spacing after breast-feeding	Continue with any method started during 'age' 3, or shift to the combined pill/injectable/implant from a progestagen-only pill for greater effectiveness. Later, an intrauterine device or system is progressively more appropriate, for a combination of the least long-term health hazards, efficacy and reversibility
5 After the (probable) last child	The first choice is an intrauterine device or system; other possibilities are the progestagen-only pill, or the combined pill, if free of arterial or venous factors, or injectable/implant according to choice
6 Family complete, family growing up	Vasectomy or female sterilization. If the woman wishes to avoid surgery, or is troubled by heavy or painful periods, it might be more logical to use the intrauterine system instead of sterilization
7 Perimenopausal (no sterilization)	Contraceptive hormone replacement therapy will become more available (continuous combined methods being the norm, such as the intrauterine system plus estrogen implant). It is important to recognize that, at this age, weaker contraceptives (e.g. foam) may be fully effective when combined with very reduced fertility

- After a planned birth.
- When there are problems with a particular method.
- When the family is complete.

Initially, while the relationship is being established, a high degree of efficacy may be considered most important. However if their sexual experience is infrequent or sporadic, barrier methods may be ideal provided they are used correctly, especially as they have the bonus of some protection against sexually transmitted diseases (STIs).

For child spacing, less efficient methods with reduced health risk may well be preferred. Once the family is established, but the couple are not sure whether it is yet complete, the IUD can have particular merit. These points are summarized in Table 8.1, which is derived from Table 15 of my book *The Pill* and also looks forward to the near *future*.

This changing pattern of reproductive desire, in the couple's total life situation, places a big responsibility on the doctor or nurse to be themselves flexible and fully informed about the whole range of methods available. *They must also be able and willing to spend time finding out who they are actually dealing with* under the headings summarized in Figure 8.1!

COMPLIANCE WITH CONTRACEPTIVE METHODS

8.2 DO NOT THE WORDS 'COMPLIANT' AND 'NON-COMPLIANT' SOUND RATHER 'BOSSY', AND AS THOUGH WE PRESCRIBE AND THEN EVERYTHING ELSE IS THOSE SILLY CONTRACEPTIVE-USERS FAULT?

Yes: but if we can ourselves agree not to mean anything of the sort, there are no simpler words alluding to the user's responsibility in avoidance of user-failure. More on the provider's responsibility follows later.

Regardless of whatever professional hat we wear, we are all consumers when it comes to thinking about or using contraception. But *how* contraception is *considered*, *discussed* and, more importantly, *delivered* will determine just how well it is accepted and used.

8.3 HOW BIG IS THE PROBLEM?

Today contraceptive choices and services are freely available, and research shows that people have the facts (in their heads) about contraception. Yet unintended pregnancy and requests for abortion remain persistently high.

Abstinence, that most effective of all methods, applies in recent surveys to less than half of all girls who were 16 at their last birthday (just 48% claimed to be virgins in a 1991 study from the South-west of England, and only 12% by age 20). Given the potential emotional and psychosocial trauma, quite apart from the risk of STIs and cervical neoplasia, this group (and the boys too), should receive our encouragement, as providers, to continue resisting peer-group pressure; i.e. that it really is worth *waiting* for 'Mr or Miss Right'. They should not be labelled a *minority* group, since this has an implication of abnormality. Yet, in the real world, the remainder do need confidential and appropriate family planning services.

Although the under 16s achieve more publicity, the older teenagers and women aged 20–25 are together responsible for far more unplanned pregnancies. A 1991 study of recent mothers by Anne Fleissig showed that in the UK as many as one in three of the last pregnancies was unplanned. In the same year it was estimated in *Population Trends* that one in five clinical pregnancies ended in legal abortion. Cumulatively, about one woman in three in the UK now has at least one termination before the age of 30.

In another 1991 study of teenage mothers 84% had no intention to become pregnant, but were using no contraception when they conceived. ... Although in some studies where there *was* good compliance, the combined oral contraceptive (COC) has had failure rates which were well below 1/100 woman-years (Table 0.2), in typical use failure rates of 3% are commonly reported, rising to up to 20% in inner city areas. Worldwide, it has been calculated that if by improved pill taking we could reduce the failure rate of this one method by 1%, at least 630 000 fewer women would have accidental pregnancies each year.

8.4 WHAT IS THE MOST IMPORTANT SINGLE REASON FOR UNWANTED CONCEPTIONS?

Sex! But not just in the obvious way. See the God–Adam joke on page 17...

1   Sex is embarrassing. Contraception is inextricably linked with emotional and sexual well-being, and it is impossible to talk about contraception without addressing sexuality – the two are inseparable. Research shows that contraception continues to be a source of considerable embarrassment and anxiety for both men and women, and this has implications for its uptake and usage. It can have an inhibiting effect on people's willingness to seek information and advice from professionals.

2   Also, in Elphis Christopher's memorable phrase (see Appendix 2), 'sex is hot, and contraception is cold'. Snowden wrote in 1990 that whil[e] it may be argued that the prevention of pregnancy is beneficial, the use of contraception is not a pleasant experience for most people, which is a[?] marked contrast to the sexual behaviour which prompts its need! Actua[l] choice results from a negative process of 'seeking the least bad' among the options. The methods not chosen are even more disliked than the method that is chosen.

3   And sex is *now*, the possible problems seem unimportant. Head knowledg[e] can be superb without affecting behaviour in the heat of the moment. The[?] brain and the genitalia are not used at the same time (page 17)!

Risk-taking and AIDS are not unlike risk-taking and pregnancy. Neither AIDS infection nor fertilization are certain, the gambler often survives, and the penalty is remote: 9 months in the case of pregnancy, maybe years in the case of AIDS.'

(Malcolm Potts, 1988)

So like safer sex the built-in problem of family planning is the 'planning bit'.

This highlights the potential advantages of the postcoital methods. But the potential may not be realized. A 1992 study by Nigel Bruce of unplanned pregnancies in North London showed that more than half of those who could have sought such emergency help because they (a) knew about it and (b) knew there had been a contraceptive risk, did not do so! Asked why, the reason given amounted to that they 'had got away with it before'. ...

So, strong in matters of sex is the gambling instinct! plus inertia. ...

4   The early years of reproductive life are not that fertile, through anovulation. In the first year after the menarche 85% of cycles are anovular, but this falls to an average of 30% after 5 years. So young people's experience of 'getting away with it' in early years is likely to catch them out a little later, as their fertility peaks in the late teens and early 20s.

5   Finally, 'the fact that contraception has to do with sex seems to set up an environment where risks are exaggerated or misunderstood' (Malcolm Potts). So 'sex' even explains some of the *risk illiteracy* of our clients about (say) the pill ... ordinary, unprotected, sex and even the cigarette that follows all seem so natural and safe by comparison!

8.5 IN THE MANY STUDIES OF COMPLIANCE IN DEVELOPED COUNTRIES, WHAT ARE THE BACKGROUND FACTORS THAT HAVE BEEN SHOWN TO CORRELATE WITH NON-USE OR POOR USE OR EARLY DISCONTINUATION OF CONTRACEPTIVE METHODS?

Here is a list, longish but doubtless not complete, relating mainly to the COC:

- Young, immature. Youth after the very first years means also optimum fertility, hence a greater likelihood of not getting away with any of the more frequent compliance errors. According to Jones and Forrest in 1989, failure rates of the pill in the first 12 months of use are more than five times higher in the under-20s compared with the 35–44 age group.
- Unmarried.
- Nulliparous.
- Early coitarche.
- Multiple sexual partners.
- Previous contraceptive failure/abortion, or:
- Perception of low personal risk of conception (especially because of previous 'scares' which resolved).
- Erratic daily timetable
- Cultural or religious opposition to birth control.
- Poor social conditions.
- Parents not married.
- Lack of parental support.
- Low evaluation of personal health.
- Low educational attainment and goals.
- Feelings of lack of personal self-worth and self-determination.
- Feelings of *fatalism* (babies happen, rather like death, 'when your number comes up').
- Cigarette smoking (unplanned conception more likely, but in several studies of young teenagers *also* likely to start sexual activity younger).
- Alcohol: 'Drink in – wits out!' 53% of 16–24 year olds in an SW England study felt they were more likely to forget about the risk of pregnancy after drinking alcohol. The same applies to other drugs of addiction.
- Media 'scare stories' and misinformation/myths.
- Fear of side-effects.
- Experience of side-effects: above all, bleeding side-effects; also other side-effects, perceived or real, especially weight gain, headaches, nausea, depression, breast tenderness, acne.

- Wrong or incomplete information (e.g. about missed or vomited pills).
- Poor service delivery/counselling/advice about the methods. This is the (*preventable*) provider contribution to compliance problems! See Qs 8.16–8.17.

NOTE: There is some considerable *overlap* between these risk factors, but more importantly and very usefully in practice, there is *synergism*. Ensure more time for counselling when combinations of the above apply! See also Appendix A2, pages 509–15.

8.6 WHAT SITUATIONS/CIRCUMSTANCES CORRELATE WITH UNPROTECTED INTERCOURSE?

Here are a few which are well documented:

- First ever intercourse (or first with a new partner).
- Around the start or the end of any relationship – another good argument therefore for *long-term relationship(s)* since there will be fewer 'bust-ups'! And for *long-term, 'forgettable', methods*.
- Times of major life stress: e.g. bereavement, unemployment.
- On holiday, or trips away from home – indeed any situation where the individual or couple feel anonymous, a bit mad, and so liable to behave out of character.

8.7 WHAT ARE THE FACTORS IN NON-COMPLIANCE AND DISCONTINUATION IN THE THIRD WORLD?

Everything above, only more so. Wrong information, for instance. In Egypt in a recent survey the commonest error of *providers*, leave alone users of the pill, was the belief (as often in the UK, see Q 8.8) that the next packet of pills should be routinely started on the 5th day of the withdrawal bleed! Fatalism, and cultural and religious obstacles to good compliance are often very strong.

But the biggest single factor is the basic one of *non-availability of the actual methods*, or the drying up of supplies once a good method like DMPA has been initiated. ... Artificial contraceptives are seen as an easily avoidable expense and inconvenience in many poor communities of the developed world, too.

8.8 WHAT DO SURVEYS SHOW ABOUT MORE SPECIFIC ASPECTS OF COC COMPLIANCE?

A 1986 general practice survey in a mainly low social class (inner city) area showed that only 28% of women were taking the pill in accordance with the makers' instructions. Much of the confusion related (most crucially, see Q 4.15!) to when to start the next packet after the pill-free interval (PFI):

- 12% believed they should wait until the 5th day of the withdrawal bleed;
- 11% thought they should start the next packet only when the bleeding stopped, or after 1 week but only if the bleeding had stopped.

Starting late with the next packet was not perceived as anything to do with missing pills! (see Qs 4.15, 4.24). Two-thirds of the pill-takers in a similar GP study thought the most contraceptively risky pills to miss were in the middle of a pack. ... There is little to suggest any improvement in the 1990s, in such settings.

By contrast, in 1988 in a semirural setting of higher social class, 89% were found to take their pills correctly. *But could this in part be because those women had much more personal attention from the providers, before and during a course of pills?* We must admit that medical error – and especially not providing enough *time* for counselling and questions – can be significant components of user failure (see Qs 8.15 and 8.16).

8.9 DO WE EXPECT A LOT FROM PILL-TAKERS?

Yes.

Correct pill use means that a healthy woman has to take a pill daily for months or years at a time, whether her intention is to delay or prevent pregnancy, and whether she is consistently sexually active or not. She must know how long to wait between pill packets, how to make up missed pills, and when to use another method as a back-up. She then must have the back-up method available and actually use it. Finally, she must be confident about the pill's effectiveness and safety, despite frequent rumours and negative reports in the press. In short, the pill is a more complex method to deliver and use than we previously thought.'

(Linda Potter, Family Health International)

According to an NOP survey in the UK in 1991, 'on average women seem to forget a pill about eight times a year'! And young teenagers seem to be late with their pills up to three times per month.

Oh! for the contraceptive pill that Ann Furedi (Birth control Trust) seeks one that (a) tastes of chocolate; (b) guarantees that you lose weight; and (c) gives you an orgasm every time!

8.10 TEENAGERS ARE MENTIONED A GREAT DEAL IN THE CONTEXT OF COMPLIANCE. WHAT ARE THE IMPORTANT MEDICAL AND LEGAL CONSIDERATIONS WHEN PRESCRIBING A MEDICAL METHOD LIKE THE PILL TO GIRLS BEFORE THE AGE OF CONSENT (16 IN THE UK)?

1 *Medical.* Although early cycles after the menarche are anovulatory, very early conceptions can still occur and are becoming ever commoner. Aside from that there is the risk of STIs, cervical neoplasia and much potential emotional trauma. But it must be made clear that the risks are those of *precocious sexual activity and multiple partners, not of the pill or other contraceptive.*

A modern low oestrogen *combined pill* is usually a suitable method, though its 'default state' (i.e. of conception if errors are made) is not ideal. As far as we know once periods are established it poses no special problems in teenagers, as compared with women in their 20s (including with respect to breast cancer or cervical cancer, see Qs 4.77 and 4.79). *Injectables* and *implants* (especially perhaps the new Implanon (Q 5.157)) are currently preferable to IUDs – because of the pelvic infection anxieties about the latter, though they too are definitely not absolutely contraindicated. Re progestagen-only injections, see also Qs 5.103–5.104

Since this age group are now the most at risk of all sexually transmitted agents including HIV it is essential to promote *use of the condom in addition*, often, to the selected main contraceptive. Reliance on the condom alone for pregnancy prevention by teenagers usually gives poor results. If it is selected, take every opportunity to mention the *emergency pill.*

2 *Legal and socio-ethical.* Sexual intercourse before the age of consent represents a major category of technical law-breaking, not by the girl but by the male partner(s). Yet prosecutions are very rare if they are about the same age.

Any general practitioner faced with an under 16 year old needs first, as appropriate, opportunely and non-patronizingly, to raise the advantage – both psychological and physical – of delaying intercourse until later.

Next, if this 'rings no bells', seek agreement by the young person that they will tell, or allow you to tell, at least one parent. This is vastly preferable.

8.11 BUT WHAT IF UNDER-16S COMPLETELY REFUSE THE INVOLVEMENT OF A PARENT/GUARDIAN?

In 1985 the House of Lords overturned an Appeal Court judgment in the celebrated case brought by Mrs Victoria Gillick. In the new ruling Lord Fraser of Tullybelton made the following points which lead to what has since become known as 'Gillick competence'. They are also in the revised DHSS *Memorandum of Guidance* (DHSS HC(FP)86). In the summary which follows, note that the highlighted initial letters spell out the words

*Un**P**rotected **SS**exual **I**nter**C**ourse*

It is good practice to proceed to prescribe a medical contraceptive without parental knowledge and consent if:

1 the girl, although under 16 years of age, will *Understand* the doctor's advice;
2 she cannot be persuaded to inform the *Parents* or allow the doctor to inform them;
3 she is very likely to begin or to continue having *Sexual intercourse* with or without contraceptive treatment;
4 her physical or mental health or both are likely to *Suffer* unless she receives contraceptive advice or treatment;
5 her best *Interests* (therefore) require the doctor to proceed without parental consent.

At all times the young woman's entitlement to 100% assurance of *Confidentiality* is the same as for any adult. This must not only be real, as goes without saying, but also it must be *explicit* to her, e.g. as she recognizes the receptionist who is a friend of her mother's!

8.12 HOW ARE COMPLIANCE, SIDE-EFFECTS AND DISCONTINUATION CONNECTED?

In a complex way. To quote Linda Potter again referring primarily to pill-users in poor communities (in inner cities of rich countries as well as in the Third World):

Poor compliance can lead directly to pregnancy. However, incorrect use can also contribute to discontinuation. Studies indicate that as many as 60% of new OC-users discontinue use before the end of the first year, most within the first 6 months, and most of these because of menstrual irregularities and other side-effects.

The side-effects may be either the cause or effect of incorrectly taken pills, and may lead to either discontinuation or failure, making the relationship a complex one. For example, nausea in the first few months may lead to intermittent use, which in turn may provoke breakthrough bleeding, which in turn may lead to discontinuation.

8.13 ACCORDING TO THE UK FPA's NATIONAL INFORMATION SERVICE, WHAT IN ORDER TO HELP THEM TO USE CONTRACEPTIVES WELL DO POTENTIAL CONSUMERS THEMSELVES CONSIDER MOST IMPORTANT?

Above all, information. Some professionals feel consumers cannot deal with 'too much information'. The FPA enquiries (about 200 000 per year) lead to the conclusion that consumers want *more* information, *not less*.

Sadly, in the FPA's experience too many professionals do not provide full information about the range of options, fully explain the side-effects or discuss risks and benefits of contraceptive methods.

Many professionals make assumptions, often underestimating a person's degree of motivation, ability or needs and 'censor' or limit information, and many use a variety of ways to pressure a woman to use certain methods. Because of this, women (quite rightly) express feelings of anger, frustration and powerlessness because they feel they are not listened to, not spoken to on equal terms and given neither time nor 'permission' to voice fears or anxieties.

Family planning advisers need to be aware of how far they might go in determining choice rather than influencing it, i.e. there is a need to consider the differences between informed consent and *informed choice*.

There are fears, worries and doubts about potential, perceived and currently known side-effects. What consumers consider important when choosing a method are:

- effectiveness – will it work? (emphasis on failure rather than success);
- suitability;

- risks and benefits;
- how to use a particular method;
- how the method works.

8.14 WHAT MNEMONIC IS A GOOD GUIDE TO COMPREHENSIVE, CLIENT-CENTRED COUNSELLING?

In US Family Planning circles the recommended word is 'GATHER'. This stands for:

G: GREET each young person warmly.

A: ASK the young person about herself (himself) and why they have come.

T: TELL the young person about each available family planning method. Then demonstrate the method(s) that most interest her.

H: HELP her to choose the method she feels will best suit her and her partner.

E: EXPLAIN how to use the chosen method, using a user-friendly leaflet to be taken away and for reference.

R: RETURN for follow-up. Agree on a time to meet again routinely OR at short notice upon request.

The very first word beautifully conveys a client-centred approach. (Note my preference for 'young person' to the word 'client' that is often used).

8.15 HOW SHOULD THE INFORMATION BE CONVEYED?

Verbally and by the written word. The onus is on providers to give information that is accurate. It should update, reassure and demythologise – all without embarrassment. *Knowledge is power.*

Providing written information, and currently the best source in the UK is the FPA leaflets, offers privacy, anonymity and *time* to absorb information at leisure. People can remember only 20% of what they hear and only 50% of what they hear and see.

The length of the text is not a barrier to communication for consumers, provided the material is well organized, well laid out and well signposted. Indeed the more comprehensive FPA leaflets which are now available should be given with the words *'keep this in a safe place for reference'*.

Contraceptive manufacturers and family planning organizations are at last actively working together to standardize and simplify the information given. Providers can already choose, selectively, to offer some of the better manufacturers' literature, which has been much improved in recent years. Possibly even more important is creative packaging, whereby user-friendly design assists compliance and some companies' packets now convey valuable information like what to do in the event of missed or vomited pills. The increasing use of video and audio recordings is also welcomed as they can save time and be discussion openers, ensuring the ground is covered fully, especially the bits the provider may find 'boring' and so forget to mention at the crucial first visit.

8.16 AS AN OVERSTRETCHED BUT WELL-INTENTIONED FAMILY PRACTITIONER, HOW MIGHT I IMPROVE MY FAMILY PLANNING SERVICE?

1 Generally, more people attend GPs for contraception than community-based family planning clinics. But you might lend support to the view that *availability of the choice* of service is paramount – including the clinic service, which is moreover an essential resource for the practical training of doctors and nurses in this field.

   Availability of complementary (not rival) and accessible services is important; at present, potential users of contraception may have to run a bit of an obstacle race in order to find the service that meets their specific needs. One of the most useful improvements that many health authorities still need to make is to implement the recommendation of the 1991 RCOG Working Party on Unplanned Pregnancy, that there should be 'a senior specialist to oversee the provision of contraception and sterilization, both by community clinics and in general practice. ...' – a coordinating *community gynecologist or Head of Reproductive Health Services*, in fact.

2 Doctors and nurses tend to put birth control methods into five main categories: barrier, hormonal, intrauterine, sterilization, termination of pregnancy. But to our clients there are primarily just two categories: those methods you can get on with yourself – and those where you have to involve (get 'permission' from) other people, possibly rather bossy people, and so lose privacy and control.

   Given that context, therefore, in our own services, we must set aside any illness-oriented style and adopt an information-providing and counselling mode for these healthy couples.

3 There are a number of very practical questions you might consider:

Family planning, the scope

In our practice, do we:

- provide a full range of contraceptive methods, on site or easily arranged, including postcoital contraception *and condoms* (discuss with the local AIDS budget-holder)?
- provide pregnancy testing and support and counselling for unplanned pregnancy?
- provide counselling and referral for male and female sterilization?
- provide advice and help with regard to 'safer sex'?
- provide help or referral for sexual and relationship problems?
- provide advice, treatment or referral for STIs?
- provide advice, help or referral for infertility?
- provide comprehensive well-woman/well-man services?

Service provision

Do we:

- work as a team (I include here receptionist, health visitor, school nurse, practice nurse, partners)?
- provide flexible clinical services, with rapid access/walk-in facility for urgent first visits (postcoitally) and adequate support to those with follow-up problems (e.g. side-effects of IUDs or pills)?
- provide *sufficient time* for all family planning consultations, especially the first or the postcoital visit? Have we fully thought through the pros and cons of a dedicated session?
- provide an assurance especially to the young of *confidentiality* in visits, communications and record keeping?
- provide (where possible) a choice of male or female doctor?

Training

Do we:

- ensure all staff (including reception/clerical staff, but most especially nursing staff) are appropriately trained?

Information

Do we:

- always provide standardized, complete, up-to-date and objective information? That is, the information we ourselves would expect to receive.

- use suitable language that both enables and informs? Thus, *do not* talk about coils, rhythm method or morning-after contraception, but do talk about *IUDs, natural family planning* and *emergency (postcoital) contraception.*
- make it clear during counselling for pills and barrier methods that there is a profound difference between the failure rates for perfect use and typical use?
- Always discuss risks *and* benefits?
- Recognize people are not always comfortable and may feel too shy to ask questions? (It may help to 'ventriloquize' some questions, and to ask certain others to check that the most important facts have been retained.)
- Always provide good *written information* that backs up and reinforces any verbal advice?
- Publicize our services so people know about them?

Ensuring compliance is, after all, not about professionals 'telling' consumers what to do – it is about enabling consumers to make informed choices through a partnership with health professionals.

(Toni Belfield)

IATROGENIC CAUSES OF UNPLANNED PREGNANCIES

8.17 HOW WRONG CAN WE, THE PROVIDERS, SOMETIMES BE? MAY A DOCTOR OR NURSE BE AN ACCESSORY IN CAUSING 'IATROGENIC' UNPLANNED PREGNANCIES?

Very much so. We have just been reviewing, in a contraceptive context, plenty of evidence for the saying: 'you can take the horse to the water but you cannot make it drink'. But is it not also clear already that we as providers may fail in the first place to 'take the horse to the water'?

Many 'sins of omission and of commission' by providers are obvious from Qs 8.13–8.16 above. The list which follows of over 30 more errors, primarily medical or prescribing errors in nature, is by no means complete. Indeed I should be interested to receive other examples, for use in my next edition! As it stands it already reveals many traps for the unwary FP provider. ...

The prescriber may be an accessory to an unwanted pregnancy in any of the following ways:

1   First and foremost, by not allowing *enough quality time* for the contraceptive consultation, backed by good literature. This leads to one of the commonest, most basic errors, which is when the practitioner simply says 'you must stop the pill' without *any* adequate discussion of the future method (see 7 below).

2   When changing methods, by not ensuring an appropriate overlap between them. For instance, when changing from progestagen-only pill (POP) or IUD to condom, failing to advise use of the condom for 7 days *before* the POP is discontinued or device removed. Or if a woman is transferring to a (for her) untried method like the diaphragm or Femidom (see Q 3.55), removing an IUD before she has found it to be satisfactory. And prior to female sterilization, failing to advise abstinence or extra care with barrier methods for the cycle leading up to the surgery risks a clip-induced ectopic *or* an intrauterine conception (see also Qs 6.13 and 6.14.)

3   Especially postpartum, if any amenorrhoeic sexually active woman wants to start using a hormonal or intrauterine contraceptive, by insisting on waiting (a) for a 6-week postnatal visit (see Q 8.22) or (b) for the next period (*which then never comes because she conceives during the wait!*) – when there other are ways of minimizing the risk of fetal exposure (see Qs 5.133–5.134 and 8.22).

Chapters 1–3

4   After a bad attack of pelvic inflammatory disease, overstressing that the woman may be infertile – so she is inefficient with subsequent contraception.

5   Overstressing the ineffectiveness of coitus interruptus (see Q 2.6) so it is not used when it would be a very great deal better than nothing in an 'emergency' situation.

6   Failure to warn about the 300+ million sperm in each man's ejaculate, and the unpredictability of sperm survival in the female genital tract. Hence failure to explain the consequences: that a tiny 'leak' of semen may cause a pregnancy, and that the postmenstrual 'safe period' is of a completely different order of potential efficacy from the properly identified postovulatory phase (see Qs 1.4–1.17).

7   With Persona®, recommending the method to the 'wrong' kind of couple ('limiters' when should be 'spacers'); failure to offer the *option* of relying only on the second infertile phase as described at Q 1.31–1.32.

and failure to explain the preliminary need for two natural cycles of barrier method use after *any* hormones (including for emergency contraception).

8 Failure to advise about effective condom use, and especially about common chemicals/prescriptions which rapidly damage rubber (see Q 2.21).

9 Regarding caps, giving such a profusion of other instructions about spermicide, etc. (most of which have never been validated), that the woman fails to get the most important message: namely that she should make a secondary check that her cervix is covered following every insertion of her diaphragm or cap, however comfortable it feels.

Chapter 7 (considered here, since regularly indicated through failed use of above methods)

10 Failure to inform male and female barrier contraceptive users about the existence of *postcoital (emergency) contraception*; and failure to offer it when appropriate (e.g. if an IUD has to be removed midcycle, see Q 6.14).

11 Use of the incorrect term 'morning after pill', and failing to stop its use by others (see Q 7.1)

12 Failure to inform women that the PC 'emergency pill' can be used up to 72 hours after exposure.

13 Not being prepared to insert an IUD postcoitally up to 5 days *after ovulation* as calculated in good faith (see Q 7.15). With exposure on day 7 this could mean, quite legally and ethically, insertion up to 12 days after unprotected intercourse! And with a solitary exposure, 5 days *after intercourse* is acceptable at any time in the cycle.

Chapters 4 and 5

14 Giving erroneous starting instructions for the combined pill (see page 123 and Q 4.49 for the correct ones).

15 Failure to explain the significance of the pill-free week in the initial pill consultation, in advance and along with the FPA's *Choosing and Using* COC leaflet (see Qs 4.15–27). [Understanding at the outset the simple idea, that the COC is bound to work least well at the end of the regular time when it hasn't been taken at all (i.e. the contraceptive-free time), helps to stop the common notion that 'being a bit late starting' is not 'missing a pill'!!]

Detailed examples:

(a) not stating clearly that starting the new packet on time is critically important, and that the first pill is the most 'dangerous' if missed;

(b) not explaining that if pills are missed at the end of a packet, the next following pill-free break should be shortened or eliminated;

(c) implicitly wrong instructions for subsequent packs, e.g. *'the doctor said* (s/he probably didn't, but was the point clarified?) *'that I should wait until the fifth day of my next period – or until it is finished – before I restart each packet'*;

(d) instructing the woman to start a *new* brand of pill on day 1 of the withdrawal bleed (WTB) following the last one, without advising her what to do if by chance she gets no WTB in that cycle. She may well then wait beyond 7 days unless otherwise instructed.

16 Failure to check at follow-up whether pill-takers still have a copy of the FPA leaflet, and replacing as necessary (this is routine at MPC).

17 Simply represcribing the COC (perhaps with a 'pep-talk' about compliance) after true pill method failures, or even when only one or two tablets missed. Instead, the *tricycle method* should be offered (see Qs 4.27 and 4.31).

18 Inadequate explanations at pill discontinuation. Examples:

(a) Failure to inform a woman that the pill-free week is *only a safe time for unprotected intercourse if she does in fact restart a new packet*. If she is discontinuing the method, it is very common for a woman to assume that the condom is unnecessary for the first week. In reality she might well ovulate early in the second week (see Qs 4.15 and 4.24).

(b) Failure to explain that calendar calculations, of even the potentially safer second phase of the safe period, are completely invalidated during the first cycle following pill discontinuation, which can be very variably prolonged.

(c) Failure to dispel the myth: *'I heard that women often take a long time to get pregnant after stopping the pill, so I thought I would be safe'*.

19 Failure to forewarn and explain that the occurrence of break-through bleeding should not be considered as a period (and the pill therefore stopped in mid-packet) – and that it may subside over time. Choosing brands which produce good cycle control is obviously helpful too.

20 Failure to demolish the myth that you should not restart with a new pack until a 'period' has occurred. Not explaining in fact that *absent withdrawal bleeding* is very rarely because a pregnancy has occurred. (Some women become pregnant through failure to restart the pill after the first episode of absent WTB, and hence become unnecessarily pregnant solely because they thought they already were. ...)

21 Ovulation induction in a woman who presents with oligoamenorrhoea but definitely does not (yet) want to be pregnant! (see Q 4.63). '*No-one ever asked me if I wanted my fertility problem treated!*'

22 Unnecessarily avoiding the COC in cases of past secondary amenorrhoea from which there has been a complete recovery (see Qs 4.62 and 4.66).

23 Unnecessarily instructing the woman to discontinue/avoid the COC because of the *medical myths* in Qs 4.232 and 4.252 and 4.253 including for minor surgery like laparoscopy (see Q 4.193).

24 In the case of a healthy woman who really wants to continue pill-taking, agreeing too readily to her 'taking a break' when idea comes only from a friend (Qs 4.247–4.248).

25 Unnecessarily instructing the woman to stop the POP (or any EE-free method) before any surgery, however major (see Qs 5.42 and 5.73).

26 Telling the woman correctly to stop the COC before major surgery (see Q 4.192), or because of migraine with focal aura or other *valid* reason but failing to discuss and organize an alternative such as DMPA!

27 Failure to explain to a woman transferring to the POP that she should cease to take 7-day breaks.

28 Failure to discuss with a lactating POP-user that her chance of breakthrough conception will greatly increase whenever she begins weaning her baby. So if efficacy is very important to a woman, she should be advised to start the COC on the first day of the first of her returning periods (see Q 8.29).

29 Failure to advise appropriately (see Qs 4.34, 5.29 and 5.91) when prescribing any of the hormone methods of Chapter 4 and 5 in the event of use of *interacting drugs*, whether short term (e.g. rifampicin just for 2 days!) or long term.

30 *Bad handwriting* (a real problem in practice). The most dangerous example of this is when Femodene is intended but Femulen is read by the person issuing the pills. I am aware of at least one pregnancy caused this way, as the woman continued to take routine pill-free breaks of a week's duration!

Preventive recommendation, as practised at the Margaret Pyke Centre: Always write: Femodene 30; Femulen POP.
Also: Marvelon 30; Mercilon 20 (these are easily misread too).

Chapter 6

31 Failure to observe the 'do not rely on the IUD for 7-days pre-removal rule' recommended at Q 6.14. Avoidable intrauterine *or* 'iatrogenic' extrauterine pregnancies in IUD-users following clip sterilization may also result. (I also warn barrier method users of the need to be exceptionally careful, or preferably abstain, during the same 7 preoperative days.)

32 Failure to insert an IUD on presentation around midcycle, if necessary up to day 5 following the most probable day of ovulation. As explained at Q 6.15, a much more generous interpretation of the phrase 'post-menstrual' could lead to a worthwhile reduction in the number of conceptions caused by clinicians who wait for the woman's elusive next period.

33 Failure to warn women that if they fail to feel the threads of an IUD, until proved otherwise, their uterine cavity is IUD-free (see Q 6.35).

CONTRACEPTION/STERILIZATION AFTER PREGNANCY

8.18 WHEN SHOULD COUNSELLING START?

It should not be an afterthought: it should be initiated antenatally. Counselling should be non-directive, with the doctor or midwife acting as an adviser and facilitator but never making the decisions. It is true that most women are more motivated towards family planning just after childbirth than at any other time, and in many parts of the world postnatal follow-up is weak or non-existent. While it may therefore be correct to 'strike while the iron is hot', caution is necessary especially regarding sterilization, and all kinds of pressure are to be avoided. For all women this is a time of emotional turmoil as well as one of rapidly changing hormonal status.

8.19 WHAT IS KNOWN ABOUT SEXUAL ACTIVITY IN THE PUERPERIUM?

See the brilliant section on this in the book by Esther Sapire, 1990. According to Masters and Johnson, writing in 1966, after delivery almost 50% of women have low levels of sexual interest for at least 3 months. In another study the same percentage had resumed sexual activity as soon as 6 weeks, but possibly with little enthusiasm on the woman's part. However that may be, the onset of sexual dysfunction reported much later can often be traced back to this time. Sleepless nights, exhaustion and limited time together may affect both partners. The man may resent exclusion from the intense bond between mother and baby, compounded by his wife's fatigue and diminished libido. In the woman, there may be multiple anxieties about the baby and about adjustment to motherhood. All these can be worse if there is a true postpartum depression.

Physical problems include breast and nipple tenderness, or dyspareunia due to pain at the site of perineal suturing, monilial vaginitis or diminished vaginal lubrication.

8.20 WHEN DOES FERTILITY RETURN AFTER PREGNANCY? WHAT IS THE EARLIEST POSTPARTUM DAY ON WHICH OVULATION MAY OCCUR, WITHOUT AND WITH BREASTFEEDING?

Despite much research it remains impossible to predict this accurately for any individual woman. This is due not only to normal biological variation, racial or genetic factors, but also to the effects of:

1 the nutritional status of the woman;
2 the stage of gestation at which the pregnancy ended;
3 whether indeed she is breastfeeding – and in that case the timing, frequency and duration of nipple stimulation, the amount of supplementary feeding and the time elapsed since delivery.

Although fertilization is the only proof that an ovulation is fertile, research suggests that *in the absence of breastfeeding fertile ovulation could possibly and very rarely occur on day 28*, and contraception of some kind should therefore be started by then (see Q 4.49).

It is even more difficult when attempting to answer the same question for *lactating women*, because the variability in intensity of baby-induced nipple stimulation is superimposed on woman-to-woman variation. But avoiding all freak ovulation events is perhaps asking too much: a better question is 'For how long can lactation be expected to provide the same kind of contraceptive protection as other acceptable birth control methods, such as the IUD?' One answer is contained in the Lactational Amenorrhoea Method (LAM), see Q 1.36.

The essential caveat is that no promise of complete efficacy of LAM is implied – as should be the case with all methods.

8.21 ISN'T THERE A TWO-WAY INTERACTION BETWEEN LACTATION AND CONTRACEPTION?

Yes. Lactation can affect contraceptives, primarily by greatly increasing the efficacy of the POP and all non-hormonal methods like barriers and spermicides. Conversely, the COC for example can affect lactation by altering the quantity and constituents of breast milk.

Breastfeeding should also be advocated and promoted by clinicians because it is so good for babies – and may give some protection against *breast cancer*.

8.22 IN AN AMENORRHOEIC WOMAN SEEN POSTPARTUM, SAY AT 6 WEEKS, IF CONTRACEPTION HAS BEEN QUESTIONABLE HOW CAN ONE AVOID STARTING A MEDICAL METHOD (E.G. FITTING AN IUD) IN EARLY PREGNANCY?

Some doctors are so paranoid about this that they insist on the arrival of a period. But they thereby risk an iatrogenic conception (see Q 8.17 (3)).

One fairly obvious practical preventive of this problem is: Why aren't routine postnatal checks arranged at or just before 4 weeks, when the risk of a fertile ovulation having occurred is negligible (see Q 8.20), even if the woman has not managed to breastfeed?

Availability of one of the ultrasensitive slide or dipstick pregnancy tests now marketed for use in the surgery is invaluable here, e.g. Clearview. On an early morning urine this will diagnose pregnancy at or before the 14th day after ovulation; but not of course one very recently conceived, due to fertilization within that time.

If that is a relevant possibility, one useful protocol is the following:

1 Request that the woman agrees to avoid all risk of conception (by abstinence, combinations of methods, whatever) for 10 or 14 days since the last intercourse (depending on whether the sensitivity of the available test is to 25 or to 50 IU/l of human chorionic gonadotrophin (hCG)).

2 She then returns with an early morning urine. If it gives a negative result this can be interpreted as 'no' conception – implanted or 'on the way':
    (a) up to 10 (or 14) days previously (this by virtue of the sensitivity of the test), *plus*:
    (b) *since then also*, on her responsibility, as she had agreed to be 'safe' during that time.

3 After discussion (recorded in the case-notes) of the tiny risk that an early conception might yet be present, the COC could be started or one might proceed at once to a DMPA injection or IUD insertion. If hormones are to be used, or an IUS inserted, for extra security the couple should use the condom for a further 7 days. And there *must* be an early follow-up visit to finally exclude conception.

8.23 CAN NATURAL FAMILY PLANNING BE USED SUCCESSFULLY AFTER CHILDBIRTH (ASIDE OF LAM, Q 1.36)?

See Q 1.35. The fundamental problem, throughout reproductive life, is how to recognize fertile ovulation far enough in advance to allow for the capriciousness of survival of the very best among the millions of sperm deposited at intercourse.

The problem is compounded after pregnancy by the very variable effects of lactation, as discussed above.

With or without breastfeeding, postpartum the oestrogenic changes of increased quantity, clarity, fluidity, slipperiness, elasticity and good spinnbarkeit occur well in advance of the first fertile ovulation. Hence, if cervical mucus is used there are numerous false alarms.

Users of natural family planning who begin mucus observations from the cessation of lochia and who do abstain or switch to another method from the very first appearance of oestrogenic mucus onwards will most probably avoid pregnancy. But they will also be avoiding unprotected intercourse for an unnecessarily long time. Changes in the cervix – dilatation, softening and elevation away from the introitus – may help (see Q 1.35).

To date newer techniques using various biochemical changes are still disappointing for ovulation prediction far enough ahead.

8.24 DO YOU RECOMMEND AN IUD FOR FAMILY SPACING?

Yes, and it is an even better choice when the family might prove to be complete but the couple aren't sure yet.

See Chapter 6 for more details. Particularly relevant points at this postpartum time are:

1   *Infection.* This can be caused by lack of screening or poor technique during insertion (Q 6.55) or exacerbated if uterine tenderness due to postpartum endometritis is overlooked. The individual's risk of sexually transmitted conditions still poses the main threat for the future, however.

2   *Perforation.* This is a particular concern in relation to postpartum IUD insertion. Heartwell and Schlesselman (in a 1983 report) found this complication to be more frequent among lactating than in non-lactating women. However, *no* significant additional risk for T-shaped IUDs was shown by Chi in 1987 (rate 1 in 1632 during lactation). Perforation in lactation seems to be primarily a problem of linear (e.g. Lippes Loop) devices and can be almost eliminated by withdrawal insertion techniques – and by extra care by an experienced inserting doctor. Ideally, postpartum clinics should not be used routinely for training purposes, since lack of expertise markedly increases this risk.

8.25 WHAT IS YOUR ADVICE ON THE TIMING OF POSTPARTUM IUD INSERTIONS?

See Qs 6.101–6.102. Good results are reported whenever this is between 4 and 8 weeks after delivery. I favour 4 weeks to avoid all the 'hassle' discussed in Q 8.22 above, though the postcoital contraceptive action of the IUD method does provide some leeway.

After lower segment caesarean section (LSCS) the scar will have healed by 4 weeks, and is situated at the level of the internal os. So there is no need to delay insertion beyond say 6 weeks. After elective LSCS the cervical canal may require gentle dilatation, often with local anaesthesia, as for nulliparae. These insertions are not for beginners.

Immediate post-placental insertion
See Q 6.102. The new GyneFIX™ IUS (Q 6.139), bearing a biodegradeable enhancement of its retaining knot, is being studied for this indication. It shows greater promise (notably with respect to expulsions) than previous designs. Follow-up arrangements should be good, so that the women may have their now elongated threads shortened, or a new device inserted if expulsion is noted.

Immediate insertion after caesarean section
Modern IUDs may similarly be inserted via the lower segment incision immediately the placenta has been delivered, with superb results reported from China. Some researchers suture the device to the fundus with chromic catgut, but this appears to be unnecessary.

Immediate post-abortion insertion
Can be appropriate: See Qs 6.103 and 6.142.

8.26 ARE COCs SUITABLE IMMEDIATELY POSTPARTUM?

Despite their efficacy, convenience and many other advantages, COCs should *not* be used during lactation. Most studies report some adverse impact on breastfeeding performance and milk volume composition. And in any case the COC cannot improve upon the near 100% efficacy of the POP plus full lactation.

8.27 WHEN SHOULD THE COC BE STARTED IN WOMEN WHO DO NOT BREASTFEED?

If a COC is started too late, some women will become pregnant before their first period. If it is started too early, there is the risk that the oestrogen content will increase the already increased risk of thromboembolism in the puerperium. So ideally COC taking should not begin until the similar changes induced by pregnancy have returned to normality. This starts dramatically with delivery of the placenta, but fibrinogen concentrations actually increase at first until a decline starts around day 5. Dahlman and others found that both blood coagulation and fibrinolysis were significantly increased during the first 2 weeks, but by 3 weeks both were in general normal.

This literature may be interpreted as implying that oestrogen-containing pills should normally not be commenced earlier than day 21 of the puerperium, and this would be the optimum time for those perceived as being at high conception risk (see Q 4.49).

Selective delay beyond 4 weeks using an alternative contraceptive may be safest where known risk factors for thrombosis apply, particularly in combination. These factors are obesity, preceding severe pregnancy hypertension, operative delivery, especially caesarean section, restricted activity, age above 35 and grande multiparity.

8.28 WHAT IF THE WOMAN DID HAVE PREGNANCY-RELATED HYPERTENSION?

It used to be thought that women with hypertension in a preceding pregnancy would be unusually prone to oral contraceptive-induced hypertension. This was disproved by Pritchard and Pritchard in 1977. It is definitely however a relative contraindication (see Q 4.133(1)), meaning judicious use of the COC method with extra careful subsequent monitoring (WHO 3, Q 4.130).

Why? Because the RCGP study showed that this past history is linked for unknown reasons with an increased risk of arterial thrombosis – and seriously so if they also smoke (risk ratio of over 40!). If no alternative to the COC as subsequent contraception is acceptable and the 'pre-eclampsia' was severe at the preceding delivery, starting the COC should be delayed for at least 8 weeks.

8.29 WHERE SHOULD THE POP FIT INTO ANY SCHEME FOR POSTPARTUM CONTRACEPTION?

Very prominently. This is discussed in detail at Qs 5.55–5.59. Unlike the combined pill, POPs have not been found to impair the quantity or the quality of breast milk.

1 *Timing of postpartum use.* Since there is no anxiety about enhancing the risk of thrombosis, it is medically safe to start the POP in the early puerperium. However, studies have shown an increased risk of puerperal breakthrough bleeding in POP users, despite the expectation

that they should have amenorrhoea during lactation. It is therefore now suggested that women (whether or not breastfeeding) should begin to take the POP after about day 21 following delivery.

Any amenorrhoeic woman in whom cyesis has definitely been excluded if necessary by the routine described above (see Q 8.22), may start the POP at any time, with 7 days additional contraceptive precautions.

2 *Efficacy*. It is important to bear in mind that since there is the additional contraceptive effect of breastfeeding, less than perfectly compliant POP-takers will 'get away with it': until, perhaps, weaning and hence fertile ovulation commences (see Q 5.58). Two successive women in one of my own clinics gave the history that their next baby came 'too soon' that way, because the suggestion that they might prefer to switch to the COC at weaning had not been made to them!

This point needs making in *advance*: if efficacy is very important to a woman, she should be prescribed the COC so she can start it at the first of her returning periods.

8.30 WHAT ABOUT INJECTABLE CONTRACEPTION? DOES THE SAME APPLY AS WITH THE POP (ABOVE)?

Most studies of DMPA show either no change or an improvement in both quantity of milk and duration of lactation. Both DMPA and NET-EN and their metabolites cross from maternal plasma into breast milk, and to a greater extent than with the POP. It has been calculated that a child would have to breastfeed for 3 years to receive as much DMPA as the mother receives in 1 day. To date, no morbidity and no adverse effects on growth have been found.

1 *Timing of the first dose.* Since in some countries contact with medical personnel may be limited to delivery, the first dose of DMPA is often given within 48 hours of delivery. Injectables do not increase the risk of puerperal thrombosis; but this is much earlier than necessary for contraception and it has been noted that such early administration increases the likelihood of heavy and prolonged bleeding. Hence in the UK the first dose is now preferably (but not always) delayed to 5–6 weeks postpartum. In a woman who is not breastfeeding I would be quite happy to give DMPA early, at any mutually convenient time before Day 21 – so it could be sure to prevent the earliest likely ovulation – but with forewarning about the increased risk of bleeding.

2   *Efficacy.* Here there is no concern that the method will become less effective as breastfeeding frequency diminishes. Instead, the woman must be warned to plan well ahead if she wants another baby, because of the well-recognized delay in return of fertility – though this has often been exaggerated (see Q 5.119).

8.31 WHAT IS THE POLICY ABOUT HORMONAL METHODS IF THERE WAS TROPHOBLASTIC DISEASE IN THE LAST PREGNANCY?

This is fully discussed at Q 4.75.

8.32 WHAT CONSIDERATIONS APPLY TO MALE OR FEMALE STERILIZATION IN THE EARLY PUERPERIUM?

It often appears convenient for all concerned if the woman is sterilized at this time, and if so earlier the better. But Professor Robert Winston showed that the decision is more commonly regretted at this time of emotional instability for many couples. So there is a welcome trend to offering laparoscopic sterilization as an interval procedure about 12 weeks postpartum. The inadvisability of routine postpartum procedures is well shown by the observation that a distinct minority, around 15%, change their minds during that 12 weeks, preferring to keep their contraceptive options open longer.

There then still remains the risk of early death of the latest child (e.g. by the sudden infant death syndrome). Many vasectomy services therefore prefer to defer the procedure until the youngest child is 6–12 months of age. It is not clear why such admirable caution is less commonly observed by obstetricians with regard to female sterilization.

For more about sterilization, see Qs 8.56–8.61 below and Further Reading.

CONTRACEPTION FOR THE OLDER WOMAN

BACKGROUND FACTORS

8.33 WHAT IS THE INTRINSIC FERTILITY OF OLDER WOMEN, ABOVE AGE 40?

The available evidence suggests as shown at the bottom of Table 0.2, Q 0.19, that the intrinsic fertility of such women is reduced to about half what it was at the age of 25, with a further decline above 45. An unknown part of this is due to reduced frequency of intercourse. Whatever the explanation, the conclusion is that a method with an accidental pregnancy rate unacceptable in a younger woman may well be satisfactory for use in the 40s. For example, the POP in the Oxford/FPA study has a failure rate (0.3 per 100 woman-years) which is indistinguishable above age 45 from that to be expected in a younger woman using the combined pill. Another example is the recommendation to use the contraceptive sponge above 50 (see Q 3.64).

Some older women, however, may have actual or potential gynaecological morbidity to weigh up against the risks of the combined pill (see Q 8.38) and so may be better off due to its beneficial effects although not really needing such a high efficacy method.

8.34 HOW MAY ONE NORMALLY DIAGNOSE PHYSIOLOGICAL INFERTILITY AFTER THE MENOPAUSE?

Despite much research, there is no simple answer to the question '*When can I stop all contraception?*' Long spells of amenorrhoea in women under 45 may indicate the arrival of a premature menopause, but they may be due to other spontaneously reversible causes. Even above that age prolonged amenorrhoea does not rule out the chance of a later ovulation, though the risk is less if there are definite vasomotor symptoms.

We now know that FSH measurements alone are most misleading – they only mean reduced feedback of ovarian hormones on the pituitary *at that time*, the ovaries may well still have potentially fertile ova to release. Occasionally women with many months of amenorrhoea, symptoms of the menopause and even elevated FSH levels subsequently ovulate and even conceive! As a rule of thumb, women above the age of 50 years who have had amenorrhoea for over 12 months, preferably also with vasomotor symptoms, may abandon alternative contraception. During the 1-year wait any simple method (e.g. contraceptive foam) is adequate. Below age 50 there is a greater risk of spontaneous late ovulations, so 2 years' of amenorrhoea with extra precautions is recommended. Below 40 this is 'secondary amenorrhoea' and needs to be investigated fully by standard tests.

The classical rule is as above; 2 years' amenorrhoea are required for the infertility diagnosis right up to 50. That age limit seems to have been arbitrarily chosen, without any hard data. Lowering it to 45 in recent years has made life easier for many women: minimally less safe, but perhaps acceptably so.

If FSH levels (preferably two) are performed it may be possible in some situations (see Qs 5.64, 5.127 and 8.44) to shorten the time of use of other contraception after the apparently last period. But it must always be made clear that the risk of a later fertile ovulation cannot be completely excluded.

8.35 WHAT ARE THE MEDICAL RISKS ASSOCIATED WITH PREGNANCY?

Although it may be easier to prevent, pregnancy at this age is in many ways a greater catastrophe. Both maternal and perinatal mortality are much higher. There is also a steady increase in the risk of chromosome abnormalities with maternal age. Hence while we should certainly avoid using too 'strong' a method, the woman needs to be reassured that any chosen method will in reality prove to be effective in her case.

8.36 WHAT IS THE BEST METHOD FOR WOMEN ABOVE 40?

There is no such thing as a single best method. Individualization is the key, as usual.

HORMONAL METHODS

8.37 IS THE TERM 'THE CONTRACEPTIVE GAP' NOW APPLICABLE TO SMOKERS ONLY?

Yes: with modern pills, available epidemiology and the relevant authorities suggest that we may now legitimately continue the ordinary COC at a woman's request to the menopause, if she is an entirely healthy, migraine-free non-smoker. *Age alone is no longer a contraindication.*

For smokers however, starting at age 35 we are left with a 'contraceptive gap' between that age and the menopause. It poses an acute problem for those many couples who have hitherto been 'spoilt' by non-intercourse-related methods. Many seek sterilization, some without being entirely ready for so permanent a step: yet it would be unnecessary if they were non-smokers.

8.38 WHAT ARE THE DESIRABLE FEATURES OF CONTRACEPTION AT THE CLIMACTERIC?

Table 8.2 summarizes the desirable features. It is clear that only some *appropriate* combination of oestrogen with progestagen is capable of providing all the first six features in that table. What is appropriate? That depends on the need for contraception, see Qs 8.39 and 8.40.

TABLE 8.2 DESIRABLE OR 'IDEAL' FEATURES OF ANY CONTRACEPTIVE FOR USE DURING THE CLIMACTERIC (BEFORE AND AS REQUIRED AFTER THE MENOPAUSE)

1 Effective in this age group
2 Improves sex life by:
   (a) perceived effectiveness and reassuring period pattern
   (b) not being an intercourse-related method
   (c) oestrogenic slowing of skin ageing, improved body image and libido, and treatment of vaginal dryness
3 Controls climacteric symptoms (especially vasomotor and psychological symptoms, and the urethral syndrome)
4 Controls symptoms of 'normal' cycle (especially the premenstrual syndrome, and irregular, heavy or painful periods)
5 Reduces incidence or manifestations of gynaecological pathology. This potential benefit applies to pelvic infection, extrauterine pregnancy, fibroids, dysfunctional haemorrhage, endometriosis, functional ovarian cysts, and carcinoma of the ovary and uterus
   (Consequent reduction in the risks of treatment for these conditions, especially hysterectomy)
6 Oestrogenic protection against osteoporosis
7 Absence of masking of the menopause
8 Absence of systemic adverse effects:
   (a) known serious conditions such as hypertension and cardiovascular disease
   (b) anxiety about possible effects on other serious conditions, for example, breast cancer, especially with long duration of use

Note: Only a combination of oestrogen and progestagen is capable of providing all the above desirable features (*excepting* numbers 7 and 8). The remaining options chiefly act as contraceptives – usually without a positive benefit on the conditions shown.

Over and above the reassurance of regular bleeds, it is now clear that there is often some symptomatic loss of ovarian function starting 5–10 year before the actual menopause. Women in these years would derive additiona *non-contraceptive* benefits if (upon *their request*) they were allowed by their physicians to use some form of combined therapy. Many of the desirable features listed in Table 8.2 can be provided, at least in theory. There is the potential to improve sexual harmony by avoiding intercourse-related methods, and by preventing oestrogen deficiency with associated skin ageing, poor vaginal lubrication and loss of libido. The first manifestations of climacteric symptoms can be suppressed. Many women suffer preventable hot flushes and in some osteoporosis may begin before they see their last period. Symptoms of the so-called 'normal' menstrual cycle (premenstrual syndrome, heavy and painful periods) are often controlled.

Perhaps most important is the reduced risk of frank gynaecological disorders which are related to the menstrual cycle, listed at (5) in the table. It follows that use of an appropriate COC – *or of course the LNG-IUS, without or as indicated with added oestrogen* – will often eliminate the need for and risk of other medical or surgical treatments.

8.39 TABLE 8.2 SUGGESTS THAT THE BENEFITS OF THE COC ARE GREATER IN THE OLDER AGE GROUP AND SO STILL OUTWEIGH THE RISKS EVEN IF THEY ARE INCREASED SOMEWHAT WITH AGE. BUT WHICH PILL SHOULD BE USED?

First, this increased permissiveness re the COC applies only to arterial and venous completely risk-factor-free women. Second, enthusiasm for the COC must be a little tempered with caution as regards breast cancer risk, which does go up with age (Qs 4.86–4.87). Third, the COC is not the only oestrogen/progestagen combined option anyway.

Ideally the minimum acceptable dose of any progestagen and the oestrogen should always be used, to produce the least possible metabolic effects on both lipids and clotting factors. At present the first choice normally lies between Mercilon and Loestrin 20, as the only 20 µg combined products available in the UK; though I understand a 20 µg gestodene product is imminent.

8.40 IS IT EVER APPROPRIATE TO GIVE A CYCLICAL HORMONE REPLACEMENT REGIMEN (HRT) BEFORE THE MENOPAUSE? AND MIGHT THIS SUFFICE FOR CONTRACEPTION?

Not for *contraception* – none of those giving oestrogen alone at some time in their cycle is reliable. There are new modalities for the perimenopause being devised which do use natural oestrogens by various routes plus continuous progestagen and are contraceptive: notably the *LNG-IUS plus HRT*.

Otherwise standard HRT products, although medically even safer (see Q 8.41), are best reserved (and then usefully) for those with oestrogen deficiency symptoms who are not at risk of pregnancy. They might be abstaining, relying on sterilization or vasectomy, or happily using some other contraceptive.

8.41 SO WHAT IS THE REAL DIFFERENCE BETWEEN THE COC AND HRT? HOW IS IT WE CAN RECOMMEND HRT TO SMOKERS OF ANY AGE, WHEREAS SMOKERS MUST STOP THE COC AT 35?

Synthetic oestrogen (ethinyloestradiol (EE)), even at the lowest practical dose for contraception plus acceptable cycle control, has a long half-life and does create significant pro-thrombotic changes in the blood. The fear is that these might facilitate superimposed arterial thrombosis in an important artery, if its wall has already been affected by atheroma. These arterial wall changes are much more likely among smokers, who also have enhanced platelet aggregation and impaired fibrinolysis. So: no COC for older smokers

After the menopause – or leading up to it if birth control is not an issue (see Q 8.40) – the 'gentler' *natural oestrogens* are sufficient as oestrogen replacement. Blocking ovulation is no longer an issue and along with intermittent progestagen they can and do give good control of endometrial shedding, especially when no longer competing with the woman's own hormones. Moreover they seem to have beneficial effects on atherogenesis in the vessel walls. This is suggested by a reduction in heart attack rates in many studies (*primary prevention*). The HERS study of 1998 fails to show a benefit in *secondary prevention*: presumably because the slight prothrombotic effect possessed even by natural oestrogen can have an adverse short-term effect greater than the beneficial longer term effect on arterial walls – once those arterial walls are already damaged (e.g. through years of smoking).

Natural oestrogens have been shown to correct unfavourable menopausal lipid changes plus they affect various non-lipid mechanisms which are believed to confer arterial disease benefit: involving arterial tonus, prostaglandins and fibrinolysis. Moreover the minimal changes in coagulation/haemostasis and the increased VTE risk, are not thought to be greater than would occur in any woman continuing to receive natural oestrogen from her own ovaries (as for example through a late menopause) Non-oral routes may be preferable in this respect, avoiding a 'bolus' peak dose via the portal vein to the liver.

8.42 WHY THEN DO WE NOT USE NATURAL OESTROGENS FOR CONTRACEPTION IN ALL WOMEN, WITH OR WITHOUT RISK FACTORS, BEFORE THE MENOPAUSE?

Mainly because of the need for contraception and cycle control, which EE does so well. Since natural oestrogens are less completely or predictably absorbed and have lower potency, they have so far not proved so effective in either capacity. This may change with further research.

Natural (opposed) oestrogens can be used for women, especially smokers, using for example sterilization or vasectomy but needing HRT before the menopause: in synchrony with their own cycle, and with forewarning about breakthrough bleeding. But in risk factor-free women a COC with only 20 µg of EE is more effective, since it 'removes' the menstrual cycle and then replaces it with a (usually) well-controlled artificial cycle.

8.43 IF THE COMBINED PILL OR CYCLICAL HRT PRODUCTS ARE USED IN A WOMAN'S LATE 40s, WILL THEY NOT MASK THE MENOPAUSE?

Yes. The 'standard' teaching has been to switch to a non-hormonal method and only discontinue all contraception after the occurrence of complete amenorrhoea for 12 months (or 2 years if under age 45). But this precludes use of HRT (whose withdrawal bleeds like those of the combined pill will indefinitely mask the menopause, and which is not safely contraceptive) at the very time when vasomotor symptoms may be most pronounced.

8.44 HOW CAN INFERTILITY AT THE MENOPAUSE BE DIAGNOSED IN WOMEN STILL USING THE COC?

The 'standard' teaching at Q 8.34 above is impossible to follow with increasing use at this age of HRT and, for healthy nonsmokers, of 'Mercilon' (since the withdrawal bleeds will indefinitely mask the true menopause). The former is not safely contraceptive, and if it can be avoided the latter is best not used (unnecessarily) when fertility is extremely low or absent. *A possible protocol for COC-users follows.* We normally use it when the woman reaches age 50 (the average age of the menopause):

1 Measure FSH at the end of the pill-free week.
2 If it is normal she still needs contraception – though above 50 the risks of the COC would in most cases be thought unjustifiable, there is no need for such a powerful contraceptive and an alternative should be offered (e.g. foam, Q 3.64 or the POP can be ideal (Q 8.46, 5.63).
3 If the FSH is high, above the 'menopausal' level specified by the laboratory, there are preliminary data that such a woman has begun – as a consequence of ovarian failure – to rely totally on the COC for her oestrogen. Therefore when it is stopped for just 7 days the FSH climbs

rapidly. She may even report 'hot flushes' at the end of each pill-free week, the situation being comparable to sudden loss of ovarian oestrogen by oophorectomy. She now switches to a simple barrier contraceptive (or just 'Delfen' foam, which is adequate at this age, or the POP) for about 6 weeks, and records any subsequent bleeds and vasomotor symptoms.

If all four of the following are true it is very suggestive of ovarian failure:

(a) a second high FSH result;
(b) no spontaneous bleeds after stopping the COC;
(c) 'hot flushes' occurring, and:
(d) above age 50.

After advice that the risk of later ovulation can even so not be completely excluded, the woman may then elect to discontinue contraception, whether or not she also chooses to commence HRT.

Or for greater peace of mind she may elect to continue contracepting for 6–12 months with e.g. the POP (Q 8.46) or foam.

8.45 HOW CAN INFERTILITY DUE TO OVARIAN FAILURE BE DIAGNOSED IN WOMEN WHO WERE STARTED ON HRT BEFORE THEIR MENOPAUSE?

A similar protocol is as follows:

1 Measure *FSH*, logically in the oestrogen-only phase.
2 A level *above 25 IU/l*, which is somewhat raised despite the HRT feedback on the pituitary, is suggestive of ovarian failure. But this should definitely be confirmed, exactly as for the COC above, after stopping exogenous hormones for 6 weeks. The same four criteria (a–d in Q 8.44) should apply before contraception is maybe stopped (with no guarantees given ...). Again, for greater peace of mind she may elect to continue some form of contraception for 6–12 months.
3 If the woman has a *normal FSH* result and/or *ever later menstruates while off either COC or HRT, she should assume some residual fertility and* (continue to) *use a contraceptive* – again, whether or not she decides to take HRT.

8.46 HOW CAN INFERTILITY DUE TO OVARIAN FAILURE BE DIAGNOSED IN POP-USERS?

Women may, if they so choose, use this ultra-low dose contraceptive well beyond age 50.

Unlike with the COC, if prolonged amenorrhoea occurs as a new phenomenon along with symptoms suggestive of the menopause, the woman may have her FSH measured while still taking the method. If it is low she still needs the POP. If it is high, the same criteria (presence and persistence of vasomotor symptoms, amenorrhoea and a repeat high FSH value 6 weeks after stopping the treatment, plus age above 50) mean that her chances of a further fertile ovulation are extremely low, and possibly nil. With all the caveats above, she may therefore discontinue contraception. See Q 5.64.

Younger women and any who want more complete reassurance may if preferred continue using a simple method, as usual until 1 year after the last non-hormonally-induced bleed.

The replies to the last three questions make it abundantly clear that we still do not have (and badly need) a simple test of complete and final ovarian failure at the menopause!

8.47 IS IT ALWAYS IMPORTANT TO ESTABLISH PRECISELY WHEN THE MENOPAUSE TAKES/TOOK PLACE?

No, not in my opinion. If contraception is not an issue and the woman is on cyclical HRT with natural oestrogen, the diagnosis of the precise time of the menopause may be considered of academic interest only. The woman simply continues seeing artificial 'periods' for as long as she chooses to use that HRT. The management of any irregular bleeding is the same.

But, for reasons of risk, the COC is not recommended after the menopause, or normally at all above age 50, since fertility is so low that a very simple contraceptive will suffice. Any who abandon contraception without having followed the strict rules of Q 8.34 above (with or without being on HRT), have to be prepared to take responsibility for their decision: *a guarantee that ovulation will not occur again cannot be given.*

8.48 ASIDE FROM A LOW DOSE COC, WHILE WE AWAIT NEW DEVELOPMENTS, WHAT *CONTRACEPTIVE* FORMS OF COMBINATION HORMONE THERAPY MIGHT BE GIVEN – ESPECIALLY IN SMOKERS ABOVE AGE 35 WHO HATE BARRIER METHODS?

This essentially means using natural oestrogens in some form. It is already not uncommon for some doctors to prescribe an *oestrogen preparation* by any standard route (e.g. percutaneously) in the years leading up to the menopause, and *combine it with a POP*. They could be said to be giving the progestagen to protect the uterus from oestrogen-induced cancer, but choosing to give it in such a way (i.e. daily) that the couple can also be told they need no longer use a barrier contraceptive. The failure rate is unknown, probably similar to that of the POP alone; though some have argued it might be higher due to interference by the oestrogen with the mucus effect of the POP.

The main problem before the menopause is that the prescriber and the woman do not have the reassurance of regular bleeding. Breakthrough bleeding and spotting are frequent. These may sometimes be suppressed by giving a second or even a third POP daily, but fear of endometrial overstimulation can lead to frequent endometrial biopsies. See Q 8.49 below.

ALTERNATIVES TO THE OESTROGEN/PROGESTAGEN COMBINATIONS FOR OLDER WOMEN

Most of these are simply contraceptives. They do not provide the gynaecological benefits, the control over climacteric symptoms nor the potential prophylaxis against osteoporosis – which are given by the combined pill or (not always with contraception) other HRT oestrogen–progestagen regimens. Yet they remain valid options when hormones are not desired or are contraindicated.

8.49 DO MANY OLDER WOMEN GET ON WELL WITH THE PROGESTAGEN-ONLY PILL?

Yes, in this age group this is highly effective and deservedly popular (see Qs 5.1–5.78) – and acceptable if desired even beyond age 50.

The problems (see Q 5.33) include erratic bleeding patterns with fear of pregnancy; and hypo-oestrogenism (see Q 5.66). The latter can be treated with (added) continuous HRT oestrogen. Anecdotally, this combination then works well as a contraceptive, though it is not licensed as such and there have been no formal trials. Because of residual ovarian function irregular bleeding is common, but is often controllable by giving additional tablets of the POP or the (licensed) Micronor-HRT tablets giving 1 mg of norethisterone.

If this combination is used as a contraceptive as well as HRT it would be wise to follow the full 'named patient' routine in Appendix 1 (page 507).

See also Qs 5.64 and 8.44 regarding diagnosis of the menopause.

8.50 WHAT ABOUT INJECTABLES AND IMPLANTS (SEE CH. 5)?

These have similar problems to the POP, related both to amenorrhoea and to irregular bleeding. Moreover, most women are looking for added oestrogen at this age, hence the ideal injection or implant regimen would again be a combination (and such are often tried by prescribers, though not licensed: therefore page 507 would apply). See also Qs 5.102–5.107, about the whole matter of possible hypo-oestrogenism with DMPA.

8.51 IS THE COPPER IUD UNDERUTILIZED AT THIS AGE?

Yes, definitely, see Q 6.20. It is suitable not only because it is about as effective as sterilization, as a result of reduced fertility, but also because infection and expulsion rates decline with age and are lowest in the 40s. In the absence of intermenstrual or very heavy bleeding it can be highly acceptable. There is no need routinely to change any copper intrauterine device fitted after the 40th birthday, until after the menopause (see Q 6.136).

8.52 HOW ABOUT THE LEVONORGESTREL-RELEASING IUS (SEE Qs 6.143–6.149)?

This is a particularly useful option. Not only can protection against most of the gynaecological problems be expected, especially menorrhagia which is so common in this age group, even due to fibroids, but also it provides local progestagen protection against endometrial hyperplasia and cancer. This also permits oestrogen hormone replacement to be given later when it is indicated, systemically, while almost completely avoiding the side-effects of systemic progestagens. It is 'PMS-free, contraceptive, no-bleed HRT'!

Remember that there is no licensing problem if the LNG-IUS is used for menorrhagia (meaning only 'heavy periods', after all) in a woman who might need contraception (Q 6.144(4)). If she herself has been sterilized, or if the LNG-IUS is used for endometrial protection as part of HRT, then for the present the criteria of Appendix 1 (page 507) should be observed.

8.53 WHAT ABOUT THE CONDOM AND VAGINAL CONTRACEPTIVES?

These options are as appropriate at this as any other age, and have their own obvious advantages. But in my experience they (especially the condom) are not sufficiently 'user-friendly' to be accepted for the first time by couples who have not used them regularly earlier in their reproductive life.

Many women introduced to the diaphragm however are surprised by its ease and convenience.

The use of spermicides alone is not recommended in the younger older years (!). But Delfen foam is in my experience sufficient contraception and very acceptable:

- above the age of 50 and
- at any age for that necessary time following what appears to be the menopause (see Qs 8.34, 8.44–8.46) – which can only ever be finally diagnosed in retrospect.

8.54 CAN THE METHODS BASED ON FERTILITY AWARENESS BE RECOMMENDED LEADING UP TO THE CLIMACTERIC?

No. At present for those whose views make this the only acceptable approach, the mucus and cervical assessment methods (see Qs 1.24 and 1.35), or Persona®, all require a lot of unnecessary abstinence by older women. This is because during the climacteric there is follicular activity with oestrogenic mucus and oestrone-3-glucuronide in the urine – but without necessarily being followed by a fertile ovulation.

In an older woman who ovulates only (say) once every 4 months, a most useful new technology would be a means to predict each actual ovulation, far enough ahead to allow for sperm survival. Just three short spells of abstinence per year and she could avoid all the risks of the artificial methods of birth control.

8.55 ISN'T POSTCOITAL CONTRACEPTION (AS IN Ch. 7) BEST AVOIDED IN THIS AGE GROUP?

Not so, it may be entirely justifiable. There should be no hesitation in using either hormonal method even above the age of 45, so long as there is actually a finite pregnancy risk. POEC would often be the better choice since it has even fewer contraindications than the Yuzpe method.

8.56 SURELY EITHER MALE OR FEMALE STERILIZATION IS THE IDEAL ANSWER, FOR MANY OLDER COUPLES ABOVE AGE 35?

It certainly can be, for many. According to recent surveys around 45% of couples above age 40 in the UK rely on sterilization of one or other partner. The methods are effective and highly convenient, free of all proven long-term risks after the initial operation.

Most authorities consider any association of bleeding problems with *female sterilization* by tubal occlusion using clips or rings is coincidental, not causal.

Female sterilization appears to give a so-far unexplained protection against ovarian cancer. Otherwise neither method gives gynaecological benefits.

There are many traps for the unwary clinician, above all marriage breakdown, now that it is so frequent. Requests for reversal are more frequent after vasectomy because the man often remarries a younger woman. Careful counselling is mandatory, including an assessment of both the general and the sexual relationship of the couple, and a consideration of relevant aspects of gynaecology even if vasectomy is the operation proposed.

8.57 WHAT IS THE RISK OF LATE FAILURE? CAN TOTAL REASSURANCE BE GIVEN AFTER SAY 2 YEARS?

Unfortunately, no. Such late failures do occur even after vasectomy with two subsequent negative sperm counts. Our estimate from the Elliot-Smith clinic in Oxford (at which I have operated since 1970) was around 1:2000.

This still makes vasectomy much more effective than female sterilization: the American CREST study (in which over 10 000 women were followed up for up to 10 years) showed a surprisingly high overall failure rate of 1.8% (*American Journal of Obstetrics & Gynecology* 1996;174:1161–70). For every sterilization method assessed, at least 50% more failures were ascertained after 2 years as had been identified before.

They did not have the more effective Filshie clip, which is standard in the UK. However, on the CREST 'model', the known 2-year failure rate of Filshie clips which is around 3:1000 would need increasing to about 5:1000 after 10 years. Currently therefore we should inform young women at counselling that the lifetime failure rate of Filshie clip sterilization is estimated at 1:200; and that 1:3 of the failures is ectopic.

Obviously all these risks decline dramatically with diminishing fertility approaching the menopause.

8.58 ARE THE ALTERNATIVES TO STERILIZATION OFFERED OFTEN ENOUGH?

I think not. Many couples would actually prefer to avoid surgery and there are plenty of ways of doing so, as outlined above. Before referral for sterilization, especially of relatively young couples, in my experience three important choices are far too often not even mentioned. These are the injectable, DMPA (see Qs 5.88–5.136), the latest implant (Implanon, Q 5.157) and modern IUDs/IUSs. The gold standard among copper IUDs is the Copper T-380 – read all about its remarkable efficacy at Q 6.10. But GyneFIX and the LNG-IUS have their own merits (Qs 6.139 and 6.143).

Certainly another method would be preferable to sterilization when the woman is past the age of about 48, since sterilization will not provide 'value for money'. (The chance of pregnancy is so low and her 'auto-sterilization' by the menopause is imminent.) Indeed, depending on the regularity or otherwise of her menstrual cycle and vasomotor symptoms, a simple method like Delfen foam might be adequate.

8.59 WHAT ABOUT HYSTERECTOMY?

A hysterectomy may *sometimes* be appropriate and indeed may be essential gynaecological treatment. Hence the vital importance of diagnosing in the female partner large fibroids, adnexal masses and stress incontinence before even vasectomy is arranged.

Even by the modern minimal access techniques the morbidity and mortality, however, greatly exceed those of the other options above.

8.60 IS TRANSCERVICAL RESECTION OR ABLATION OF THE ENDOMETRIUM FOR MENORRHAGIA CONTRACEPTIVE?

Unfortunately, not so. After all, blastocysts can even implant sometimes in the ovary or on the peritoneum, so the absence of (most of) the endometrium is not enough. Younger women conceive with surprising ease. Moreover important risks are emerging:

1 The pregnancy has a high chance of being a tubal ectopic.
2 The fetus may have a major malformation.
3 There may be serious intrauterine growth retardation.
4 There may be varying degrees of placenta accreta.

8.61 SO WHAT CONTRACEPTION IS RECOMMENDED FOR A WOMAN HAVING ENDOMETRIAL RESECTION/ABLATION?

It is normally preferable that laparoscopic sterilization is performed under the same anaesthetic. Otherwise one of the above effective methods may and should be initiated, not excluding an IUD.

However, according to the experts in this field IUDs are relatively contraindicated (WHO 3), and if used are best fitted immediately, with great care and antibiotic cover. And it must be understood that the device can sometimes be almost impossible to remove, stuck among adhesions in a shrunken uterine cavity.

The levonorgestrel-IUS (see Q 6.143), of course, might prevent the need for this surgery in the first place – especially as it often helps *pain*, which is not usually improved by the ablative techniques. Alternatively, the gynaecologist may insert it as an adjunct at the time of ablation, or after resection of submucous fibroids, or at follow-up hysteroscopy if the problems do not resolve.

8.62 SO WHAT IS YOUR CONCLUSION – WHAT PRACTICAL GUIDELINES ARE THERE REGARDING CONTRACEPTION FOR THE OLDER WOMAN?

1 As usual, the choice will depend on the outcome of non-directive counselling, considering all the options discussed briefly here and more thoroughly earlier in this book. It begins to look as though no contraceptive method is absolutely contraindicated on the basis of age alone.
2 One of the very best modern options to emerge, though, is the levonorgestrel-releasing IUS – *alone, or with oestrogen if needed for relevant symptoms.*

8.63 WHAT ELSE IS IMPORTANT IN DISCUSSING CONTRACEPTION AROUND THE CLIMACTERIC?

It is important to remember that contraception is often a 'ticket' to see the doctor. In reality there may be many basic anxieties concerned with sexuality, the woman's relationship to her partner, the 'empty nest' syndrome, new health problems, ageing, and low self-esteem with the 'finality' of the approaching menopause. Moreover, even if as so often the woman tries to assume sole responsibility, her partner's caring involvement should be sought, and promoted if found! See also Appendix 2, pages 509–15.

THE FUTURE

8.64 WILL WE EVER HAVE A PILL FOR MEN?

At long last, a marketed systemic male contraceptive looks promising within the next 5 years – though it will most probably not be a simple pill.

The most promising approaches are a long-acting testosterone ester by injection, probably every 3 months, coupled with an oral or injectable or implanted progestagen, or possibly a prolactin analogue.

The concept is one of suppressing spermatogenesis by pituitary suppression (similar to the effect of the COC in women) but maintaining masculinity and libido though the androgen content. A careful balance needs to be struck between efficacy and the risk of promoting aggression, prostatic hypertrophy and the already-present male susceptibility to arterial disease.

Although some women say they would never trust a man to use such methods effectively, I am confident they would in fact be a useful addition to choice in stable relationships. It would be good if I could be on the 'pill' for a while, then my wife perhaps also, *sharing* the risks and side-effects of contraception for a change!

8.65 WHAT SHOULD BE THE DIRECTION OF FUTURE CONTRACEPTIVE RESEARCH?

Figure 8.2 displays elegantly, though simply, the primary sites of action both of the existing methods and those currently under study. Those which are most likely to become available within the next 10 years have been discussed in detail in the appropriate earlier chapters.

Inspection of the figure confirms an obvious fact: that the major scientific interest in birth control research has been directed at relatively high-technology, interventionist methods which have the potential or the reality of systemic side-effects. Returning to a theme with which we began the book (see Table 0.1, Q 0.16), the main choice for women is between the efficacy and convenience of systemic methods like the COC but the associated risk of both annoying and serious side-effects; and the relative lack of efficacy and inconvenience of methods like the diaphragm, coupled with their virtual absence of risk. ('Inconvenience' primarily indicates that the method is coitally related.)

Regrettably, most contraceptive researchers have concentrated on attempts to improve the existing pill and devising similar systemic agents but they are always trying to make the effective, convenient but *potentially dangerous* methods safer. It is my view (and one that is shared by the majority of the women and their partners that I meet) that the researchers would do better to concentrate their resources on making the *safe methods which also help to protect against STIs* more effective and more independent

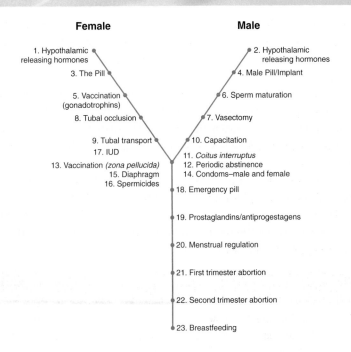

Figure 8.2 Possible points of intervention to control fertility. Q 8.64. For existing methods, the figure shows the *main* sites of action of each. Updated from *People* (IPPF) 1981 8(4): 6–7.

of intercourse. This indeed is the orientation of the research programme at the Margaret Pyke Centre.

It is impossible to contradict the following statement: 'no chemical can be devised which, whether given to women or to men, and whether used by the oral, nasal, retinal, cutaneous, subcutaneous, rectal or vaginal route, will be totally free of all risk'. Try as we will (and indeed must, since the urgency of world birth control demands research along every possible avenue) with new steroid compounds by slow-release and innovative routes, or using releasing hormone analogues, immune methods, or whatever; anything that gets into the bloodstream gets everywhere in the body and must therefore be capable of causing harmful effects, somewhere.

This is the heart of the problem to which Carl Djerassi drew attention in his classic book *The Politics of Contraception*. How do we prove that the unwanted effects of a systemic agent are acceptable or (hopefully) do not exist? It is because this process is so difficult, so expensive and so time-consuming that Djerassi was so pessimistic about the future of contraceptive research.

Perhaps we should be starting somewhere else. Far more research should concentrate on producing a method, empowering women and acting probably at the vaginal or cervical level, which is as effective and 'user friendly' as the levonorgestrel IUS but as medically safe and STI protective as the condom.

This approach is surely at least as important as the conventional wisdom of the scientific establishment, which starts with current or innovative systemic methods (now for men as well as women) which are effective and convenient, and then strives diligently towards making them risk free.

Success down that road – though it must be travelled as well – will be nearly as impossible to prove as it ever will be to achieve! And even then, in view of the world shortage of monogamy ... for safer sex many couples will still need to use a condom or equivalent as well.

Appendix 1
Use of licensed products in an unlicensed way
A1

This is quite often necessary for optimal contraceptive care, and is legitimate provided certain criteria are observed. These are well established (Reference: Mann R. In: Goldberg A, Dodds-Smith I eds, *Pharmaceutical medicine and the law*. London: RCP, 1991: 103–110).

The prescribing physician must:

1. Adopt an evidence-based practice, endorsed by a responsible body of professional opinion.
2. Ensure good practice including follow-up, to comply with professional indemnity requirements. *NB. This will often mean the doctor providing dedicated written materials because the manufacturer's insert does not apply.*
3. *Explain to the individual that it is an unlicensed prescription.*
4. Give a clear account of the risks and the benefits.
5. *Obtain informed (verbal) consent and record this and the discussion in full.*
6. *Finally, keep a separate record of the patient's details.*

This is generally termed 'Named patient prescribing'.

SOME COMMON EXAMPLES

... but there are certainly others which you may well identify in your own contraceptive practice

- Long-term omission or shortening of the pill-free interval as in the bicycle/tricycle regimens of pill-taking – for any reason (Q 4.31).
- Advising use of more than one pill per day: when enzyme-inducers are being used with COC (Qs 4.37–4.38) or POP (Q 5.29), or hormonal EC (Q 7.30); or two POPs daily in the overweight young woman (Qs 5.13–5.15).

- Use of 'add-back' oestrogen along with Depo Provera (Q 5.107) or the POP (Qs 5.66–5.67), to treat diagnosed hypo-oestrogenism.
- Use of copper IUDs for longer than licensed, particularly above age 40. (Qs 6.134, 6.136).
- Insertion of the LNG-IUS in a woman who has been sterilized (if the woman herself currently needs or may some time in the future need contraception it is already licensed, even if her main current problem is menorrhagia, Q 6.144).
- Use of the LNG-IUS as part of hormone replacement therapy (Qs 6.149, 8.52)
- Use of the progestagen-only method of emergency contraception (Qs 7.5, 7.10) – but licensing is imminent.
- Use of any hormonal EC beyond 72 hours after the earliest exposure or more than once in a cycle (Qs 7.8 and 7.42).
- Use of the POP with HRT together – as contraception in the older woman (Q 8.49).

Appendix 2
Factors to be considered in giving contraceptive advice

Some notes in a handout prepared by Dr Elphis Christopher for the Margaret Pyke Centre Doctors' Courses in Basic Family Planning, edited and used here with her kind permission.

THE FACTORS WHEEL (See Fig. 8.1, Q. 8.1)

INTRODUCTION

Although divided into equal segments in Figure 8.1, the different factors are not compartmentalized but rather overlapping and interlocking. Some factors are obviously more important than others for individuals, couples and societies and will vary over time: changing with increasing knowledge and experience both about contraception and abortion and the reality of pregnancy, child-rearing and population pressures. Altered socioeconomic circumstances and changing relationships (separation, divorce) will also have differing consequences for the use of contraception. Running like a leitmotif through all the aspects of family planning is the *status of women* and how their role is perceived: whether they are seen principally as child-bearers and -rearers.

Attitudes towards sexuality and its expression – e.g. whether regarded mainly for procreation or pleasure – can have profound consequences for the sustained use of contraception and the planning of families.

Sexual activity is often impulsive and not planned for, tied up as it is with powerful and often overwhelming drives and emotions (*sex is hot*) whereas the use of contraception requires forethought and conscious effort (*contraception is cold*).

At some level most couples would really prefer *not* to be bothered about contraception. ...

1 SOCIETY, CULTURE AND RELIGION

Societal attitudes towards reproduction, fertility, sexuality and family planning are important in so far as they create the general climate in which arise the decisions about whether to have children, how many, and whether to use contraception.

All religions are pro-natalist and anti-abortion. Some may allow a pregnancy to be terminated for specific reasons, e.g. where the woman's life is at risk.

Religions may not be adverse to planning or limiting one's family but may be divided as to the means to do it, e.g. restricted to abstinence or natural family planning for strict *Roman Catholics*.

There is a notion shared by some Catholics and some from an Afro-Caribbean background that there are a certain number of souls/children waiting 'out there' and it would be wrong to prevent their arrival. ...

Orthodox Jews: the man must not impede the sperm hence male methods are not used though the woman may use contraception.

For *Muslims* both husband and wife must agree to the use of birth control; abortion may be allowed to prevent a handicapped child. Strict Moslem women can only be examined by female doctors and touch their own vulva with the left hand. Somewhat of a problem for female barrier users!

Both Jews and Muslims must avoid sexual relations during and for a specified time after any menstrual bleeding – a major perceived obstacle to intrauterine and some hormonal methods.

Cultural factors rather than religious ones appear more significant among *Caribbean* women. Birth outside of wedlock is not considered a social stigma. Fertility (or the proof of it) is considered very important:

How seriously people take their religion and their perception and knowledge of what it actually says with regard to family planning obviously varies. Some may have rejected their background. Thus in giving contraceptive advice it is essential to ascertain the particular person's views (today) and to avoid making assumptions about their beliefs and attitudes.

NOTE: Treat the person not the culture.

SOME ASPECTS OF 'SUBCULTURE'

Feelings of:

Apathy	Those for whom birth control is
Fate	anathema may feel they have little
God's Will	control over other areas of their lives. Their sexual
	relationships are the one free area of their lives.

Especially among the socially deprived (of whatever ethnic background) in the inner cities, such vulnerable individuals find it difficult to seek advice about sexual or contraceptive matters due to fear of professional attitudes; they are highly suspicious about loss of confidentiality. Sex however is free and available within a relationship. It is private and satisfying. Sex may provide a positive counterbalance to the idleness of unemployment and low self-esteem. Motherhood may seem the only source of fulfilment in an otherwise gloomy picture.

They often lead chaotic disordered lifestyles with frequent change of partners and may be poorly motivated to sustain their use of contraception and need much support, e.g. by a domiciliary family planning service.

2 CLASS, EDUCATION AND KNOWLEDGE

Generally speaking those in long-term education and from a higher socioeconomic class tend to have similar family sizes, regardless of cultural/societal/religious influences, and are more motivated to use contraception.

Included in education is *sex education*. For years there has been a belief that teaching teenagers about contraception will be giving them a licence to have sex. Sexual ignorance is seen as bliss. The adolescent is often caught in a double bind. There is a loss of face for a teenager to admit to ignorance on sexual matters though he/she may desperately need help.

There is considerable anxiety about sex education and its effects among certain ethnic groups in Britain, particularly the *Cypriot* and *Asian* minorities.

3 FAMILY, PARENTS, PEER GROUP

In patriarchal cultures such as *Asian* and *Cypriot*, marriages are arranged or semi-arranged. A marriage is not considered a true one unless there are children, especially sons, who increase the status of women within those societies.

Peer group pressure can be significant among certain teenage groups especially girls who have been in local authority care.

4 THE COUPLE

The balance and quality of the relationship can effect the use of contraception. *Consider*:

- Trust, mutuality, sharing good communication.
- Humour.
- Consideration and care can cope with the vicissitudes of contraception.

Erratic use of contraception:

- Anger, disappointment, resentment with the partner: the woman may stop the pill and try to withhold sex.
- The question of who is in *control*, who is in charge, can get acted out in whether contraception is used and who is the one who uses it.
- Resentment of the other's sexuality demands/needs.
- Conflict about pregnancy: where one partner wants a pregnancy but the other does not and sabotages the use of the method (pills thrown away, IUDs removed without telling the partner).
- A pregnancy may be 'arranged' to hold on to the partner.
- When relationships are beginning or ending this often leads to erratic or non-use of contraception.

THE SEXUAL RELATIONSHIP – ATTITUDES TO SEX ITSELF

Whether attitudes are positive or negative can be revealed at the contraceptive consultation and whether there is sexual self-confidence. *Vaginal examination is very pertinent here; reveals much.*

Sexual problems can present *covertly*, and can be shown by: *Ambivalence towards contraceptive methods*:

- Nothing is suitable; reluctance to be examined.
- Sex is really for procreation.
- Giving in to sexual desires – losing control – may not fit in with image of nice clean upright woman.
- Inability to give oneself permission to enjoy sex.

Sexual abuse may lead to:

- Promiscuity ('acting out').
- Masochistic behaviour.

- Repeated terminations.
- Repeated sexually transmitted infections.
- Cold, unresponsive.
- Vaginismus.
- Avoidance of vaginal examination.
- 'Sex made good by having babies.'

Sexual problems can influence the use and choice of contraception. If the man has premature ejaculation or the woman has no sexual desire or if there is infrequent sex, the couple may feel the use of contraception is pointless.

Or the methods themselves may cause sexual problems, e.g. man may lose his erection with the condom.

5 THE INDIVIDUAL

Attitudes to concepts of male/female, femininity/masculinity. Equated with possibility of having children. Obtain sexual identity and self-esteem from that. Pertinent for teenage girls with nothing else in their lives. For the man who feels inadequate and unable to compete with other men, getting a woman pregnant may satisfy a need to prove himself.

Unconscious factors:

- The need for a baby.
- Testing the relationship.
- Unresolved conflict about the future of the relationship.
- Sex is 'disgusting' though consciously saying it is a good thing.
- After birth 'mothers can't be lovers' (altered body image; real and imagined damage).
- Bad birth experience. } exacerbates sexual and
- Abnormal birth, stillbirth. } contraceptive problems
- Post abortion – grief and dismay about the need for a termination may lead to erratic use of contraception despite consciously saying do not want to get pregnant.
- Post diagnosis of sexually transmitted disease or abnormal cervical smear/colposcopy (feelings of anger, grief, shame, past secrets, sexual abuse may all be revealed; woman may not want to continue with her sexual relationship but be unable to talk about it, she may complain of loss of libido, blaming the pill).

6 CHILDREN

Importance and value of children. Confer adult status, carry on the family name, insurance for old age, keep you young, ensure some kind of immortality, keep the marriage or relationship together, prevent boredom and loneliness, provide interest/entertainment, satisfy the need to be needed, define a role in life and provide stability.

- They can be used as a bastion against an unfriendly world 'me and my baby' (certain teenage mothers), or as creating one's own tribe (can be seen in families with many social problems).
- Can lead to non-use or poor use or fault finding with all contraceptive methods.

7 METHODS THEMSELVES AND SERVICES

Truism – we do not have the perfect method = MAGIC.

8 ABORTION SERVICES

Need for good abortion service as supplement to family planning services because methods fail, couples fail to use methods conscientiously and women should not have to have a child they feel they cannot care for properly. But abortion interacts in many ways: e.g. with conscientiousness of use of methods, effects of guilt feelings, etc.

How are emotional factors revealed?

1 Ambivalence about methods.
2 Dissatisfaction with methods.
3 Reluctance to be examined – psychosomatic examination, vaginismus, *always* menstruating.
   Vagina = private area, frightening, vulnerable dangerous, dirty, messy, blood and discharge comes from it, not owned as a nice pleasurable place, symbol of messy sexual desires, exposed is shameful
4 Reluctance to involve partner.
5 Not keeping subsequent appointments.
6 Running out of supplies.

Vulnerable groups who need special support:

1 The young.
2 The young single mother.

3   Where different fathers for pregnancies/children.
4   Chaotic lifestyle, unstable relationships.
5   Mentally and physically handicapped.
6   Mental illness.
7   Families with children 'in care' and/or on the non-accidental injury register.
8   Women who have repeated abortions.
9   Women with five or more children especially with poor spacing and achieved by a young age.

Some defences:

1   Chaos creator in waiting room. Diverts you from the problem. Patient wants you to get rid of her at one level; at another, cry for help.
2   Hostility, aggression, hides anxiety.
3   Chatty, friendly, doesn't let you get a word in, de-doctors you.
4   Jokiness.
5   Tears. Real/imaginary. Hostile 'keep out'.
6   Sexualizes interview. 'Easier to relate to me sexually than work with me as a doctor.'
    Denial; avoidance; hidden communication – secret code you need to decipher; non-verbal clues.

Treatment:

1   Awareness on part of doctor about problems and how they present.
2   Listen carefully (what lies behind patient's words) – overt, covert. May need to *confront* – 'nothing on offer seems right for you'. 'Perhaps angry that you have to take responsibility, prefer partner to.'
3   Use of doctor's own feelings with this patient provides powerful clues, for example: Anger; sympathy, or seduced; feeling put down; on a pedestal, preening with pride 'only you can help, doctor.'

Above all:

4   Reactions to suggestion of vaginal examination and to the actual examination.

MAIN SOURCES OF REFERENCES AND QUOTATIONS

Carter Y, Moss C, Weyman A (1998) *RCGP handbook of sexual health in primary care.* RCGP, London.

Evans I, Huezo, C (1997) *Family planning handbook for health professionals.* IPPF, London.

Filshie M, Guillebaud J (1989) *Contraception: science and practice.* Butterworths, London.

Guillebaud J (1999) *Contraception today. A pocketbook for general practitioners.* Martin Dunitz, London.

Kubba A, Sanfilippo J, Hampton N (1999) *Contraception and office gynaecology: choices in reproductive healthcare.* WB Saunders, London.

McPherson A, Waller D (eds) (1997) *Women's Health* (Formerly Women's problems in general practice) 4th edn. Oxford University Press, Oxford.

Potts M, Diggory P (1983) *Textbook of contraceptive practice.* Cambridge University Press, Cambridge.

Sapire E (1990) *Contraception and sexuality in health and disease.* McGraw-Hill, Isando.

IMPORTANT BACKGROUND READING – PLUS TITLES FOR A GENERAL READERSHIP

Djerassi C (1981) *The politics of contraception: birth control in the Year 2001,* 2nd edn. Freeman, Oxford.

Ehrlich P, Ehrlich A (1991) *The population explosion.* Arrow Books, London.

Guillebaud J (1997) *The pill,* 5th edn. Oxford University Press, Oxford.

Montford H, Skrine R (1993) *Psychosexual Medicine Series 6. Contraceptive care: meeting individual needs.* Chapman & Hall, London.

Szarewski A, Guillebaud J (1998) *Contraception – a user's handbook,* 2nd edn. Oxford University Press, Oxford.

A4

Appendix 4
World Directory of Pills – equivalent brand names

Below are listed details of some equivalent brand names used worldwide, identical with or very similar to currently marketed UK low-dose combined pills. It is based, with permission, on the *Directory of Contraceptives* published by the International Planned Parenthood Federation, 1996, edited by Ronald Kleinman. See this for a list of names for different but related formulations arranged by country of availability, and for POPs. The pill brands currently available in Britain are in *italics*.

> **NOTE:** Beware that sometimes the same or a very similar name is used in different countries for quite different formulations, e.g. Gynera vs Genora.

PHASIC PILLS

For comparison with monophasic brands, the *average* daily doses given in the British phasic brands are shown below:

Tri-Minulet, Triadene	EE 32.4 + GSD 78.6
Logynon, Trinordiol	EE 32.4 + LNG 92
Binovum	EE 35 + NET 833
Trinovum	EE 35 + NET 750

ABBREVIATIONS

Oestrogens: EE, ethinyloestradiol. Progestagens: NGM, norgestimate; GSD, gestodene; DSG, desogestrel; LNG, levonorgestrel; NET, norethisterone (norethindrone in North America). Also relatives of NET: NEA, norethisterone acetate.

GROUP A (NORGESTIMATE, NGM)

EE 35 µg + NGM 250 µg Anele, *Cilest*, Effiprev, Effiprev 35, Ortho-Cyclen

GROUP B (GESTODENE, GSD)

EE 30 µg + GSD 75 µg Ciclomex, Evacin, Femodeen, Femoden, *Femodene*, *Femodene ED*, Femovan, Ginera, Ginoden, Gynera, Gynovin, *Minulet* Minulette, Moneva, Myvlar.

Triphasic formula (EE 30 µg + GSD 50 µg; EE 40 µg + GSD 70 µg; EE 30 µg + GSD 100 µg) Milvane, Phaeva, *Triadene*, Triciclomex, Tri-Femoden, Trigynera, Tri-Gynera, Trigynovin, *Tri-Minulet*, Triodeen, Trioden, Triodena, Triodene

GROUP C (DESOGESTREL, DSG)

EE 30 µg + DSG 150 µg Cycléane-30, Desogen, Desolett, Frilavon, *Marvelon*, Marviol, Microdiol, Novelon, Ortho-Cept, Planum, Practil, Prevenon, Varnoline

EE 20 µg + DSG 150 µg Cycléane-20, Lovelle, Marvelon 20, *Mercilon*, Microdosis, Myralon, Securgin, Segurin

GROUP D (LEVONORGESTREL, LNG)

EE 30 µg + LNG 150 µg Ciclo, Ciclon, Combination 3, Contraceptive LD, Duofem*, Egogyn, Egogyn 30, Femigoa, Femranette mikro, Follimin, Gynatrol, Levlen, Levonorgestrel Pill, Levora, Lo-Femenal*, Lo-Gentrol*, Lo-Ovral*, Lo/Ovral*, Lo-Rondal*, Lorsax, Mala D, Microgest, Microginon 30, Microgyn, *Microgynon 30*, *Microgynon 30 ED*, Microvlar, Minibora, Minidril, Minigynon 30, Minivlar, Min-Ovral*, Mithuri, Neo-Gentrol 150/30, Neomonovar, Neovletta, Nordet, Nordette 150/30, Norgestrel Pill*, Norgylene, Norvetal, Ologyn-Micro, Ovoplex 30/150, Ovoplexin, Ovral L*, Ovranet, *Ovranette*, Riget, Rigevidon, Sexcon, Stediril-d 150/30, Stediril-30, Stediril-M, Suginor

EE 20 µg + LNG 100 µg Alesse, Balancelle, Loette, Leios, *Microgynon 20 (new)*, Micro-Levlen, Miranova

Triphasic formula (EE 30 μg + LNG 50 μg; EE 40 μg + LNG 75 μg; EE 30 μg + LNG 125 μg) Fironetta, Levordiol, *Logynon*, *Logynon ED*, Modutrol, Triagynon, Triciclor, Triette, Trigoa, Trigynon, Trikvilar, Tri-Levlen, *Trinordiol*, Trionetta, Triovlar, Triphasil, Triquilar, Triquilar ED, Tri-Regol, Trisiston, Tri-Stediril, Triviclor, Trolit

GROUP E (NORETHISTERONE, NET)

EE 35 μg + NET 1000 μg Brevicon 1, Brevinor-1, Genora 1/35, Gynex 1/35E, Intercon 1/35, Jenest, Kanchan, Membrettes, NEE 1/35, Nelova 1+35E, Neocon, Neo-Norinyl, Norcept-E 1/35, Norethin 1/35E, *Norimin*, Norimin-1, Norinyl 1/35, Norquest, Ortho 1+35, Ortho Novum 1/35, Ovysmen 1/35, Secure

EE 35 μg + NET 500 μg Brevicon, *Brevinor*, Conceplan mite, Genora 0.5/35, Gynex 0.5/35E, Intercon 5/35, Mikro Plan, Moda Con, Modacon, Modicon, NEE 0.5/35, Nelova 0.5/35E, Neo-Ovopausine, Nilocan, Norminest, Orthonett-Novum, Ovacon, *Ovysmen*, Ovysmen 0.5/35, Perle LD

EE 30 μg + NEA 1500 μg *Loestrin 30*, Loestrin 1.5/30, Logest 1.5/30, Minestril-30, Zorane 1.5/30

EE 20 μg + NEA 1000 μg Loestrin, *Loestrin 20*, Loestrin 1/20, Lostrin 1/20, Minestril-20, Minestrin 1/20, Norgest, Zorane 1/20

Triphasic formula (EE 35 μg + NET 500 μg; EE 35 μg + NET 750 μg; EE 35 μg + NET 1000 μg) Ortho 777, Ortho-Novum 777, Triella, *TriNovum*

Triphasic formula (EE 35 μg + NET 500 μg; EE 35 μg + NET 1000 μg; EE 35 μg + NET 500 μg) Improvil, Synfase, *Synphase*, Tri-Norinyl

---

*These pills also contain dextronorgestrel (non-contraceptive).

Index

IUD

abortion 352, 392, 419
advantages 348–9
airports, security devices 424
alkalosis 399
antibiotics 384
antisepsis 396
asthmatic attack 399
benign trophoblastic disease 383
bimanual examination 394–5
bleeding and pain 379
bleeding pattern 377–8
caesarean section 391, 486
cancer 420
cervical
  erosion 421
  smears 375
  stenosis 383
choice of 386–90
contraindications 380–6
copper
  absorption 419
  allergy 384, 420–1
  devices 341–2
counselling 367, 400–1
device design 345–6
diabetes 383, 385–6
disadvantages 349–50
drugs 425
duration of use 354, 405–16
EC 431–2
ectopic pregnancies 353
effectiveness 344–8
embedding 364
endometriosis 383
epilepsy 421
expulsion 360–2, 424
  rate 347
extrauterine pregnancy 353–5
failure rate 344–5
fibroids 383
first choice 387–8
follow-up 400–5
genital tract 341–2
grand mal 399
heavy periods 423
history 340–1, 342
hump of infection 368, 370, 371
iatrogenic pregnancy 346–7
immunosuppressive drugs 384
increased bleeding 378–9
inert devices 344
insertion 390–9, 401
  crises 397
  EC 448–9
  emergency tray 399
  interval 390–1
  pain 421

patient position 395
practical requisites 393
time 368–9
instructions after fitting 421–3
interval insertion 390–1
intrauterine pregnancy 351–3
lesions of heart 385
local anaesthesia 395
long term 344
lost 352–3
lost threads 356–60, 422–3
male dyspareunia 404
Medical Devices Agency 418–19
menstrual flow 379–80
miscarriages 351
mode of action 343
multiloads 389
NMR 404–5
nulliparous woman 389
older women 392, 499
partial perforation 364
partner's agreement 420
past tubal pregnancy 355
pelvic infection 364–77, 373, 374
perforation 362, 422–3
persistent bradycardia 398
post delivery 391
post-abortion insertion 486
post-insertion visit 370–1
post-placental insertion 486
postpartum 391, 485–6
preinsertion analgesia 395
primary dysmenorrhoea 383
prior screening 370
problems 371
progestagen-releasing 342
prosthesis 385
removal 351–2, 373–4, 403–4, 425
  hooks 360
reversibility 408–9
safety 419–20
sanitary protection 424
scarred uterus 383
self-removal 419
sexual partners, number of 420
shape of uterus 361
short-wave diathermy 404
size of uterus 361
spermicide 422
STIs 369–70, 383
strings 422
suitable patients 349
sunbed 424
systemic effects 343
threadless 372
tilted womb 421
time of insertion 347–8
uterine fibroids 386